T0328899

Biomarkers in Cardiovascular Disease

Biomarkers in Cardiovascular Disease

EDITED BY

VIJAY NAMBI, MD, PhD
Staff Cardiologist, Associate Professor of Medicine
Michael E DeBakey Veterans Affairs Hospital
Baylor College of Medicine
Houston, TX, United States

ELSEVIER

ELSEVIER

3251 Riverport Lane
St. Louis, Missouri 63043

Publisher: Dolores Melani
Acquisition Editor: Robin R Carter
Editorial Project Manager: Jaclyn A. Truesdell
Project Manager: Poulouse Joseph
Designer: Alan Studholme

List of Contributors

Mahmoud Allahham, MD
Resident, Internal Medicine
Baylor College of Medicine
Houston, TX, United States

Kelly Arps, MD
Johns Hopkins Division of Cardiology and Ciccarone
Center for the Prevention of Heart Disease
Johns Hopkins University
Baltimore, MD, United States

Christie M. Ballantyne, MD
Professor of Medicine and Genetics
Chief
Sections of Cardiovascular Research and Cardiology
Department of Medicine
Director
Center for Cardiometabolic Disease Prevention
Baylor College of Medicine
Houston, TX, United States

Agastya D. Belur, MD
National Heart
Lung & Blood Institute
National Institutes of Health
Bethesda, MD, United States

Pavan Bhat, MD
Department of Cardiovascular Medicine
Heart and Vascular Institute
Cleveland Clinic
Cleveland, OH, United States

Teresa L. Carman, MD
Director
Vascular Medicine
Division of Cardiovascular Medicine
University Hospitals Cleveland Medical Center
Cleveland, OH, United States

Anna Marie Chang, MD, MSCE
Director of Clinical Research Operations
Emergency Medicine
Thomas Jefferson University
Philadelphia, PA, United States

Razvan T. Dadu, MD, PhD
Houston Methodist DeBakey Heart and Vascular
    Institute
Houston, TX, United States

Weill Cornell Medical College
Newyork, NY, United States

Amit K. Dey, MD
National Heart
Lung & Blood Institute
National Institutes of Health
Bethesda, MD, United States

Aditya Goyal, MD
National Heart
Lung & Blood Institute
National Institutes of Health
Bethesda, MD, United States

Ron Hoogeveen, PhD
Associate Professor
Medicine
Baylor College of Medicine
Houston, TX, United States

Hani Jneid, MD
Associate Professor of Medicine
Cardiology
Baylor College of Medicine
Houston, TX, United States

Peter H. Jones, MD
Associate Professor of Medicine
Division of Atherosclerosis and Vascular Medicine
Section of Cardiovascular Research
Department of Medicine
Baylor College of Medicine
Houston, TX, United States

Neal S. Kleiman, MD
Director
Cardiac Catheterization Laboratory
Houston Methodist DeBakey Heart and Vascular
 Center
Houston, TX, United States
Professor of Medicine
Weill Cornell Medical College
New York, NY, United States

John W. McEvoy, MB, BCh, MHS, FRCPI
Professor of Preventive Cardiology
National University of Ireland
Galway Campus
National Institute for Preventive Cardiology
Galway, Ireland

Nehal N. Mehta, MD, MSCE
Chief
Section of Inflammation and Cardiometabolic disease
Cardiology
NHLBI
NIH
Bethesda, MD, United States

M. Wesley Milks, MD
Assistant Professor of Clinical Medicine
Division of Cardiovascular Medicine
The Ohio State University College of Medicine
Columbus, OH, United States

Lem Moyé, MD, PhD
Professor of Biostatistics
UTHealth School of Public Health - Houston
Houston, TX, United States

Vijay Nambi, MD, PhD
Staff Cardiologist, Associate Professor of Medicine
Michael E DeBakey Veterans Affairs Hospital
Baylor College of Medicine
Houston, TX, United States

Ian J. Neeland, MD
Assistant Professor of Medicine
Department of Medicine/Division of Cardiology
University of Texas Southwestern Medical Center
Dallas, TX, United States

Morgan Oakland, MD
Thomas Jefferson University
Department of Emergency Medicine
Philadelphia, PA, United States

Kershaw V. Patel, MD
Division of Cardiology
Department of Internal Medicine
University of Texas Southwestern Medical Center
Dallas, TX, United States

W. Frank Peacock, MD, FACEP, FACC
Associate Chair and Research Director
Emergency Medicine
Baylor College of Medicine
Houston, TX, United States

Kayla A. Riggs, MD
Department of Internal Medicine
University of Texas Southwestern Medical Center
Dallas, TX, United States

Anand Rohatgi, MD
Associate Professor
Internal Medicine/Cardiology
University of Texas Southwestern Medical Center
Dallas, TX, United States

Anum Saeed, MD
Fellow, Lipids and Atherosclerosis
Baylor College of Medicine
Houston, TX, United States

Navdeep Sekhon, MD
Assistant Professor
Emergency Medicine
Baylor College of Medicine
Houston, TX, United States

Mohita Singh, MD
Resident, Internal Medicine
Baylor College of Medicine
Houston, TX, United States

Zhe Wang, MSc
Department of Epidemiology
Human Genetics and Environmental Sciences
School of Public Health
University of Texas Health Science Center at Houston
Houston, TX, United States

W.H. Wilson Tang, MD
Professor of Medicine
Cleveland Clinic Lerner College of Medicine
Director, Center for Clinical Genomics
Cleveland Clinic
Cleveland, OH, United States

Bing Yu, PhD
Department of Epidemiology
Human Genetics and Environmental Sciences
School of Public Health
University of Texas Health Science Center at Houston
Houston, TX, United States

Biomarkers: A Preface to Cardiovascular Disease?

Although we have made significant progress in the identification and management of cardiovascular diseases (CVDs), it remains the leading cause of death in the western world. Furthermore, although the management of traditional risk factors for atherosclerotic CVD continues to improve the residual risk of CVD, it remains high and in fact the incidence and prevalence of heart failure continues to increase. Hence there is a continued need not only for better diagnostics but also for identification of novel pathways and targets for therapy.

Biomarkers have been used for a long time to aid diagnosis and direct management in many disease processes, and their value and use continue to evolve and expand. The advances in technology and emergence of newer fields such as genomics, proteomics, and metabolomics have provided novel insights and exciting opportunities in the management of CVD. In this book an outstanding group of authors review and provide their expertise on the use of biomarkers in the management of various aspects of CVD.

The topics covered include statistical approaches in the evaluation of biomarkers; laboratory standards and approaches; biomarkers and traditional cardiovascular risk factors; evaluation of symptoms in the emergency room; management of various common CVDs including acute coronary syndromes, heart failure, and venous thromboembolism; and antiplatelet therapy monitoring. Then we also introduce the readers to the proteomics, genomics, and metabolomics and look into the future of what is coming. As the field continues to evolve with the significant advances in technology, throughput, and approaches, it is highly likely that novel treatment and diagnostic approaches will emerge. Biomarkers will be integrated in the day-to-day assessment of not only disease but also health and may provide us with the first clues of changes in our bodies before the onset of symptoms.

A sincere thanks to all the wonderful authors who have contributed to this book and made it a comprehensive review of the value of biomarkers in CVD and, of course, my family—mom, dad, in-laws, wife, and kids—without whom I could not achieve anything in life!

Contents

The views presented in this book represent those of the authors and not necessarily of the Department of Veterans Affairs.

CHAPTER 1

Lab Standards: A Practical Guide for Clinicians

RON HOOGEVEEN, PHD

BIOMARKERS: DEFINITION AND UTILITY IN CLINICAL PRACTICE

Biomarkers have been broadly defined as biological characteristics that can be objectively measured and evaluated as an indicator of normal biological processes, pathogenic processes, or pharmacological responses to a therapeutic intervention.[1] Using this broad definition, biomarkers can include measurements of proteins (i.e., proteomics), metabolites (i.e., metabolomics), genetic variants such as single-nucleotide polymorphisms (SNPs) commonly identified in genome-wide association studies, and RNA (e.g., microRNAs and messenger RNAs). Furthermore, imaging techniques to identify and quantitate biological markers of pathogenic processes are also considered biomarkers.

From a clinical perspective, biomarkers can be of use in risk assessment for a variety of factors related to health or disease, such as exposure to environmental factors, genetic exposure or susceptibility, markers of subclinical or clinical disease or surrogate endpoints to evaluate safety and efficacy of different therapies.[2] Therefore biomarkers are generally classified according to different stages in the development of a disease. Screening biomarkers are markers used for screening of patients who have no apparent disease, diagnostic biomarkers can assist in the care of patients who are suspected to have disease, and prognostic biomarkers are used in patients with overt disease to aid in the categorization of disease severity and prediction of future disease course, including recurrence and monitoring of treatment efficacy.[3] Biomarkers may be used to enhance clinical trials to support both more efficient drug development and use of new therapeutics entering the market. For example, predictive biomarkers may allow specific targeting of patients who are likely to respond positively to treatment (aka enrichment strategy), thereby potentially reducing the cost of drug development by reducing the size of the study population required to demonstrate a drug's safety and efficacy. Furthermore, by demonstrating that a drug will only have clinical utility for a particular subpopulation of patients, biomarker-based enrichment strategies can reduce the adverse effects and unnecessary costs associated with the administration of drugs to patients in the biomarker-negative population, who are less likely to benefit from such treatment.

Novel biomarkers such as cardiac troponins (e.g., cTn-T and cTn-I) and natriuretic peptides (e.g., B-type natriuretic peptide [BNP] and amino-terminal proBNP [NT-proBNP]) have shown their efficacy in the diagnosis and risk stratification of patients with suspected acute coronary syndrome (ACS) and heart failure (http://www.aacc.org/AACC/members/nacb). Because prevention of cardiovascular events in patients at increased risk is likely to have a significant impact on the overall public health burden, the development of novel biomarkers for screening is currently an active area of investigation. In particular, the identification of biomarkers to monitor the efficacy of new treatments for heart failure is emerging as a critical priority to enhance translational research in heart failure drug development.

BASIC PRINCIPLES OF WHAT MAKES FOR USEFUL BIOMARKER CHARACTERISTICS
Sensitivity and Specificity

It is important to consider a number of issues that influence the clinical utility of potential novel biomarkers for cardiovascular risk assessment. One of the major considerations is whether a novel biomarker can improve upon the cardiovascular risk prediction that can be attained with existing well-established cardiovascular risk markers. To this end, a potential marker needs to exhibit sufficient sensitivity and specificity to allow for risk classification.

A new era of high-sensitivity assays represent an important advance in the use of diagnostic and prognostic markers for cardiovascular risk stratification. As the name implies, high-sensitivity assays detect

Biomarkers in Cardiovascular Disease. https://doi.org/10.1016/B978-0-323-54835-9.00001-6

1

concentrations of the same biomarkers but at much lower concentrations. With the development of high-sensitivity assays, various terms such as limit of the blank (LoB), limit of detection (LoD), and limit of quantitation (LoQ) used to describe the smallest concentration of a biomarker that can be reliably measured by an analytical procedure are becoming increasingly important as medical decision levels may approach the lower analytical limits of these tests. The Clinical and Laboratory Standards Institute has published the EP17 guideline[4] to provide a standard method for determining LoB, LoD, and LoQ. EP17 defines LoB as the highest apparent analyte concentration expected to be found when replicates of a sample containing no analyte (i.e., blank sample) are tested. Note that a blank sample devoid of analyte can produce an analytical signal that might otherwise be consistent with a low concentration of analyte. $LoB = mean_{blank} + 1.645\ (SD_{blank})$. LoD represents the lowest analyte concentration that can be reliably distinguished from "analytical noise" or the LoB. As defined in EP17, LoD is determined by using both the measured LoB and test replicates of a sample known to contain a low concentration of analyte. The mean and SD of the low concentration sample is then calculated. EP17 defines LoD as $LoD = LoB + 1.645\ (SD_{low\ conc.\ sample})$. LoQ is the lowest concentration at which the analyte can not only be reliably detected but also at which limit predefined goals of bias and imprecision are met. Typically, LoQ (aka "functional sensitivity") is defined as the concentration that results in a coefficient of variance ($CV = [SD/mean] * 100\%$) of 20% and is thus a measure of an assay's precision at low analyte concentrations. The LoQ may be equivalent to the LoD, or it could be at a much higher concentration, depending on whether the estimated bias and imprecision at the LoD meet the requirements for total error for the analyte (i.e., LoD = LoQ) or not (i.e., LoQ > LoD).

In particular, high-sensitivity assays for cardiac troponins have shown added sensitivity for cardiac myocyte necrosis,[5–7] but there remains a need for careful interpretation of these tests by the practicing clinician.[8] According to expert consensus, high-sensitivity troponin assays should have a CV of <10% at the 99th percentile value of the population of interest.[5] Furthermore, to be classified as a high-sensitivity assay, concentrations below the 99th percentile should be detectable above the assay's LoD for >50% of healthy individuals in the population of interest. A number of manufacturers are currently producing high-sensitivity troponin assays, but there is wide variability in assay characteristics (Table 1.1, adapted from Sherwood et al.[9]), which prevents direct comparisons between the assays and poses a challenge with the advent of high-sensitivity troponin testing. Establishing the 99th percentile value in the general population, for each assay, will be critical in optimizing the sensitivity and specificity of high-sensitivity troponins and can serve to minimize false-positive testing.[10]

TABLE 1.1
Analytic Comparisons of Contemporary High-Sensitivity Cardiac Troponin Assays

	Limit of Detection (ng/L)	99% CV (ng/L)	10% CV (ng/L)
Hs-cTn-T			
Roche Elecsys	5.0	14 (13%)	13
Hs-cTn-I			
Abbott ARCHITECT	1.2	16 (5.6%)	3.0
Beckman Access	2–3	8.6 (10%)	8.6
Mitsubishi Pathfast	8.0	29 (5%)	14
Nanosphere	0.2	2.8 (9.5%)	0.5
Radiometer AQT90	9.5	23 (17.7%)	39
Singulex Erenna	0.09	10.1 (9.0%)	0.88
Siemens Vista	0.5	9 (5.0%)	3
Siemens Centaur	6.0	40 (10%)	30

CV, coefficient of variance; *Hs-cTn-I*, high-sensitivity cardiac troponin I; *Hs-cTn-T*, high-sensitivity cardiac troponin T.
Adapted from Sherwood MW, Kristin Newby L. High-sensitivity troponin assays: evidence, indications, and reasonable use. *J Am Heart Assoc.* 2014;3:e000403, with permission.

The receiver operating characteristic (ROC) curve is typically used to evaluate the clinical utility of a biomarker for both diagnostic and prognostic purposes.[11] More specifically, evaluation of a novel biomarker is generally based on its capability to improve the area under the ROC curve (AUC).[12] However, even strong independent risk predictors can have a very limited impact on the AUC. Therefore calibration, i.e., measuring how well the predicted probability agrees with the observed proportions in a population, is essential in the assessment of the accuracy of prediction models.[13] Reclassification can directly compare the clinical impact of two prediction models by determining how many individuals would be reclassified into clinically relevant risk strata (e.g., low, intermediate, or high), which may form the basis for treatment decisions. The percent reclassified can thus be used as a measure of the clinical impact of a new marker when added to an existing prediction model.

Variability

A number of aspects related to the biophysical and/or structural features of a specific biomarker can also greatly influence its utility. For example, it is important to understand how circulating levels of a particular biomarker are influenced by factors such as diet, diurnal variation, day-to-day variation within an individual, half-life in circulation, and dynamic range within a population. Information regarding the intraindividual variation in biomarker levels as well as the analytical variation of biomarker assays at medical decision levels can be particularly useful to the practicing clinician in interpreting test results. Biomarkers that have a relatively long half-life in circulation (i.e., at least several hours) and a relatively small intraindividual variation in circulating levels compared with the dynamic range within a population are better suited as potential markers for risk prediction.

Assay Standardization

It is highly desirable that a proposed marker can be measured accurately using standardized and cost-effective methods in a routine clinical laboratory setting. For most well-established risk factors, methods are eventually adapted so that these biomarkers can be measured using standardized assays on specialized automated chemistry analyzers in routine clinical laboratories. The development of standardized reference methods and standard reference materials (SRMs) containing known amounts of the analyte of interest is a crucial component of assay standardization.

Immunoaffinity assays are most commonly used to evaluate emerging risk factors. Immunoassays use monoclonal or polyclonal antibodies to capture targeted proteins through establishment of diverse noncovalent bonds (e.g., electrostatic or hydrophobic interactions, van der Waals forces, or hydrogen bonds), specific to the individual antigen-antibody pair. Target proteins are then indirectly quantified based on the signal intensity of luminescent (e.g., electrochemiluminescence immunoassay [ECLIA]), fluorescent (fluorescent immunoassay [FIA]), enzymatic (e.g., enzyme-linked immunosorbent assay [ELISA]), or radioactive (radioimmunoassay [RIA]) antibody-labeled reporter molecules or via light scattering of antigen-antibody complexes (e.g., immunoturbidimetry and nephelometry). ELISA methods in particular are considered the "work horse" of novel biomarker research. ELISA methodology generally provides sufficient sensitivity, is relatively cost-effective, does not require advanced instrumentation, and can be performed in routine laboratories.[14] However, ELISA methods are notoriously difficult to standardize, even when monoclonal antibodies are used, and can be subject to interfering factors such as antibody-specific cross-reactivity, complexity of the sample matrix, autoantibodies, and genetic mutations or polymorphisms which can alter epitope recognition by monoclonal antibodies.

Mass spectrometry (MS) is the most common technology used in proteomics biomarker research because of its unique ability to identify proteins in a nonbiased manner. The mass-to-charge (m/z) ratio of a molecule is the principal measurement obtained from MS analysis, and data from a specific sample are usually displayed as a "spectrum," which is a plot of the m/z ratio on the x-axis versus the level of intensity on the y-axis. Currently a number of different instruments are being manufactured which use MS sometimes combined with a chromatographic technique to aid in the separation of molecules in a complex sample matrix. The two most common chromatographic techniques used in combination with MS are liquid chromatography (LC) and gas chromatography (GC). Using LC combined with tandem mass spectrometry, captured ions are subjected to sequential ionization, and fragmented products of these ions can be analyzed, which allows for the identification of different peptides. Methods based on the combination of chromatography and MS techniques (e.g., gas chromatography-mass spectrometry [GC–MS] and liquid chromatography/tandem mass spectroscopy [LC-MS/MS]) are generally considered "the gold standard" because they are not affected by the same interfering factors as ELISA methods. However, GC–MS and LC-MS/MS are generally less cost-efficient and, because they require a higher level of operator expertise, are generally not well suited for routine clinical laboratories. The recent advancements in GC–MS and LC-MS/MS technologies will almost certainly improve their clinical utility in the near future.

Biomarker Stability

Specialized sample processing and storage requirements can also affect the clinical utility of a biomarker. In particular, the effect of long-term storage on biomarker stability varies greatly among analytes and is dependent on storage conditions, sample matrix, and the addition of specific preservatives. Large prospective epidemiological studies are ideally suited to assess the predictive value of novel risk factors. Because most epidemiological studies measure biomarkers in biological samples that have been stored for long time periods, it is important to investigate what impact long-term storage may have on biomarker levels. The Atherosclerosis Risk in Communities study recently reported that the impact of long-term biospecimen storage (up to 25 years) on circulating levels of established cardiovascular lipid risk factors may be minimal.[15] However, there is a paucity of data regarding the potential impact of long-term biospecimen storage on novel biomarkers.

Causality

Issues related to the need for a causal relationship between a marker and the pathogenesis of a certain disease remain a controversial topic among biomarker researchers. Markers that have proven to be valuable in risk assessment without a clear causal relationship as well as markers that are established mediators of disease but fail to predict risk for disease have been described.

PROTEOMICS-BASED DEVELOPMENT OF CARDIOVASCULAR BIOMARKERS

The human proteome is far more complex than the human genome and has been estimated to include anywhere from 20,000 (based on the number of protein-coding genes) to millions of proteins resulting from alternative splicing, posttranslational modification, and proteolytic processing (Fig. 1.1). Although a number of different proteomic approaches have been applied to identify new biomarkers for cardiovascular diseases, the principle underlying all proteomic approaches is the comparative analysis of protein expression profiles in normal versus diseased tissues. A growing number of studies have used proteomic analysis of different types of tissues including vascular cells, atherosclerotic plaques, heart, and blood to identify potential novel protein biomarkers associated with the pathogenesis of cardiovascular disease.[17–20] Furthermore, the Human Proteome Organization (www.HUPO.org) initiatives have been created to aid in the development of a human protein reference database derived from different biological compartments, including plasma, urine, brain, heart, and liver.

Proteomic approaches using plasma have gained in popularity because plasma samples, unlike other biospecimens, are usually collected and stored as part of clinical examinations in large epidemiologic studies and clinical trials. Furthermore, the plasma proteome is believed to constitute a complex mixture of proteins

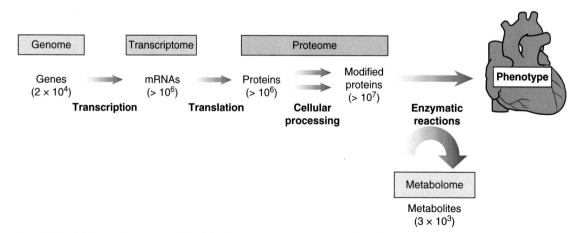

FIG. 1.1 Increasing complexity of the human proteome compared with the human genome. (Adapted from Gerszten RE, Wang TJ. The search for new cardiovascular biomarkers. *Nature*. 2008;451:949–952.)

derived from all tissues, which makes plasma an attractive medium for clinical analysis as it represents the molecular states of diverse systems.[21] The measurement of circulating biomarkers has long been central in decision-making in cardiovascular medicine, most prominently for the diagnosis of myocardial infarction (e.g., creatine kinase and troponins) and heart failure (e.g., natriuretic peptides) and for cardiovascular risk stratification (e.g., lipids and lipoproteins). However, it is clear that the complexity of cardiovascular disease requires a more complete and systematic assessment of the entire range of proteins measurable in plasma (the plasma proteome) to further our understanding of the underlying pathogenesis of cardiovascular disease. The systematic investigation of the plasma proteome may lead to unbiased discovery of novel biomarkers to improve diagnostic and predictive accuracy and identify therapeutic targets. The recent advent of novel multiplexing methods, including nucleotide-labeled immunoassays and aptamer reagents, and other proteomic approaches allows for a more systematic investigation of complex human diseases and provides new tools for biomarker development.

Tools Used in Proteomics

The diversity in protein abundance of the plasma proteome, which spans more than 11 orders of magnitude, can greatly influence the identification of potential biomarkers, particularly those that are present at extremely low concentrations.[22]

MS is the most powerful tool for systematic and unbiased investigation of proteins present in tissues and cells, including posttranslational protein modifications.[23-25] However, the complexity of the plasma proteome requires multiple sample preparation stages, including depletion of high-abundance proteins, concentration of low-abundance proteins, protein separation (e.g., LC or GC), and protein identification (e.g., trypsin digestion).[26]

A large number of different methods for sample preparation and protein separation and identification have been described.[27] Sample processing usually include protocols to solubilize proteins in chaotropic agents (e.g., urea) or nonionic detergents (e.g., 3-[(3-cholamidopropyl)dimethylammonio]-1-propanesulfonate [CHAPS]). These types of reagents do not substantially alter protein charge, which affects the chromatographic properties of proteins during fractionation.

The most widely used technique for proteomic protein separation is two-dimensional electrophoresis (2-DE).[28,29] Proteins are amphoteric molecules that carry a negative, positive, or zero net charge, which is determined by their amino acid composition and the pH of their environment (molecular charge). In 2-DE proteins are first separated based on their differences in molecular charge, a process known as isoelectric focusing. The proteins are then separated according to their molecular weight by sodium dodecyl sulfate-polyacrylamide gel electrophoresis in the second dimension. After separation by 2-DE, the proteins can be visualized via a number of different techniques, such as staining, radiolabeling, and immunodetection. The final step in the proteomic analysis is protein identification, which almost always involves some form of MS as mentioned previously.

Although 2-DE and MS have been the methods of choice for proteomic analysis, other methodologies that use multiplexing of immunoaffinity assays are currently being developed. Protein microarray technology generally uses a platform for capturing proteins by immobilizing potential ligands (binding partners) on a solid surface, followed by detection and identification of the bound protein.[30] Potential ligands include antibodies and nucleic acids among other molecules. A specific example of microarray technology has been developed by the Luminex Corporation (Austin, TX). The Luminex xMAP system is a multiplexed microsphere-based suspension array platform for high-throughput protein and nucleic acid detection.[31] This platform is unique in that it combines flow cytometry with conventional ELISA technology, which makes it relatively cost-effective and accessible to routine laboratories. Several studies have demonstrated its use as an efficient tool for both genetic and proteomic biomarker discovery.[32-34] Multiplex analysis can be very useful to examine the effects of an intervention on numerous biomarkers in clinical research studies, particularly when there may be small sample volume of stored plasma or serum.[33] However, some multiplex assays may require validation before selection in a clinical research protocol because low assay sensitivity and relatively poor correlation to conventional ELISA methods may be problematic, particularly for some analytes with very low plasma concentrations.[33] Furthermore, a major obstacle for affinity proteomic technologies is that multiplexing is limited because of cross-reactivity of affinity reagents.[35]

Other proteomic approaches currently under development include systems for (1) ultrasensitive detection of single molecules, (2) nucleotide-labeled immunoassays, (3) aptamer reagents for efficient multiplexing at high sample throughput, and (4) coupling of affinity capture methods to MS for improved specificity (see Fig. 1.2).

1. Ultrasensitive detection of single molecules by immunoaffinity assays is typically accomplished by using highly sensitive detectors, antibodies labeled with fluorescent or luminescent reporters for signal amplification, and preanalytical enrichment steps.[37,38]

2. Labeling of antibodies with nucleic acids can significantly improve assay sensitivity because nucleic acids can be amplified and quantified by Watson-Crick base pairing to fluorescently labeled primers based on the polymerase chain reaction (PCR).[39] One specific development of this principle technique, referred to as a proximity extension assay, has shown particularly useful in multiplexing by significantly reducing the problem of cross-reactivity.[40,41]

3. An alternative strategy to address the limitations of current immunoassays is the development of affinity reagents other than antibodies, such as synthetic molecules or aptamers. Aptamers can include engineered antibody fragments, synthetic peptides, or oligonucleotides.[42,43] Oligonucleotide-based aptamers are particularly attractive because they are simple and cost-efficient to design and have the major advantage that they can be amplified for improved sensitivity and easy detection using PCR and hybridization arrays. Large libraries of random oligonucleotides are mixed with target proteins in an iterative process to test for binding, whereas other oligonucleotides that bind to other targets are depleted from the pool. The nucleotide aptamers will physically interact with the protein surface and display high-affinity binding that can be altered via sequence modifications.[44] A commercial platform using this aptamer technology has been developed by SomaLogic Inc.[45]

4. The target specificity of affinity-based assays can be improved by coupling them to MS methods. The affinity reagents are used to capture protein targets in a pull-down assay which are then eluted from the

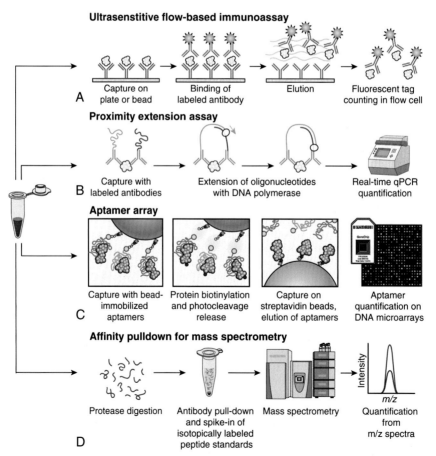

Ultrasensitive flow-based immunoassay

A — Capture on plate or bead → Binding of labeled antibody → Elution → Fluorescent tag counting in flow cell

Proximity extension assay

B — Capture with labeled antibodies → Extension of oligonucleotides with DNA polymerase → Real-time qPCR quantification

Aptamer array

C — Capture with bead-immobilized aptamers → Protein biotinylation and photocleavage release → Capture on streptavidin beads, elution of aptamers → Aptamer quantification on DNA microarrays

Affinity pulldown for mass spectrometry

D — Protease digestion → Antibody pull-down and spike-in of isotopically labeled peptide standards → Mass spectrometry → Quantification from m/z spectra

FIG. 1.2 Use of emerging affinity-based proteomics methods. (Adapted from Smith JG, Gerszten RE. Emerging affinity-based proteomic technologies for large-scale plasma profiling in cardiovascular disease. *Circulation*. 2017;135:1651–1664.)

reagent, digested to peptides, and sequenced to detect captured proteins by using unbiased MS. Captured protein targets can then be quantified using isotopically labeled synthetic peptides by targeted MS.

ADVANCES IN MICRORNA RESEARCH FOR CARDIOVASCULAR RISK PREDICTION

MicroRNAs (miRNAs) are short (~19–25 nucleotides in length) noncoding RNA molecules that modulate the stability and/or the translational efficiency of target messenger RNAs (mRNA) by base pairing with complimentary sites within these target mRNAs. Generally miRNAs act as negative regulators of gene expression because miRNA:mRNA duplex formation leads to degradation or translational inhibition of the target mRNA, although examples of a few exceptions to this have been reported.[46,47] More than 2500 miRNAs have been identified, and it is estimated that more than 50% of the human genome is under miRNA control.[48,49]

Evidence from a number of recent studies highlight the important role of miRNAs in regulating key biological pathways related to lipid metabolism,[50] oxidative stress, and systemic inflammation,[51] all of which are known to be involved in the etiology of cardiometabolic disease. A number of miRNAs have been shown to control the expression of genes affecting lipoproteins and the reverse cholesterol transfer pathway

(see Rayner and Moore[52] for review and Fig. 1.3). Particularly, miR-33a and miR-33b have been shown to repress the expression of ABCA1, ABCG1, and NPC1, thereby inhibiting cellular cholesterol efflux.[50,53] Interestingly, both miR-33a and miR-33b are embedded in the intronic regions of the genes that encode the nuclear transcription factors sterol regulatory element–binding proteins SREBP1 and SREBP2, which control the expression of a number of genes involved in cholesterol and fatty acid synthesis. Inhibition of miR-33 results in increased cholesterol efflux from hepatocytes to apo A-I in vitro and raises high-density lipoprotein cholesterol (HDL-C) levels in mice.[50,53] Furthermore, miR-33a/b inhibition also has been shown to raise HDL-C and lower very-low-density lipoprotein triglycerides in nonhuman primates.[54] Although miRNAs act intracellularly, extracellular miRNAs can be detected in the circulation bound to proteins,[55] on lipoproteins,[56] or within vesicles such as microparticles, exosomes, and apoptotic bodies.[57–59] Interestingly, miRNAs are remarkably stable in circulation and share many of the essential characteristics of a good biomarker, such as noninvasive measurability, a long half-life in the sample, a high degree of sensitivity and specificity, and cost-effective laboratory testing. A number of recent studies have investigated the use of circulating miRNAs as biomarkers for the diagnosis and prognosis of cardiovascular diseases (see Condorelli et al.[60] for review),

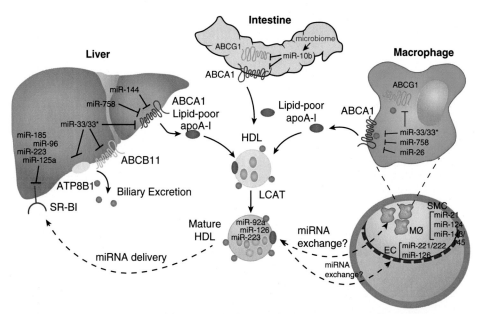

FIG. 1.3 Role of miRNAs in the regulation of HDL metabolism. (Modified from Rayner KJ, Moore KJ. MicroRNA control of high-density lipoprotein metabolism and function. *Circ Res*. 2014;114:183–192.)

including acute myocardial infarction,[61,62] heart failure,[63] cardiomyopathy,[64] and atherosclerosis.[65] Despite these promising findings, the use of miRNAs as biomarkers of cardiovascular disease will have to be validated in large population-based studies. Furthermore, the potential for miRNAs as therapeutic targets for the treatment of cardiovascular disease remains an active topic of research.

IMPACT OF NEW BIOMARKERS ON CURRENT GUIDELINES

With the rapidly emerging biomarker discoveries, clinicians need advice on the clinical validity and utility of new tests and whether they improve clinical, patient-centered, or economic outcomes. Biomarker tests initiate a cascade of decisions which subsequently determine the course and costs of patient management. Recognizing the importance of testing in medical decisions and given the limited healthcare resources, it is now generally viewed that clinical utilization and reimbursement of diagnostic tests should move from a cost-based toward a value- and evidence-based approach. Evidence-based clinical practice guidelines (CPGs) may be best suited in conveying this message to practicing clinicians and their patients. Careful evaluation of new biomarker tests should be carried out in a step-wise fashion before any recommendations can be made regarding their clinical utility or incorporation into the patient management pathway (Fig. 1.4 adapted from Horvath et al.[66]). High-quality CPGs are systematically developed statements that provide recommendations about the management of specific diseases and should be outcome oriented, reliable (i.e., developed in a transparent and reproducible manner free from commercial influence or bias), multidisciplinary, clinically applicable, clearly written, regularly reviewed and updated, appropriately disseminated and implemented, cost-effective, and amenable to measurement of their impact in clinical practice.[67,68] Furthermore, in good CPGs the overall quality or strength of the

evidence and the strength of the recommendations should be graded separately. Unfortunately, there are currently a large number of CPGs for the management of cardiovascular diseases available on the internet (WWW), sometimes with seemingly contradicting recommendations for the same condition. Obviously this complicates matters for practicing physicians trying to understand which guideline to choose in everyday practice. Therefore it is of critical importance that a more transparent process for CPG development is adopted to aid physicians in harmonizing the approaches and standards of care.

CONCLUSIONS

Biomarkers play important diagnostic and prognostic roles in cardiovascular disease risk assessment and can serve as surrogate endpoints to evaluate safety and efficacy of therapeutic interventions. With the emergence of high-sensitivity assays, it is imperative that clinicians, researchers, and laboratorians learn about the unique characteristics of these assays which will enable their implementation into clinical practice. In particular, high-sensitivity troponin assays have shown added sensitivity for cardiac myocyte necrosis, but this greater sensitivity requires careful interpretation of these tests by the practicing clinician. Continued advancements in proteomics methodologies, such as MS and novel multiplexing methods using nucleotide-labeled immunoassays and aptamer reagents, allow for a more systematic investigation of the plasma proteome which may lead to unbiased discovery of novel biomarkers to improve diagnostic and predictive accuracy and identify new therapeutic targets. Research studies into the use of miRNAs as biomarkers of cardiovascular disease risk show promise but will need further validation in large population-based studies. Despite the significant progress in biomarker research, assay standardization remains a major hurdle in the assessment of the clinical validity and utility of new biomarker tests and their implementation into evidence-based CPGs.

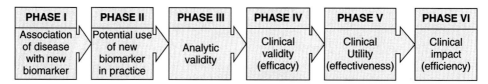

FIG. 1.4 Phases of biomarker evaluation. (Adapted from Horvath AR, Kis E, Dobos E. Guidelines for the use of biomarkers: principles, processes and practical considerations. *Scand J Clin Lab Invest Suppl.* 2010;242:109–116.)

REFERENCES

1. Naylor S. Biomarkers: current perspectives and future prospects. *Expert Rev Mol Diagn*. 2003;3:525–529.
2. Vasan RS. Biomarkers of cardiovascular disease: molecular basis and practical considerations. *Circulation*. 2006;113:2335–2362.
3. Biomarkers Definitions Working Group. Biomarkers and surrogate endpoints: preferred definitions and conceptual framework. *Clin Pharmacol Ther*. 2001;69:89–95.
4. Institute CaLS. Protocols for Determination of Limits of Detection and Limits of Quantitation, Approved Guideline. In: CSLI, ed. *CLSI Document EP17*. PA, USA: Wayne; 2004.
5. Apple FS, Collinson PO. Biomarkers ITFoCAoC. Analytical characteristics of high-sensitivity cardiac troponin assays. *Clin Chem*. 2012;58:54–61.
6. Jaffe AS. The 10 commandments of troponin, with special reference to high sensitivity assays. *Heart*. 2011;97:940–946.
7. Twerenbold R, Jaffe A, Reichlin T, Reiter M, Mueller C. High-sensitive troponin T measurements: what do we gain and what are the challenges? *Eur Heart J*. 2012;33:579–586.
8. Newby LK, Jesse RL, Babb JD, et al. ACCF 2012 expert consensus document on practical clinical considerations in the interpretation of troponin elevations: a report of the American College of Cardiology Foundation task force on Clinical Expert Consensus Documents. *J Am Coll Cardiol*. 2012;60:2427–2463.
9. Sherwood MW, Kristin Newby L. High-sensitivity troponin assays: evidence, indications, and reasonable use. *J Am Heart Assoc*. 2014;3:e000403.
10. Thygesen K, Alpert JS, Jaffe AS, et al. Third universal definition of myocardial infarction. *J Am Coll Cardiol*. 2012;60:1581–1598.
11. Zou KH, O'Malley AJ, Mauri L. Receiver-operating characteristic analysis for evaluating diagnostic tests and predictive models. *Circulation*. 2007;115:654–657.
12. Hanley JA, McNeil BJ. The meaning and use of the area under a receiver operating characteristic (ROC) curve. *Radiology*. 1982;143:29–36.
13. Cook NR. Statistical evaluation of prognostic versus diagnostic models: beyond the ROC curve. *Clin Chem*. 2008;54:17–23.
14. Oellerich M. Enzyme-immunoassay: a review. *J Clin Chem Clin Biochem*. 1984;22:895–904.
15. Parrinello CM, Grams ME, Couper D, et al. Recalibration of blood analytes over 25 years in the atherosclerosis risk in communities study: impact of recalibration on chronic kidney disease prevalence and incidence. *Clin Chem*. 2015;61:938–947.
16. Gerszten RE, Wang TJ. The search for new cardiovascular biomarkers. *Nature*. 2008;451:949–952.
17. Donners MM, Verluyten MJ, Bouwman FG, et al. Proteomic analysis of differential protein expression in human atherosclerotic plaque progression. *J Pathol*. 2005;206:39–45.
18. Jang WG, Kim HS, Park KG, et al. Analysis of proteome and transcriptome of tumor necrosis factor alpha stimulated vascular smooth muscle cells with or without alpha lipoic acid. *Proteomics*. 2004;4:3383–3393.
19. Jungblut P, Otto A, Zeindl-Eberhart E, et al. Protein composition of the human heart: the construction of a myocardial two-dimensional electrophoresis database. *Electrophoresis*. 1994;15:685–707.
20. Mateos-Caceres PJ, Garcia-Mendez A, Lopez Farre A, et al. Proteomic analysis of plasma from patients during an acute coronary syndrome. *J Am Coll Cardiol*. 2004;44:1578–1583.
21. Ping P, Vondriska TM, Creighton CJ, et al. A functional annotation of subproteomes in human plasma. *Proteomics*. 2005;5:3506–3519.
22. Anderson NL, Anderson NG. The human plasma proteome: history, character, and diagnostic prospects. *Mol Cell Proteomics*. 2002;1:845–867.
23. Aebersold R, Mann M. Mass spectrometry-based proteomics. *Nature*. 2003;422:198–207.
24. Mertins P, Qiao JW, Patel J, et al. Integrated proteomic analysis of post-translational modifications by serial enrichment. *Nat Methods*. 2013;10:634–637.
25. Udeshi ND, Mertins P, Svinkina T, Carr SA. Large-scale identification of ubiquitination sites by mass spectrometry. *Nat Protoc*. 2013;8:1950–1960.
26. Gerszten RE, Accurso F, Bernard GR, et al. Challenges in translating plasma proteomics from bench to bedside: update from the NHLBI Clinical Proteomics Programs. *Am J Physiol Lung Cell Mol Physiol*. 2008;295:L16–L22.
27. Blanco-Colio LM, Martin-Ventura JL, Vivanco F, Michel JB, Meilhac O, Egido J. Biology of atherosclerotic plaques: what we are learning from proteomic analysis. *Cardiovasc Res*. 2006;72:18–29.
28. Klose J. Protein mapping by combined isoelectric focusing and electrophoresis of mouse tissues. A novel approach to testing for induced point mutations in mammals. *Humangenetik*. 1975;26:231–243.
29. O'Farrell PH. High resolution two-dimensional electrophoresis of proteins. *J Biol Chem*. 1975;250:4007–4021.
30. Kingsmore SF. Multiplexed protein measurement: technologies and applications of protein and antibody arrays. *Nat Rev Drug Discov*. 2006;5:310–320.
31. Dunbar SA. Applications of Luminex xMAP technology for rapid, high-throughput multiplexed nucleic acid detection. *Clin Chim Acta*. 2006;363:71–82.
32. Binder SR, Hixson C, Glossenger J. Protein arrays and pattern recognition: new tools to assist in the identification and management of autoimmune disease. *Autoimmun Rev*. 2006;5:234–241.
33. Liu MY, Xydakis AM, Hoogeveen RC, et al. Multiplexed analysis of biomarkers related to obesity and the metabolic syndrome in human plasma, using the Luminex-100 system. *Clin Chem*. 2005;51:1102–1109.
34. Tozzoli R. Recent advances in diagnostic technologies and their impact in autoimmune diseases. *Autoimmun Rev*. 2007;6:334–340.

35. Ellington AA, Kullo IJ, Bailey KR, Klee GG. Antibody-based protein multiplex platforms: technical and operational challenges. *Clin Chem*. 2010;56:186–193.

36. Smith JG, Gerszten RE. Emerging affinity-based proteomic technologies for large-scale plasma profiling in cardiovascular disease. *Circulation*. 2017;135:1651–1664.

37. Jarolim P, Patel PP, Conrad MJ, Chang L, Melenovsky V, Wilson DH. Fully automated ultrasensitive digital immunoassay for cardiac troponin I based on single molecule array technology. *Clin Chem*. 2015;61:1283–1291.

38. Todd J, Freese B, Lu A, et al. Ultrasensitive flow-based immunoassays using single-molecule counting. *Clin Chem*. 2007;53:1990–1995.

39. Sano T, Smith CL, Cantor CR. Immuno-PCR: very sensitive antigen detection by means of specific antibody-DNA conjugates. *Science*. 1992;258:120–122.

40. Assarsson E, Lundberg M, Holmquist G, et al. Homogenous 96-plex PEA immunoassay exhibiting high sensitivity, specificity, and excellent scalability. *PLoS One*. 2014; 9:e95192.

41. Lundberg M, Eriksson A, Tran B, Assarsson E, Fredriksson S. Homogeneous antibody-based proximity extension assays provide sensitive and specific detection of low-abundant proteins in human blood. *Nucleic Acids Res*. 2011;39:e102.

42. Binz HK, Amstutz P, Pluckthun A. Engineering novel binding proteins from nonimmunoglobulin domains. *Nat Biotechnol*. 2005;23:1257–1268.

43. Stoevesandt O, Taussig MJ. Affinity proteomics: the role of specific binding reagents in human proteome analysis. *Expert Rev Proteomics*. 2012;9:401–414.

44. Gold L, Ayers D, Bertino J, et al. Aptamer-based multiplexed proteomic technology for biomarker discovery. *PLoS One*. 2010;5:e15004.

45. Rohloff JC, Gelinas AD, Jarvis TC, et al. Nucleic Acid Ligands With Protein-like Side Chains: Modified Aptamers and Their Use as Diagnostic and Therapeutic Agents. *Mol Ther Nucleic Acids*. 2014;3:e201.

46. Graff JW, Dickson AM, Clay G, McCaffrey AP, Wilson ME. Identifying functional microRNAs in macrophages with polarized phenotypes. *J Biol Chem*. 2012;287:21816–21825.

47. Lee S, Vasudevan S. Post-transcriptional stimulation of gene expression by microRNAs. *Adv Exp Med Biol*. 2013; 768:97–126.

48. Kozomara A, Griffiths-Jones S. miRBase: integrating microRNA annotation and deep-sequencing data. *Nucleic Acids Res*. 2011;39:D152–D157.

49. Pasquinelli AE. MicroRNAs and their targets: recognition, regulation and an emerging reciprocal relationship. *Nat Rev Genet*. 2012;13:271–282.

50. Rayner KJ, Suarez Y, Davalos A, et al. MiR-33 contributes to the regulation of cholesterol homeostasis. *Science*. 2010; 328:1570–1573.

51. Magenta A, Greco S, Gaetano C, Martelli F. Oxidative stress and microRNAs in vascular diseases. *Int J Mol Sci*. 2013;14:17319–17346.

52. Rayner KJ, Moore KJ. MicroRNA control of high-density lipoprotein metabolism and function. *Circ Res*. 2014; 114:183–192.

53. Najafi-Shoushtari SH, Kristo F, Li Y, et al. MicroRNA-33 and the SREBP host genes cooperate to control cholesterol homeostasis. *Science*. 2010;328:1566–1569.

54. Rayner KJ, Esau CC, Hussain FN, et al. Inhibition of miR-33a/b in non-human primates raises plasma HDL and lowers VLDL triglycerides. *Nature*. 2011;478:404–407.

55. Turchinovich A, Weiz L, Langheinz A, Burwinkel B. Characterization of extracellular circulating microRNA. *Nucleic Acids Res*. 2011;39:7223–7233.

56. Vickers KC, Palmisano BT, Shoucri BM, Shamburek RD, Remaley AT. MicroRNAs are transported in plasma and delivered to recipient cells by high-density lipoproteins. *Nat Cell Biol*. 2011;13:423–433.

57. Diehl P, Fricke A, Sander L, et al. Microparticles: major transport vehicles for distinct microRNAs in circulation. *Cardiovasc Res*. 2012;93:633–644.

58. Valadi H, Ekstrom K, Bossios A, Sjostrand M, Lee JJ, Lotvall JO. Exosome-mediated transfer of mRNAs and microRNAs is a novel mechanism of genetic exchange between cells. *Nat Cell Biol*. 2007;9:654–659.

59. Zernecke A, Bidzhekov K, Noels H, et al. Delivery of microRNA-126 by apoptotic bodies induces CXCL12-dependent vascular protection. *Sci Signal*. 2009;2:ra81.

60. Condorelli G, Latronico MV, Cavarretta E. microRNAs in cardiovascular diseases: current knowledge and the road ahead. *J Am Coll Cardiol*. 2014;63:2177–2187.

61. Devaux Y, Vausort M, Goretti E, et al. Use of circulating microRNAs to diagnose acute myocardial infarction. *Clin Chem*. 2012;58:559–567.

62. Fiedler J, Thum T. MicroRNAs in myocardial infarction. *Arterioscler Thromb Vasc Biol*. 2013;33:201–205.

63. Vogel B, Keller A, Frese KS, et al. Multivariate miRNA signatures as biomarkers for non-ischaemic systolic heart failure. *Eur Heart J*. 2013;34:2812–2822.

64. Gupta MK, Halley C, Duan ZH, et al. miRNA-548c: a specific signature in circulating PBMCs from dilated cardiomyopathy patients. *J Mol Cell Cardiol*. 2013;62: 131–141.

65. Fichtlscherer S, Zeiher AM, Dimmeler S. Circulating microRNAs: biomarkers or mediators of cardiovascular diseases? *Arterioscler Thromb Vasc Biol*. 2011;31:2383–2390.

66. Horvath AR, Kis E, Dobos E. Guidelines for the use of biomarkers: principles, processes and practical considerations. *Scand J Clin Lab Invest Suppl*. 2010;242:109–116.

67. Grol R, Dalhuijsen J, Thomas S, Veld C, Rutten G, Mokkink H. Attributes of clinical guidelines that influence use of guidelines in general practice: observational study. *BMJ*. 1998;317:858–861.

68. Lin KW, Slawson DC. Identifying and using good practice guidelines. *Am Fam Physician*. 2009;80:67–70.

CHAPTER 2

Statistical Interpretation of the Utility and Value of a Biomarker

LEM MOYÉ, MD, PHD

INTRODUCTION

Biomarkers, or biologic markers,[1] are molecules produced by organ systems and tissues, whose measurement provides knowledge concerning the state of the organism. When tracked over time, biomarkers can provide early evidence of a fundamental change in the body's ability to function in several domains. Molecules (e.g., creatinine and kidney function) have guided the practice of clinicians for many years, and cardiology has recently experienced a biomarker explosion, fueled by advances in biochemistry and molecular biology, greater measurement precision, and ubiquitous high-speed computing. This chapter will discuss the role of biostatistics and computing in the comprehension and use of contemporary biomarker knowledge and some directions for the future.

SCOPE OF THE PROBLEM

Studying biomarkers presents several challenges. The first is the putative link between a biomarker signal and the pathology that signal may represent. The biomarker signal must be both accurate (the measurement is close to the actual level in the subject) and precise (measurements of the biomarker in the same environment provides similar readings). These traits are required to ensure that an elevation or depression in the biomarker level represents an actual change in the biomarker as opposed to instrument error or chance of variation.

Then, the excursion in the cardiac biomarker's value must be related to organ pathology. Measures that change under nominal organ state and also change in the presence of pathology are of limited clinical value, as are measures that change in neither normal nor pathological conditions. Epidemiologists in concert with biostatisticians have developed the quantitative tools required to assess each of these characteristics, leading to the generation of some ubiquitous implements such as receiver–operator curves. These tools have been historically used when one is dealing with a single biomarker–disease relationship.

However, hampered by an incomplete understanding of molecular biology, immature measurement engineering, and the absence of all but the most rudimentary statistical analyses, the study of biomarkers has proceeded at a slow rate. Now, not only are new biomarkers identified on a regular and frequent basis but cardiologists also recognize the complexity of these molecules and the dynamic environment in which they are both produced and operate. These twin observations challenge the use of biostatistics to determine the use of biomarkers.

The number of potential biomarkers is theoretically overwhelming. The protein manufacturing process of the nucleus–ribosome complex (of which there are up to 10 million per cell) can generate tens of thousands of peptides in a single hour. Even though each cell (excepting the rare spontaneous mutation) contains the same complete genome, the differing microenvironments of cells in the same tissue lead to activation of different regions of the DNA complex, producing different peptides.

Many of these peptides experience only intracellular utilization and perhaps could be successfully used as indicators of intracellular pathophysiology when the measurement tools for within-cell assessment become available. Other biomarkers are transported to the cell's elaborate membrane where they are released upon and into the cell membrane of a contiguous cell, producing a reaction in this neighboring cell before denaturing. The promise of these difficult-to-detect peptides as biomarkers is difficult to gauge using present-day technology.

Still other peptides are released into the extracellular environment. Bound to complex protein–lipid entities in the plasma, they are transported to the intercellular environment of distant organs where the peptide is released. This peptide may be inert until it is in proximity to other peptides with a different tissue of origin,

Biomarkers in Cardiovascular Disease. https://doi.org/10.1016/B978-0-323-54835-9.00002-8

at which time they enter distant cells and activate their nucleic acid complexes and protein-generating machinery.

In addition, this rich process of biomarker production, elaboration, transport, and reaction is dynamic. Time and events change the complex intracellular and extracellular environments, driving the cells to continually alter both the spectrum and level of peptide production. Thus the richness of the intracellular-extracellular-temporal dynamic has the potential of generating many uncountable peptides and an equal number of cellular reactions.

When confronted with this rich environment, it is fair to ask what the goal of biostatistics is in this arena. Stepping back, we see that life's complexity has generated not just a single peptide to be sought by cardiologists like a Holy Grail but instead has revealed an internal world of biomarkers. This world, with its intense intercellular communication grid and rhythmic ebbs and flows, is a network of expression between cells in the body, from which each cell derives information and in which each cell contributes to the ceaseless chemical dialogue. Proteomics is a language that is 2 billion years old, developed by the organism to communicate with itself as it assesses and reacts to changing external and internal environments.

If this is the case, then our job is to understand enough of this language to be able to prevent or extirpate disease. Thus we must borrow the tools of the linguist who after learning basic words, begins to assemble them in varying sequences and collections to create more complex constructs and ultimately to communicate. Consideration of multiple biomarkers simultaneously through the implementation of the tools of biostatistics[2] is a first attempt to understand the structure of this dialect.

QUALITY CONTROL

Understanding the relationship between biomarker data and clinical end points requires attention to data collection and data quality. The poor quality of data, either through the entry of error-laden data points to the data set or the presence of missing data can reduce the precision of statistical estimates, increase their variance, and degrade the investigator's ability to draw meaningful conclusions. If the researcher is willing to invest time in these straightforward efforts, data correction, published errata, and manuscript retractions can be avoided. Missing data are commonly accepted as a fact of life and can be especially important for biomarker assessments.[3] Imputation procedures that permit more

than one set of replacements for the missing data, and therefore multiple data sets for analysis,[4] are preferred. Procedures for managing the analysis of missing data are now well described,[5] and score functions that are based on the Wilcoxon test[6,7] specifically deal with the inability to collect follow-up data because of intervening serious adverse events or clinical outcomes.

STUDYING BIOMARKER RELATIONSHIPS

Traditionally, the challenge of applying biostatistics to understanding relationships between findings and clinical events (e.g., heart failure) is dwarfed by the epidemiologic metrics that must be met to demonstrate a risk factor–end point causal relationship. However, in the biomarker arena, this requirement is relaxed when the investigator replaces an interest in causality with one of the secure associations, i.e., the biomarker is an accurate indicator of an organism's state without having excited the production of that state, as demonstrated by Cogle et al.[8] Investigators understand that troponin levels do not excite the production of heart attacks and are instead most interested in the degree to which troponin levels inform them of whether a heart attack has taken place. Examining the standard Bradford Hill criteria[9] from this perspective, the investigator's emphasis is on temporality, response gradient, biologic plausibility, coherency, and consistency. We must keep these in mind as we work to understand the interrelationships between cardiac biomarkers and then relate biomarkers to clinical measures that we know how to interpret. The latter has been the most comprehensively explored, requiring the concept of surrogacy.

Relationships with Clinical Outcomes—Surrogacy

Surrogacy is the process by which biomarkers are linked to a well-recognized clinical state of the organ or organism. An example of such a relationship is serum creatinine level and renal function. With the knowledge that higher levels of creatinine correspond to deteriorating kidney function and reduced levels with more normal renal function, clinicians monitor creatinine function with the well-supported hope that by doing so, they are monitoring the health of the kidney. Physicians also understand limitations of this approach, for example, serum creatinine levels are not a marker of early renal cancer. Although creatinine is not the cause of renal function (in fact quite the reverse is true), it gives a simple and direct measure of kidney function. Examples in cardiology are creatine kinase-muscle/brain (CK-MB) bands and troponin for the diagnosis of acute myocardial infarction (MI) and probrain natri-uretic peptide for the identification of heart failure.

What is therefore necessary for examining the rela-tionship between the biomarker and a clinical end point (e.g., heart failure) is the need to first identify then explicate the relationship. The exploration begins with the use of standard statistical models, e.g., regression models. In these cases, the dependent variable is the clinical end point to which the investigator believes the biomarker is linked. The predictor variable is the bio-marker level itself or the change in the biomarker, e.g., Schutt et al.[10] However, typical regression analysis can-not usually be conducted in this circumstance because the clinical state (the occurrence of a heart attack or the occurrence of heart failure) is itself not a continuous variable but is dichotomous (it either occurs or not). In this case, there are several useful options.

One is logistic regression.[11] Because the dependent variable is dichotomous, considering the probability of its occurrence makes sense. In logistic regression, we begin not with the probability of the event, but with the odds (the ratio of the probability of the event to the probability that the event does not occur). This is written as "O" reflecting the odds of the disease. We are interested in the log of the odds ratio or $ln(O)$ which permits some linearization of the risk factor. In the absence of the biomarker, the $ln(O_0) = \beta_0$, reflecting that without the knowledge of the value of the bio-marker, the log of the odds is β_0. We signify $ln(O_B)$ to reflect the odds in the presence of the biomarker, and thus the odds of the event are $O_o = e^{\beta_0}$. However, we signify the odds of the event in the presence of the biomarker as $ln(O_B) = \beta_0 + \beta_1 x_i$, where the term $\beta_1 x_i$ reflects the contribution of the biomarker x_i. Its odds ratio is $O_B = e^{\beta_0 + \beta_1 x_i}$. Then the odds ratio R is simply,

$$R = \frac{O_B}{O_0} = \frac{e^{\beta_0 + \beta_1 x_i}}{e^{\beta_0}} = e^{\beta_1 x_i}.$$ Using data and standard

statistical procedures, the parameters β_0 and β_1 are esti-mated by b_0 and b_1. Hypothesis tests and 95% confi-dence intervals are available for these estimates from standard statistical packages.

This approach has been implemented to evaluate the relationship between bone marrow mononuclear cell phenotypes and the occurrence of heart failure in patients receiving cell therapy[12] and in the evaluation of changes in acute area of left ventricular injury after MI.[10]

One can isolate, identify, and remove the influence of confounders (e.g., race, gender, and ethnicity) by con-ducting adjusted logistic regression. If the organism's state is related to a time component, the Cox propor-tional hazards regression analysis permits one to take time into account.[13] An example of such an approach is given in the study by Lupon et al.[14] and Zethelius et al.[15]

However, building this relationship between biomarker and the end point is not sufficient for its use-fulness in determining surrogacy. In current practice, this requires a demonstration of its use, which is com-monly conducted through the development of a sen-sitivity and specificity analysis. Here, we dichotomize the disease state as D^+ and D^- and the proteomic result as T^+. For example, the state in which the biomarker is believed to indicate the disease to be present is T^+, with T^- pointing to the absence of the disease. With this nomenclature, we define sensitivity as the probability of disease given the biomarker reaches the threshold or $P[T^+|D^+]$. Note that probability presumes knowledge of the disease state initially; we know the disease state initially and ask, "given that the disease is present, how likely is it that the biomarker be positive?" Analogously, specificity (the probability that the biologic marker is below the threshold given the absence of the disease) is $P[T^-|D^-]$. These probabilities are of course related to the threshold value of the biomarker itself, and one can adjust these quantities by carrying out a receiver opera-tor curve (ROC) analysis, which is simply graphing $P[T^+|D^+]$ and $1 - P[T^-|D^-]$ as a function of the threshold value of the biomarker. What is of greater interest to the clinician is the predictive value of the test.

Biomarker Assessment for Utility

A useful tool for assessing biomarkers is to check the degree to which they predict clinical outcomes. Statis-tical models can produce statistically significant rela-tionships between biomarkers and clinical variables of interest such as mortality. However, clinicians are inter-ested in determining the degree to which these bio-markers can usefully predict outcomes of clinical merit such as death, reinfarction, or worsening heart failure.

There are several statistical tools that can provide the predictive value of these biomarkers. These are each based on the preliminary completion of logistic regression or Cox hazard analysis. An important, tradi-tional measure is the area under the curve (AUC). AUC assesses the area under the receiver operational curve and is a measure of the degree to which the biomarker-based decision rule improves over random chance. The range of the AUC is between 0 and 1, a simple random selection rule producing an ROC of 0.5.

A newer implement is the integrated discrimina-tion improvement (IDI). This tool requires a multi-step approach. It begins with computing the slope of the linear regression of the predicted probabilities of events, which is known as the discrimination slope. The

IDI is simply the difference in the slopes of two different predictive models. The greater the difference in the slopes, the greater the IDI of one model over the other. Working with these models assumes that they are appropriately calibrated.

Net reclassification improvement is an assessment of whether a new model changes the reclassification of patients from one model, demonstrating how many patients are shifted into different clinical risk categories (low, moderate, or high) by using a different model. This tool is of particular interest because it can provide an easily understood estimate of the ability of two different models to separate individual patients based on risk.

These aforementioned tools are particularly useful as quantitative prediction models increase in complexity.[16] The model-building procedure begins with the evaluation of univariate relationships between commonly assessed "risk factors" and the clinical end point of interest. This is followed by a second round of models in which the separate prognostic value of the variable of interest is compared with other known important prognostic variables in a multivariable model. This is conducted either deterministically or by a statistical algorithm in a stepwise fashion. At this point, the AUC and c-statistic can be assessed to determine the "predictive value" for each of the models. Comparing predictive accuracy between two models using Net reclassification improvement (NRI) and IDI can provide an additional perspective on the ability of the models to improve upon each other.

In 2013, Candell-Riera et al.[17] used the IDI and NRI procedures in assessing the incremental prognostic value of myocardial perfusion–gated single-photon-emission computed tomography (MPGS) compared with exercise test, concluding that IDI and RCI for both exercise and MPGS were high. However, there was only improvement in the prediction of major cardiovascular adverse events (MACE) events, not death. This is similar to comparing the R^2 or the percent of variability explained between two regression analyses.[18] There are, however, some concerns about underestimation of the variability of the standard error of an IDI estimate.[19]

Another approach to assessing the predictive power of the test is through Bayes procedures. This is available by reversing the conditions of the probability. Specifically, the positive predictive value is the probability of disease given that the test is above the threshold, $P[D^+|T^+]$, and the negative predictive value or $P[D^-|T^-]$ is the probability that the patient does not have the disease given the test is below the threshold. Note that these are related to but are separate from the computations for sensitivity and specificity.

If one has a simple two-by-two table with counts of patients who meet each of the criteria such as $T^- \cap D^-$, $T^- \cap D^+$, $T^+ \cap D^-$, and $T^+ \cap D^+$,[a] then all four probabilities are easily calculable. However, typically, one is provided simply with the sensitivity and specificity. To compute the positive and the negative predictive value from these quantities, the investigator simply needs Bayes Theorem[20] which states that the positive predictive value $P[D^+|T^+]$ is

$$P[D^+|T^+] = \frac{P[T^+|D^+]\,P[D^+]}{P[T^+|D^+]\,P[D^+] + P[T^+|D^-]\,P[D^-]}.$$

And, for negative predictive value $P[D^-|T^-]$,

$$P[D^-|T^-] = \frac{P[T^-|D^-]\,P[D^-]}{P[T^-|D^-]\,P[D^-] + P[T^+|D^+]\,P[D^+]}.$$

Note that the computation for predictive value includes the likelihood of the disease, $P[D^+]$ and $P[D^-] = 1 - P[D^+]$. The introduction of this quantity loosens the link between sensitivity and specificity on the one hand and predictive values on the other. Just because of the observation that acute MI symptoms include left-arm numbness, it does not imply that every case of left-arm numbness indicates an evolving MI, and high sensitivity and specificity does not *prima facie* imply high predictive values.

Examining Relationships Between Biomarkers

The foregoing discussion of the overwhelming number of proteins and their impact on the production of other proteins diminished our enthusiasm for identifying the one single biomarker that produces, for example, the best possible prognostic information on the changing status of a patient in heart failure. Investigators should therefore focus their attention to studying the influences of combinations of biomarkers by asking how does one assemble the most predictive collection of biomarkers that predict the organism's clinical state.

The investigator retains the choice of how these relationships are first generated. Perspicacious scientists who have studied the field may already, for example, understand the relationship between CD34 and CD133/CD134, and their impact on the change in left ventricular ejection fraction[21] can build this relationship into a larger ensemble of biomarkers which may be even more predictive.

A standard approach in generating these relationships is through management of the correlation matrix **R**.

---

[a]The simple $\cap$ simply means "and".

This is a $p \times p$ matrix, whose diagonal elements are one and whose off-diagonal elements represent the correlations between the p biomarkers, such that the element in the ith row and jth column contains the correlation between the ith and jth biomarker. We assume that there is a large collection of subjects from whom this set of biomarkers has been collected.

As the mathematics quantities such as those that appear in biochemical kinetics, relationships in biology that are of higher order also have strong linear components. Thus the confinement of classical statistics consideration to linear relationships is defensible, although we will see later that this is not the only assumption available to us. With this in mind, the correlations identified in the R matrix reflect the interrelatedness of these sets of variables, i.e., the degree to which the different biomarkers measure the same thing. In fact, the larger the correlations between the different biomarkers, the more prominent the central theme that they point to becomes.

The notion of interrelatedness is the root argument for assembling from the original collection of p biomarkers a collection of r new variables that summarize the overlap among the original biomarkers. The success in naming these new variables is the degree to which the "same thing" can be identified and categorized. Thus this process is one of identification and categorization. The three statistical procedures of interest are as follows: (1) principal components, (2) canonical correlation, and (3) discriminant analyses.[22]

Each of these three procedures is based on the principal axis theorem from linear algebra[23,24] which permits the partitioning of the correlation matrix R by writing $R = P'\Lambda P$, where Λ is the $p \times p$ diagonal matrix of eigenvalues and P is the $p \times p$ nonsingular matrix of eigenvectors. The necessary presumption that R is invertible is tantamount to the assumption that each of the original biomarkers makes some contribution separate and apart from the others.

Principal Components

The simplest of the three procedures, principal components, simply uses the columns of the matrix P as coefficients to create a new variable from the original variables. The diagonalization of the correlation matrix R permits us to associate with each column (denoted by $\underline{P}_j$) of P an eigenvalue λ_i, and then use of Lagrange multipliers demonstrates that this repartitioning of R reduces the overall variability in system.[25] Because the total variance in the original system is the sum of the diagonal elements of $R = tr(R) = p$ and $tr(R) = tr(\Lambda)$, no information contained in the original variables is

lost by the transformation. Thus λ_i/p is the fraction of variability explained by the ith new variable. In addition, the columns of the matrix Λ can be reordered so that $\Lambda = \text{diag}(\lambda_{[1]}, \lambda_{[2]}, \lambda_{[3]}, \ldots \lambda_{[p]})$, where $\lambda_{[1]}$ is the largest eigenvalue, $\lambda_{[2]}$ is the largest eigenvalue, $\ldots \lambda_{[p]}$ is the smallest eigenvalue. The order the columns of P can be rearranged accordingly as well so that

$$P = \left[\underline{P}_1, \ \underline{P}_2, \ \underline{P}_3, \ \cdots \underline{P}_p \right],$$ where $\underline{P}_1$ is the eigenvalue

corresponding to $\lambda_{[1]}$. With this as foundation, the investigator creates a new matrix $S = \Lambda^{-\frac{1}{2}} P$ $y_i = \sum_{j=1}^{p} s_{ij}x_j$.[b]

Thus the first principal component has variance $\lambda_{[1]}$, explains $100\frac{\lambda_{[1]}}{p}$ percent of the total variability of the system, and is created by computing $y_{[1]} = \sum_{j=1}^{p} s_{1j}x_j$.

Similarly, the second principal component has variance $\lambda_{[2]}$, explains $100\frac{\lambda_{[2]}}{p}$ percent of the total variability of the system, and is created by computing $y_{[2]} = \sum_{j=1}^{p} s_{2j}x_j$.

The investigator continues in this fashion until all p components are generated.

Principal components offer two advantages to the investigator. The first is the percent of the variance explained by the earlier principal components with the largest variance explaining most of the variability of the system. For example, if the variance of the first r principal components (where $\frac{100}{p} \sum_{i=1}^{r} \lambda_{[i]}$) where $1 < r < p$ is substantial, then the system may be adequately summarized by these first r components. Collapsing a system of 40 biomarkers down to a subsystem of nine principal components explains that most of the variability in the system is a substantial dimensionality reduction.

The second advantage is that the components are independent of each other. Thus there is less confounding and more stability in any regression analyses conducted on the subset of principal components. They are, in addition, amenable to statistical hypothesis testing using such tests, e.g., the sphericity criterion.[19]

A disadvantage of principal components is that commonly one cannot helpfully provide a meaning for

---

[b] S_{ij} is the element in the ith row and jth column of the matrix S.

the new variables produced in this reduced-dimension environment. Discerning the meaning of each new variable takes experience and skill. Proceeding one step further to factor analysis in which the principal components are rotated can be of considerable advantage here. Principal components analysis is a procedure commonly found in widely used statistical computing packages, e.g., SAS.

An example of the use of this function in cardiology is the generation of a composite cardiac impairment score (CCIS).[26] Beginning with six measures of left ventricular function, a complete principal components analysis was used to identify and encapsulate what the original variables measured in common and produced new variables that were uncorrelated. This first principal component was calculated as:

CCIS = −0.4766 * LVEF + 0.4353 * LVEDVI + 0.5080 * LVESVI − 0.3679 * WMIZ − 0.1087 * WMBZ + 0.4119 * In farct Size,

where LVEF is left ventricular ejection fraction, LVEDVI is left ventricular end diastolic volume index, LVESVI is left ventricular end systolic volume index, WMIZ is wall motion in the infarct zone, and WMBZ is wall motion in the border zone. The units of the constants were such that the resulting score was unitless.

The CCIS was higher when the values of LVEDVI, LVESVI, and infarct size were large and when the values of LVEF, WMIZ, and WMBZ were low. This might be described as myocardial flaccidity. It explains 56.2% of the total variability in the system, i.e., one variable contains half of the information that the original six variables held.

Canonical Correlation

Canonical correlation is related to principal components analysis. Principal components analysis focuses on one data set with p variables, whereas canonical correlation focuses on a data set with two collections or classes of variables. Principal components analysis is focused on creating new variables from the original collection of variables that would explain as much of the information in the data set as possible and be uncorrelated with each other. In canonical correlation the investigator is focused on identifying new variables in the first class of variables that are highly correlated with new variables generated from the second class of variables. Just as in principal components evaluation, one conducts these evaluations in sequence, first finding a new pair of variables that are highly correlated with each other (a high between class correlation), then finding a second pair of new variables (one from each of the classes of variables) that are also highly

correlated with the stipulation that these two new variables (one from each class) are uncorrelated with the first new pair. Here canonical refers to identifying relationships between variables that are latent (or not directly observed) by building these latent variables from multiple variables that are observed.

An example of the use of canonical correlation is the study of cell phenotypes from the bone marrow and the peripheral blood. In a sample of individuals, three phenotypes are measured from the bone marrow and three from the blood. Although one could examine the relationship between the same phenotype comparing its value in the bone marrow to that of the blood, the investigators proceed under the assumption that the phenotype levels in the bone marrow signify a concept characterized as "state of the bone marrow". Similarly, the "state of the peripheral blood" is characterized by the peripheral blood phenotypes. The answer to the questions, "what are these states" and "how are they related to each other," is provided by the implementation of canonical correlation.

Because there are two batteries of variables, the overall correlation matrix is partitioned as $\mathbf{R} = \begin{bmatrix} \mathbf{R}_{11} & \mathbf{R}_{12} \\ \mathbf{R}_{21} & \mathbf{R}_{22} \end{bmatrix}$, where $\mathbf{R}_{11}$ is the $p \times p$ matrix for the first battery of variable, $\mathbf{R}_{22}$ is the $q \times q$ matrix for the second battery of variables, and the matrixes $\mathbf{R}_{12}$ and $\mathbf{R}_{21}$ are the $p \times q$ and $q \times p$ correlations of products between the batteries, respectively. In this formulation, the formula is focused on identifying the eigen structure of the $q \times q$ matrix $\mathbf{R}_{22}^{-1} \mathbf{R}_{21} \mathbf{R}_{11}^{-1} \mathbf{R}_{12}$.

When applied to the abovementioned example of phenotypes, 72% of the information that both the bone marrow–derived and peripheral blood–derived phenotypes contained was explained by the first canonical correlate, and a total of 99% of the variability was explained by two.

Discriminant Analysis

An additional statistical analysis tool that is based on the correlation matrix is discriminant analysis. In this case a cohort of subjects has a collection of p biomarkers measured and in addition has an end point measurement (e.g., the presence or absence of heart failure). In this case the investigator is interested in developing a function of biomarkers that are most predictive of heart failure. As we have seen, logistic regression can also play a role in answering this question. However, an advantage of discriminant analysis over logistic regression is that discriminant analysis is readily interpretable if there are more than two categories of clinical outcomes.

There are two forms of discriminant analysis that have been traditionally deployed. As an example, we will consider a battery of proteomic assays for participants in the first clinical category 1 (with correlation matrix R_1) and the same battery of proteomics in the second clinical category 2 with correlation matrix R_2. Assume that all these biomarkers are normalized to mean 0 and variance 1. Then, if the battery of proteomics for the ith individual is collected into a column vector with p element $\underline{x}_i$, the quadratic form function $D_Q = \underline{x}_i' R_1^{-1} \underline{x}_i - \underline{x}_i' R_2^{-1} \underline{x}_i$ is the operative function, classifying this individual into class one if $D_Q \le t$ and into class two if $D_Q > t$. If we assume that the correlation matrix for the biomarkers of the individuals in the two different clinical states is the same, i.e., $R_1 = R_2 = R$, then the function simplifies to the linear function $D_L = \underline{x}_i' R \underline{x}_i$, and linear discriminant analysis is carried out. An advantage of this procedure is that when individuals are so classified, the a priori knowledge of the group in which they actually reside leads to a straightforward classification analysis that produces sensitivity and specificity estimates, from which predictive values can be generated if one knows the likelihood of the disease states (vide supra).

When there are many biomarkers for consideration, it is possible to conduct stepwise discriminant analysis, in which biomarkers are individually considered for their discriminant ability and added one at a time in the order in which discriminating capability is optimally increased in each step. However, it is most important during this maneuver to have a data set on which the automatic procedure is created (the training set) separate and apart from the data on which the data are to be used (testing or validation set). This introduces an assessment of the reproducibility of the finding.

An example of this approach is that of Li et al.[27] who examined genome-wide methylation of whole blood in 102 participants with acute coronary syndrome and 101 controls using HumanMethylation450 array. Their external replication of discoveries in 100 patients and 102 controls identified new blood methylation alterations associated with this syndrome and provided an important new collection of biomarkers with potential clinical and therapeutic significance. Another example is that of DeFilippis et al.,[28] in which 1032 plasma metabolites were examined. A clinical state assessment revealed that 11 subjects experienced a thrombotic MI, 12 subjects suffered from nonthrombotic MI, and 15 subjects had stable coronary artery disease (CAD). Biomarker assays were conducted at both the time of catheterization,

6 h after catheterization, and a final point at more than 3 months after catheterization. A statistical classifier related to discriminant analysis was constructed, suggesting high sensitivity and specificity in differentiating thrombotic from nonthrombotic MI and stable CAD. In this evaluation, 19 metabolites promise as discriminators between these disease states.

BAYES ANALYSES AND MACHINE LEARNING

The process of combining what was learned and or believed with the current information is the crux of learning. Bayes procedure encompasses this, and to a degree, machine learning is an automation of this process.

Bayes procedures are the mathematical personification of learning. One starts with prior information then collects data (called conditional information). The prior information is combined with conditional information to produce posterior information. This posterior information is used to draw inferences about the question at issue. Mathematically, if one is interested in the value of a parameter (for example, the mean value of CD09 phenotype in the peripheral blood mononuclear cells in the post-MI setting), denoted as θ going into the experiment, then one should have prior information about this value (e.g., from previous experiments or previous ideas). This information is reflected in the prior distribution for CD09 or $\Pi_\Theta (\theta)$. This can be as simple as saying the value must be positive, or it could be made more complicated by stating that it is normally distributed. Then, one collects data $f(x_1, x_2, x_3, \ldots, x_n | \theta)$. In the end, one combines these conditional data (i.e., data that are conditional on the value of θ) with the prior information to identify the posterior distribution of θ given the data or $\Pi_\Theta (\theta | x_1, x_2, x_3, \ldots, x_n)$ as

$$\Pi_\Theta (\theta | x_1, x_2, x_3, \ldots, x_n) = \frac{f(x_1, x_2, x_3, \ldots, x_n | \theta)\, \Pi_\Theta (\theta)}{\int_{\Omega_\theta} f(x_1, x_2, x_3, \ldots, x_n | \theta)\, \Pi_\Theta (\theta)}.$$

A simplification of this concept is Bayes theorem that was used earlier to convert sensitivity and specificity into predictive values. In this somewhat more advanced paradigm, if the prior information was that the CD09 concentration followed a normal distribution and the conditional distribution is also normal, then the posterior distribution $\Pi_\Theta (\theta | x_1, x_2, x_3, \ldots, x_n)$ is normal as well with mean and variance related to the parameters of both the prior and conditional distribution.[29] This posterior distribution can be used much as normal distributions are used in the non-Bayesian context.

Historically steeped in controversy,[30-32] the development of both a solid theoretic construct (Jeffries) and advanced computations has allowed Bayes procedures to play more prominent roles in statistical analyses. However, the recognition that the posterior information from one computation becomes the prior distribution for the next computation permits these Bayes procedures to sequentially connect. This is one of the concepts of machine learning.

Machine learning is the process by which machines can learn without being explicitly programmed. It is a combination of statistics, information theory, theory of algorithms, and functional analysis.[33] An early example of this procedure using cardiac metabolomics is available.[34] This includes the regular updating of current information on a cyclical basis to convert a prior probability to a posterior probability, monitoring the probability of events as they either decrease or increase with each iteration of new information.

THE FUTURE

Although the support of biomarker research by traditional biostatistics has been reliable, there is a realization that the assumptions underlying these long-standing approaches require expansion. Rosner et al.[35] have been able to relax the normality assumptions in correcting ROCs for measurement, and Tang et al. have developed an expansion of least square methods to estimate receiver operator characteristics for biomarkers.[36] The development by Gao et al.[37] of an algorithm for pattern mixture model in the setting where a biomarker can be treated as a missing covariate is particularly instructive.

An important new component to these investigations is the "big data" concept. The "analytics" (quantitative tools that explore data sets looking for patterns) and large data sets represent a new biomarker research vista. When analytics return with results that sharpen the computer's ability to fashion a yet more incisive analytics, the process of "machine learning" has commenced. Contemporary examples of this approach are the work of Crabtree, who has applied the concept of a computational evolution system or a computing engine that identifies subtle, synergistic relationships between biomarkers in large data sets.[38] In addition, tool kits developed and made freely available by Li et al. permit characterization of transcriptomes and epigenomes for individual cells.[39] Mikacenic et al. identified two biomarker panels for sepsis,[40] and Tayefi et al.[41] have developed a data-dredging approach within a case–control design to link clinical biomarkers with traditional risk factors.

However, the future is even more promising, particularly if the field is sincere in its willingness to release itself from the assumptions of parametric modeling and the Riemann integral functions of classic calculus. Currently, the role of functions that are "barely" continuous, along with similar Brownian technologies, is focused principally on the production of metabolomics.[42] This can lead to the introduction of "genmarkers" or artificially generated peptides that, through nanotechnology, have evaluative properties. These "genmarkers" would be introduced intracellularly to assess their effects on the quantity and quality of natural biomarker production. Nanotechnology would transmit the reaction of the rich peptide-production environment to the probe as a discontinuous function over the large subset of biomarkers. Lebesgue integration theory permits the worker to assess this measurable function, integrating it over the "biomarker space" to learn the complete impact of the genmarker on the production and fate of naturally occurring biomarkers. Thus the impact of the genmarker on the intracellular environment could be quantitatively assessed, with specific attention to the reaction of peptide production. This reaction would lead to the production of other more sophisticated genmarkers, engaging the intracellular environ of peptide production in a "chemical dialogue". In this fashion, we would begin to speak and understand the language of biomarkers.

REFERENCES

1. Strimbu K, Tavel JA. What are biomarkers? *Curr Opin HIV AIDS.* 2010;5(6):463–466. https://doi.org/10.1097/COH.0b013e32833ed177.
2. Pascual-Figal DA, Ordoñez-Llanos J, Tornel PL, Vázquez R, Puig T, Valdés M, Cinca J, de Luna AB, Bayes-Genis A, MUSIC Investigators. Soluble ST2 for predicting sudden cardiac death in patients with chronic heart failure and left ventricular systolic dysfunction. *J Am Coll Cardiol.* 2009;54(23):2174–2179. https://doi.org/10.1016/j.jacc.2009.07.041.
3. Aittokallio T. Dealing with missing values in large-scale studies: microarray data imputation and beyond. *Brief Bioinform.* 2009;11(2):253–264.
4. Rubin DB. *Multiple Imputation for Nonresponse in Surveys.* New York: Wiley; 1987.
5. Kumar N, Hoque MA, Shahjaman M, Islam SM, Mollah MN. Metabolomic biomarker identification in Presence of outliers and missing values. *Biomed Res Int.* 2017;2017:2437608. https://doi.org/10.1155/2017/2437608. [Epub 2017 Feb 14].
6. Moyé LA, Davis BR, Hawkins CM. Analysis of a clinical trial involving a combined mortality and adherence dependent interval censored endpoint. *Statistics in Medicine.* 1992;11:1705–1717.

7. Moyé LA, Lai D, Jing K, Baraniuk MS, Kwak M, Penn MS, Wu CO. Combining censored and uncensored data in a U-statistic: design and sample size implications for cell therapy research. *Int J Biostat.* 2011;7: Article 29.

8. Cogle CR, Wise E, Meacham AM, et al. Detailed analysis of bone marrow from patients with ischemic heart disease and left ventricular dysfunction: BM CD34, CD11b, and clonogenic capacity as biomarkers for clinical outcomes. *Circ Res.* 2014;115(10):867–874. https://doi.org/10.1161/CIRCRESAHA. [115.304353. Epub 2014 Aug 18].

9. Hill B. Observation and experiment. *N Engl J Med.* 1953;248:995–1001.

10. Schutt RC, Trachtenberg B, Cooke JP, et al. Bone marrow characteristics associated with changes in infarct size after STEMI: a biorepository evaluation from the CCTRN TIME trial. *Circ Res.* November 18, 2014. [pii:CIRCRESAHA.114.304710. Epub ahead of print].

11. Hosmer DW, Lemeshow S. *Applied Logistic Regression.* 2nd ed. John Wiley & Sons.

12. Taylor DA, Perin EC, Willerson JT, et al. Identification of bone marrow cell subpopulations associated with improved functional outcomes in patients with chronic left ventricular dysfunction: an embedded cohort evaluation of the FOCUS-CCTRN Trial. *Cell Transplant.* 2015. [Epub ahead of print. PMID:26590374].

13. Hosmer DW, Lemeshow S, May S. *Applied Survival Analysis: Regression Modeling to Time to Event Data.* 2nd ed. John Wiley & Sons, Inc.; 2008.

14. Lupón J, de Antonio M, Galán A, et al. Combined use of the novel biomarkers high-sensitivity troponin T and ST2 for heart failure risk stratification vs conventional assessment. *Mayo Clin Proc.* 2013;88(3):234–243. https://doi.org/10.1016/j.mayocp.2012.09.016. [Epub 2013 Feb 4].

15. Zethelius B, Berglund L, Sundström J, et al. Use of multiple biomarkers to improve the prediction of death from cardiovascular causes. *N Engl J Med.* 2008;358(20):2107–2116. https://doi.org/10.1056/NEJMoa0707064.

16. Ladenheim ML, Kotler TS, Pollock BH, Berman DS, Diamond GA. Incremental prognostic power of clinical history, exercise electrocardiography and myocardial perfusion scintigraphy in suspected coronary artery disease. *Am J Cardiol.* 1987;59:270–277.

17. Candell-Riera J, Ferreira-González I, Marsal JR, et al. Usefulness of exercise test and myocardial perfusion–gated single photon emission computed tomography to improve the prediction of major events. *Circ Cardiovasc Imaging.* 2013;6:531–541.

18. Pencina MJ, Fine JP, D'Agostino RB. The integrated discrimination improvement (IDI) index is a popular tool for evaluating the capacity of a marker to predict a binary outcome of interest. *Stat Med.* 2016. https://doi.org/10.1002/sim. [7139. Epub ahead of print].

19. Kerr KF, McClelland RL, Brown ER, Lumley T. Evaluating the incremental value of new biomarkers with integrated discrimination improvement. *Am J Epidemiol.* 2011;174(3):364–374. https://doi.org/10.1093/aje/kwr086. [Epub 2011 Jun 14].

20. Moyé LA. *Elementary Bayesian biostatistics.* Boca Raton: Francis and Taylor/ Chapman Hall; 2007.

21. Perin EC, Willerson JT, Pepine CJ, et al. Effect of transendocardial delivery of autologous bone marrow mononuclear cells on functional capacity, left ventricular function, and perfusion in chronic ischemic heart failure: the FOCUS-CCTRN Trial. *JAMA.* 2012;307(16):1717–1726. [PMCID:PMC 22447880].

22. Cooley W, Lohnes P. *Multivariate Data Analysis.* John Wiley & Sons; 1971.

23. Graybill FA. *Theory and Applications of the Linear Model.* Duxbury Classic Series.

24. Seber GAF. *Multivariate Observations.* John Wiley & Sons; 1984.

25. Anderson TW. *An Introduction to Multivariate Statistical Analyses.* 3rd ed. John Wiley & Sons; 2004.

26. Bhatnagar A, Bolli R, Johnstone BH, et al. Bone marrow cell characteristics associated with patient profile and cardiac performance outcomes in the LateTIME-cardiovascular cell therapy research network (CCTRN) trial. *Am Heart J.* 2016;179:142–150. https://doi.org/10.1016/j.ahj.2016.06.018. [Epub 2016 Jul 6].

27. Li J, Zhu X, Yu K, Jiang H, et al. Genome-wide analysis of DNA methylation and acute coronary syndrome. *Circ Res.* March 27, 2017. https://doi.org/10.1161/CIRCRESAHA.116.310324. [pii:CIRCRESAHA.116.310324. Epub ahead of print].

28. DeFilippis AP, Trainor PJ, Hill BG. Identification of a plasma metabolomic signature of thrombotic myocardial infarction that is distinct from non-thrombotic myocardial infarction and stable coronary artery disease. *PLoS One.* 2017;12(4):e0175591. https://doi.org/10.1371/journal.pone.0175591. [eCollection 2017].

29. Berger JO. *Statistical Decision Theory. Foundations, Concepts, and Methods.* New York: Springer-Verlag; 1980.

30. Jeffreys H. On the prior probability in the theory of sampling. *Proceedings of the Cambridge Philosophical Society.* 1933;29:83–87.

31. Jeffreys H. *Scientific Inference, Reprinted With Additions in '37 and With New Editions in '57 and '73.* Cambridge: Cambridge University Press; 1931.

32. Savage LJ. *The Foundations of Statistics.* New York: Wiley; 1954 (1972 edition).

33. Munoz A. *Machine Learning and Optimization.* https://www.cims.nyu.edu/munoz/files/2014-cims.nyu.edu.

34. Forssen H, Patel R, Fitzpatrick N et al. Evaluation of machine learning methods to predict coronary artery disease using metabolomic data. *Stud Health Technol Inform.* 2017;235:111–115.

35. Rosner B, Tworoger S, Qiu W. Correcting AUC for measurement error. *J Biom Biostat.* 2015;6(5). https://doi.org/10.4172/2155-6180.1000270. Epub 2015 Dec 28.

36. Tang LL, Yuan A, Collins J, Che X, Chan L. Unified least squares Methods for the evaluation of diagnostic tests with the gold standard. *Cancer Inform.* 2017;16. https://doi.org/10.1177/1176935116686063. eCollection 2017.

37. Gao F, Dong J, Zeng D, Rong A, Ibrahim JG. Pattern mixture models for clinical validation of biomarkers in the presence of missing data. *Stat Med*. 2017:7328. https://doi.org/10.1002/sim. [Epub ahead of print].

38. Crabtree NM, Moore JH, Bowyer JF, George NI. Multiclass computational evolution: development, benchmark evaluation and application to RNA-Seq biomarker discovery. *BioData Min*. 2017;10:13. https://doi.org/10.1186/s13040-017-0134-8. eCollection 2017.

39. Li J, Smalley I, Schell MJ, Smalley KSM, Chen YA. SinCHet: a MATLAB toolbox for single cell heterogeneity analysis in cancer. *Bioinformatics*. May 4, 2017. https://doi.org/10.1093/bioinformatics/btx297. [Epub ahead of print].

40. Mikacenic C, Price BL, Harju-Baker S, et al. A Two Biomarker Model Predicts Mortality in the Critically Ill with Sepsis. *Am J Respir Crit Care Med*. April 18, 2017. https://doi.org/10.1164/rccm.201611-2307OC. [Epub ahead of print].

41. Tayefi M, Tajfard M, Saffar S, et al. hs-CRP is strongly associated with coronary heart disease (CHD): a data mining approach using decision tree algorithm. *Comput Methods Programs Biomed*. 2017;141:105–109. https://doi.org/10.1016/j.cmpb.2017.02.001. Epub 2017 Feb 3.

42. Altadill T, Campoy I, Lanau L, Gill K, Rigau M, Gil-Moreno A, Reventos J, Byers S, Colas E, Cheema AK. Enabling metabolomics based biomarker discovery studies using molecular phenotyping of exosome-like vesicles. *PLoS One*. 2016;11(3):e0151339. https://doi.org/10.1371/journal.pone.0151339. eCollection 2016.

CHAPTER 3

Hypertension: Key Biomarkers of Injury and Prognosis

KELLY ARPS, MD • JOHN W. MCEVOY, MB, BCH, MHS, FRCPI

ABBREVIATIONS

ACE   Angiotensin converting enzyme inhibitor
ADM   Adrenomedullin
Ang II   Angiotensin II
ARB   Angiotensin receptor blocker
ARIC   Atherosclerosis risk in communities
ARR   Aldosterone:renin ratio
AT-1   Angiotensin II receptor type 1
BNP   B-type natriuretic peptide
BP   Blood pressure
CCB   Calcium channel blocker
CKD   Chronic kidney disease
CRP   C-reactive protein
CT-1   Cardiotrophin-1
CVA   Cerebrovascular accident
ESRD   End stage renal disease
ET-1   Endothelin 1
HFpEF   Heart failure with preserved ejection fraction
HFrEF   Heart failure with reduced ejection fraction
hsCRP   High-sensitivity C-reactive protein
hs-troponin   High-sensitivity troponin
IL-1   Interleukin 1
IL-6   Interleukin 6
IMT   Intimal-medial thickness
LV   Left ventricle
LVH   Left ventricular hypertrophy
LVMI   Left ventricular mass index
MESA   Multi-Ethnic Study of Atherosclerosis
MI   Myocardial infarction
MR-proADM   Mid-region prohormone adrenomedullin
NO   Nitric oxide
NT-proBNP   Amino-terminal pro B-type natriuretic peptide
PAI-1   Plasminogen activator-inhibitor 1
PRA   Plasma renin activity
PRC   Plasma renin concentration
PTH   Parathyroid hormone
RAAS   Renin-angiotensin-aldosterone system
ROS   Reactive oxygen species
SBP   Systolic blood pressure
SD   Standard deviation
TGF-β   Transforming growth factor beta
TNF-α   Tumor necrosis factor alpha
UACR   Urinary albumin to creatinine ratio
XO   Xanthine oxidase

INTRODUCTION: THE PATHOPHYSIOLOGY OF HYPERTENSION AND WHY BIOMARKERS MATTER

Hypertension is a complex systemic disease, with important genetic and environmental drivers. Hypertension is diagnosed solely according to blood pressure (BP) thresholds, which have shifted downward over time based on evolving evidence in the field. Emphasizing this point, Sir Geoffrey Rose remarked that "hypertension is merely the value of BP above which net benefits of antihypertensive treatment had been established in randomized trials."[1] Therefore throughout the present chapter, we ask the reader to recognize that hypertension is a "man-made" designation and to bear in mind that what we really care about is abnormally elevated BP.

Elevated BP is associated with maladaptive neurohormonal responses, inflammatory and oxidative pathway aberrations, and vascular endothelial dysfunction. The kidneys have a dominant role in BP homeostasis by regulating volume status and influencing peripheral vascular resistance. A visual summary of the underlying pathophysiology of elevated BP is useful to review because it informs the choice of biomarkers that may guide the management of hypertension (Fig. 3.1).

Briefly, renal production of renin in response to apparent or actual volume depletion leads to downstream conversion of angiotensinogen to angiotensin II (Ang II), which activates Ang II receptor type 1 (AT-1) in systemic vasculature, resulting in vasoconstriction, vascular remodeling, and synthesis of aldosterone—a

Biomarkers in Cardiovascular Disease. https://doi.org/10.1016/B978-0-323-54835-9.00003-X

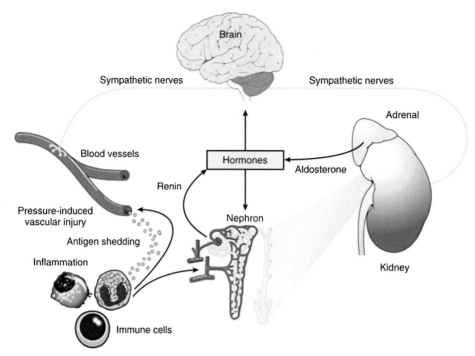

FIG. 3.1 Multisystem pathophysiology of hypertension. (From Bakris GL, Sorrentino MJ. *Hypertension: a companion to Braunwald's heart disease.* 3rd ed. Philadelphia, PA: Elsevier; 2018; with permission.)

primary regulator of systemic BP and volume status. Consequently, elevated intraglomerular pressures trigger a maladaptive cycle of hyperfiltration, glomerular injury, and sodium retention. Some patients, particularly those with preceding renal disease, have overactivity of the sympathetic system that further exacerbates vasoconstriction and renin release.

There is also increasing evidence that hypertension reflects an inflammatory condition. In parallel, oxidation of serum proteins and the resultant state of oxidative stress depletes nitric oxide (NO), leading to loss of protective properties of the endothelium and generating vasoconstriction and a prothrombotic state. These inflammatory and oxidative states interfere with the renin-angiotensin-aldosterone system (RAAS); for example, Ang II activates proinflammatory signaling, and reactive oxygen species (ROS) stimulate the mineralocorticoid receptor in an aldosterone-independent process.

In summary, hypertension is a state characterized by maladaptive vasoconstriction, volume overload, oxidative stress, and inflammation—all of which may be interrogated using various biomarkers. This chapter will describe the current and future utility of serum biomarkers in predicting the onset of hypertension in

healthy individuals, identifying subclinical target organ damage among hypertensive patients, and guiding the personalization of antihypertensive therapy. Based on the review of the literature, we have organized each main section of this chapter into subsections covering (1) RAAS markers, (2) indicators of cardiovascular stress and hemodynamic perturbation, and (3) biomarkers consistent with aberration in the inter-related inflammatory, oxidative stress, and endothelial dysfunction pathways (Table 3.1).

PREDICTING INCIDENT HYPERTENSION

Hypertension can be considered a disease of aging; in the National Health and Nutrition Examination Survey (NHANES) population, systolic BP (SBP) increased an average of 0.2 mmHg per year in the early adult years with acceleration to 0.8 mmHg per year after the age of 35 years, with similar findings in other cohorts.[2] However, there is also marked inter-individual variability and up to 12% of otherwise healthy young adults may develop hypertension before the age of 40 years.[3] Analysis of epidemiologic data has uncovered different trajectories of BP change over time, with steeper BP trajectories associated with accelerated atherosclerosis

TABLE 3.1
Biomarkers With Demonstrated and Potential Utility in the Prediction and Management of Hypertension

	Predicting Hypertension	Identifying Subclinical Organ Damage	Individualizing Therapy
Renin-angiotensin-aldosterone system	Aldosterone:renin ratio Parathyroid hormone Vitamin D	Renin Aldosterone:renin ratio Urinary angiotensinogen	Renin Urinary renin Urinary angiotensinogen Urinary sodium
Cardiovascular stress	Troponin NT-proBNP	Troponin NT-proBNP Adrenomedullin ST2	
Inflammatory/oxidative cascade	CRP Uric acid PAI-1 Urinary albumin Gamma-glutamyl transferase	CRP Uric acid Homocysteine Urinary albumin	CRP TNF-α IL-6 Endothelin 1 Uric acid
Other			Urinary metabolites of antihypertensive agents Brain-derived neurotrophic factor

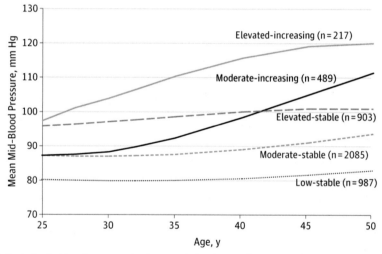

FIG. 3.2 Trajectories in blood pressure in the population-based Coronary Artery Risk Development in Young Adults (CARDIA) Study. (From Allen NB, Siddique J, Wilkins JT, et al. Blood pressure trajectories in early adulthood and subclinical atherosclerosis in middle age. *JAMA.* 2014;311(5):490–497; with permission.)

in middle age (Fig. 3.2).[4] Prediction of incident hypertension would enable clinicians to target at-risk individuals for more frequent screening or perhaps more aggressive lifestyle interventions to delay the onset of hypertension.

The only current screening and diagnostic tool for hypertension is the measurement of BP itself, which requires serial healthcare office visits or home measurement equipment.[5] Biomarker science holds the potential to identify those individuals (particularly younger adults in low-risk categories by traditional risk stratification) who are on "sinister" BP trajectories and who would benefit from efforts to prevent the development of hypertension and its sequelae.

Biomarkers Associated With Incident Hypertension

RAAS markers of incident hypertension

Inappropriate overactivation of RAAS signaling contributes to hypertensive disease, so it is reasonable to conclude that abnormal RAAS markers may predate pathologically elevated BP. In the Framingham cohort a log-linear relationship was demonstrated between increasing aldosterone-renin ratio (ARR) and hypertension incidence.[6] In the Multi-Ethnic Study of Atherosclerosis (MESA) cohort, those with subclinical hyperaldosteronism progressed faster from normotension to hypertension than others, supporting the potential of elevated ARR as a predictor of hypertensive disease.[7]

It is also theorized that chronic hyper aldosteronism leads to parathyroid hormone (PTH) activation, perhaps via renal calcium wasting. Cohort analysis of the independent predictive value of elevated PTH for incident hypertension has been mixed.[8,9] Because PTH signaling appears to activate RAAS, vitamin D deficiency may trigger both systems subsequent to secondary hyperparathyroidism. A pooled metaanalysis found an association between vitamin D deficiency and incident hypertension, and vitamin D supplementation in deficient patients can improve BP, suggesting a potential role for vitamin D biomarker testing and replacement in prehypertensive individuals, although this theory needs more testing.[10,11]

Markers of cardiovascular stress and incident hypertension

Circulating levels of troponin (measured as high-sensitivity troponin or hs-troponin) and B-type natriuretic peptide (BNP or the more frequently measured amino-terminal proBNP [NT-proBNP]) represent cardiac myocyte response to hemodynamic stress and injury. Abnormalities of these markers are present before clinically apparent hypertension; therefore such abnormalities may raise suspicion of out-of-office BPs in hypertensive range (masked hypertension), abnormalities in diurnal BP patterns, or even a subgroup in whom BP levels otherwise considered "normal" may be harmful at the individual level. Abnormalities in these biomarkers may also distinguish a population with subclinical coronary or structural disease that would be at higher risk of target organ damage should hypertension develop. In the MESA cohort 10-year risk of incident hypertension was increased for those above an NT-proBNP cutoff of 135 pg/mL.[12] The Atherosclerosis Risk in Communities (ARIC) cohort demonstrated independent risk of incident hypertension with baseline

elevation of either proBNP or hs-troponin.[13,14] There is evidence that extreme shift in pro-BNP from low-normal to elevated level confers additional risk of incident hypertension.[12] ST2, another biomarker of cardiac stress, has also been linked to incident hypertension.[15] Results of other prospective studies for these markers have been mixed, suggesting that more research is needed examining the link between subclinical myocardial strain and undiagnosed (pre) hypertensive physiology.[16,17]

Inflammatory and oxidative stress markers of incident hypertension

Evidence of inflammation and oxidative stress may be useful signs of evolving vascular dysfunction with attendant risk for incident hypertension. C-reactive protein (CRP), the most well-studied marker of inflammation, has been implicated in the development of endothelial dysfunction, vascular stiffness, and elevated BP.[18] Although some cohorts, particularly the large multiethnic Coronary Artery Risk Development in Young Adults study, failed to correlate CRP with incident hypertension, multiple prospective population-based studies have identified elevated CRP as an independent predictor of incident hypertension.[19–22] In particular, the Women's Health Study demonstrated a significant linear trend between CRP level and incident hypertension which extended to those with very low baseline blood pressure and those without traditional cardiovascular risk factors.[23]

Uric acid is a byproduct of the xanthine oxidase (XO) mediated degradation of purines, a pathway that produces ROS and is upregulated in hypertension. Uric acid itself reduces NO levels in renal endothelium, triggering activation of the RAAS pathway and enhancing the response of systemic vasculature to Ang II. Hyperuricemia has been correlated with the presence and progression of arterial stiffness and is predictive of incident hypertension in large cohorts of various ethnicities, with a metaanalysis establishing 15% increased risk of incident hypertension per 1 mg/mL increase in uric acid level.[24–27] In animal models, treating hyperuricemia reduces BP, which adds weight to the potential value of this marker.[28]

Other inflammatory mediators may also add predictive value for incident hypertension. Elevation in plasminogen activator inhibitor-1 (PAI-1), a marker of reduced fibrinolytic potential involved in the pathogenesis of vascular fibrosis, has been linked with incident hypertension, particularly in conjunction with the metabolic syndrome.[29–31] Albuminuria has been prospectively correlated to incident hypertension—a remarkable finding given that many of these studies excluded patients with urinary albumin above the accepted cutoff for normal level, suggesting that detection of high-normal albuminuria should prompt frequent BP screening and lifestyle intervention.[32–35]

Multimarker Models for Predicting Incident Hypertension

We believe that the aforementioned list of markers may hold the most clinical value via incorporation into a multibiomarker panel that can be used, along with traditional clinical risk factors, to identify candidates for frequent BP screening or for intensified preventive treatment of contributing comorbidities (e.g., obesity or hyperuricemia). A multimarker panel covering distinct physiologic pathways would appear most valuable given the multifactorial nature of incident hypertension and the inherent limitations of individual markers to predict hypertension in any one given person (inferred from the often conflicting reports for individual markers in the published literature).

A biomarker panel comprised of CRP, ARR, NT-proBNP, PAI-1, fibrinogen, and homocysteine was independently correlated in the Framingham Offspring Cohort with increased vascular stiffness, a formes fruste of hypertension.[36] In the Women's Health Study, a panel comprised of both demographic and serologic markers was predictive of incident hypertension but only marginally more so than simply using age, BP, ethnicity, and body mass index alone.[37] In another cohort a panel of seven markers, predominantly driven by the power of CRP, PAI-1, and urine albumin-creatinine ratio (UACR), was linked to incident hypertension. Elevation of ≥2 of these three was associated with incidence of 9.9 cases/100 person-years; using this threshold for prediction of hypertension had 92% specificity but only 15% sensitivity.[31] These studies demonstrate an opportunity for future groups to refine the use of blood-based biomarker panels to identify those at high risk of hypertension.

IDENTIFYING SUBCLINICAL ORGAN DAMAGE AND PREDICTING RISK OF ADVERSE OUTCOMES

Brief Summary of Target Organ Damage in Hypertension

Hypertension is a well-known risk factor for cardiovascular mortality due to coronary and cerebral arterial disease leading to myocardial infarction (MI), ischemic heart disease, heart failure (HF), and cerebrovascular accident (CVA). Left ventricular hypertrophy (LVH) is a form of target organ damage that is a major HF risk

factor. It is well established that concentric remodeling, in particular, leads to higher morbidity and mortality than other abnormal forms of left ventricular (LV) geometry, even in the absence of frank LVH. Biomarkers may play a role in allocating more costly resources (i.e., imaging) to identify structural remodeling among persons at highest risk. Renal dysfunction is another major manifestation of hypertensive end-organ damage. Hypertension accelerates the decline in renal function inherent to the aging process, and the two processes have an interrelated and deleterious relationship.

Because early damage to target organs is reversible, demonstration of subclinical organ damage in hypertensive patients represents an opportunity to perform additional screening for comorbid disease or justify intensification of BP therapy or lower BP goals (Fig. 3.3). The latter is of importance because aggressive lowering of BP, particularly diastolic blood pressure, is not without risk and may be associated with cerebral hypoperfusion in the elderly and with subclinical myocardial damage among persons with baseline LVH.[38]

Biomarkers Associated with Target Organ Damage and Adverse Clinical Outcomes

Markers of RAAS activation

It is reasonable to conclude that RAAS abnormalities suggest the presence or risk of target organ damage. For example, ARR is predictive of LV geometry and concentric hypertrophy in the same graded relationship as BNP, independent of hypertension status.[39] Renin may be measured in the form of plasma renin concentration (PRC) and plasma renin activity (PRA). PRA is independently predictive of MI and mortality and results in improved discrimination of 10-year cardiovascular risk stratification compared with the Framingham calculation in hypertensive patients.[40–42] In HF studies, risk attributed to renin elevation was most strong in the setting of chronic renal dysfunction, although it is yet to be shown whether this is true in the hypertensive population.

Urinary angiotensinogen is a newly identified biomarker specific to inappropriate renal (rather than systemic) RAAS activation. Urinary angiotensinogen is higher on average in hypertensive patients and decreases in response to antihypertensive therapy.[43] In addition, urinary angiotensinogen was identified in diabetic patients to increase from normal before patients developed albuminuria, making it possibly the earliest marker of diabetic nephropathy.[44] Therefore urinary angiotensinogen has substantial potential as a very early marker of tubuloglomerular kidney dysfunction in hypertension.

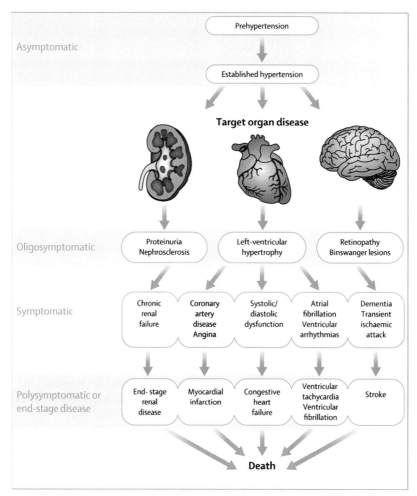

FIG. 3.3 Target organ damage in essential hypertension. The ideal utility of blood-based biomarkers is in detection of these processes before symptomatic stage. (From Messerli FH, Williams B, Ritz E. Essential hypertension. *Lancet*. 2007;370(9587):591–603; with permission.)

Markers of cardiovascular stress

BNP is released as a protective agent—it counteracts the abnormal physiology of HF by increasing glomerular filtration and promoting natriuresis, RAAS inhibition, and vasodilation. Cardiac troponins, highly specific indicators of cardiac myocyte damage, serve as markers of subclinical myocardial ischemia associated with coronary vessel and ventricular remodeling in response to high arterial pressures and other insults.

Elevated troponin and BNP may signal ventricular remodeling before it is clinically apparent; serum BNP in particular has been tied to intracardiac markers of remodeling and fibrosis and to low aortic elastic property.[45,46] Cross-sectional studies associate both cardiac troponins and BNP with echocardiographic

findings of LVH and impaired myocardial performance in asymptomatic patients.[14,47,48] More importantly, both are markedly increased in cases of concentric LVH, relative to eccentric hypertrophy and concentric remodeling. NT-proBNP is independently associated with both LV mass index (LVMI) and LV geometry.[48,49] Mueller et al. reported that a cutoff of 39 ng/mL for NT-proBNP reached 90% sensitivity and 32% specificity for detecting underlying structural damage in asymptomatic hypertensive patients.[50] Conen et al. designed a combined algorithm using CRP and BNP thresholds of 2.5 mg/L and 35 pg/mL, respectively, to reach 99% negative predictive value for the presence of echocardiographic LVH in hypertensive patients.[51]

BNP in particular has been correlated with incident HF and future HF admissions.[52] To rule out diastolic dysfunction in hypertensive patients, Ceyhan et al. used NT-proBNP cutoff of 119 ng/mL to achieve 87% sensitivity and 100% specificity.[53] In a Japanese hypertensive cohort with preserved ejection fraction (EF) and high cardiovascular risk, NT-proBNP and hs-troponin were each independently predictive of HF admission with 13.5 times greater risk in those with both biomarkers elevated than in those with normal levels.[54]

Troponin and BNP are also predictive of cardiovascular and cerebrovascular events in hypertensive patients.[55,56] In the ARIC cohort, risk stratification of stable outpatients by troponin level was more predictive of adverse vascular events than stratification by BP value.[57] Therefore NT-proBNP and hs-troponin have potential for use in risk stratification of hypertensive patients. Whether these biomarkers have a role in selecting personalized BP goals is of interest based on knowledge from other fields but to date remains untested in clinical trials.[58]

Adrenomedullin (ADM) is a hormone with natriuretic, vasodilatory, and hypotensive effects that is released by cardiac myocytes and vascular smooth muscle cells in response to sympathetic drive and volume overload. It is measured as midregion prohormone ADM (MR-proADM). In hypertensive patients, MR-proADM was associated with intracardiac markers of remodeling, echocardiographic findings of LVH, and renal damage.[59,60] Additionally, this marker was identified as an independent predictor of major cardiovascular events in the general population and of long-term mortality in a HF population, raising its potential for risk stratification in the hypertensive subset.[61,62]

ST2 is a member of the interleukin 1 (IL-1) family released in response to volume overload and cardiac remodeling, and cardiotrophin 1 (CT-1) is an interleukin 6 (IL-6) cytokine which induces myocyte growth and contractile dysfunction in response to RAAS and inflammatory signaling. Both have established value for risk prediction in the HF population and have the potential to be biomarkers for subclinical LV remodeling.[52] In hypertensive patients, ST2 and CT-1 associate with LVH, specifically with concentric hypertrophy, and ST2 elevation is associated with the presence of HF with preserved ejection fraction (HFpEF).[63–65] Unlike NT-proBNP, CT-1 is not influenced by kidney function, indicating that this marker is likely more specific than BNP in patients with renal impairment.[66]

Markers of inflammation, oxidative stress, and endothelial dysfunction

Atherosclerosis, perhaps the ultimate form of end-organ damage among hypertensive patients, is in large part an inflammatory disease. CRP has a well-established association with endothelial dysfunction, plaque formation and destabilization, thrombosis, and resulting atherosclerotic disease outcomes.

CRP elevation is correlated in hypertensive patients with vascular stiffness as measured by aortic and brachial pulse wave velocity and augmentation index, increased carotid intimal medial thickness (IMT), and progression of IMT (where CRP was more discriminatory than SBP).[67–70] A large population-based meta-analysis demonstrated nearly log-linear relationship of CRP to clinical ischemic vascular disease, with 1.5–1.7 times greater risk of major cardiovascular events associated with 1–standard deviation (SD) increase in high-sensitivity CRP (hsCRP) after adjustment for BP.[70] Although a few small studies have not demonstrated this correlation, evidence supports CRP as a predictive marker for atherosclerotic morbidity and mortality, making it a key target for further validation in cohorts comprised solely of hypertensive patients.[40]

Inflammatory pathways may also contribute to the maladaptive process of concentric remodeling in conjunction with the traditional mechanism of myocardial hypertrophy due to increased afterload. For example, increasing hsCRP levels correlates in a stepwise fashion with LVMI and adds prognostication to LVH for predicting event-free survival.[39,71]

Some studies suggest that the role of CRP in the inflammatory cascade is as a downstream protective agent as opposed to that of IL-6 and tumor necrosis factor alpha (TNF-α), which are upstream pathologic markers. IL-6 release is triggered by Ang II, and its signaling pathway results in the expression of endothelin 1 (ET-1), one of the most powerful vasoconstrictors.[72,73] TNF-α is an inflammatory cytokine that causes vascular immune cell infiltration and compensatory renal natriuresis in response to hypertension.[74] In a large metaanalysis, each 1-SD increase in IL-6 and TNF-α, respectively, were predictive of 25% and 17% increased risk for MI or coronary heart disease.[75] In a large general population cohort study, IL-6 and TNF-α (and not CRP) were also predictive of incident chronic kidney disease (CKD) over 15 years follow-up, inviting similar studies specific to hypertensive individuals.[76]

Uric acid levels, associated with the metabolic syndrome, RAAS activation, and endothelial dysfunction, are prognostic of worse clinical outcomes (Fig. 3.4). In large prospective studies of hypertensive patients,

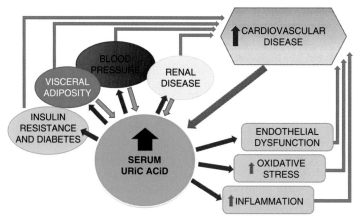

FIG. 3.4 Correlation of uric acid with hypertension and downstream conditions. (From Kanbay M, Jensen T, Solak Y, et al. Uric acid in metabolic syndrome: from an innocent bystander to a central player. *Eur J Intern Med*. 2016;29:3–8; with permission.)

uric acid is predictive of total and fatal cardiovascular events and all-cause mortality.[77] Uric acid promotes renal inflammation and impairs renal autoregulation. In hypertensive patients, elevated baseline uric acid predicts prevalent renal impairment and greater progression of renal dysfunction.[78]

Excessive urinary albumin excretion (UAE) represents dysfunction of the glomerular filtration barrier, an important metric of physiologic health in persons with hypertension. Correlation to active inflammation and decreased fibrinolysis suggests an inflammatory component to the damage inflicted on the glomerular basement membrane and renal vasculature. Albuminuria may provide the most accurate window in to the health of the vasculature and is now thought to be a very early indicator of endothelial damage and marker for widespread endothelial dysfunction.[79] Indeed, albuminuria has been associated with nearly all forms of vascular target organ damage.

Microalbuminuria is defined as >30 mg/24 h, and macroalbuminuria is >300 mg/24 h. Spot UACR provides a good estimate of the degree of albuminuria. Microalbuminuria is common in hypertensive patients, but highly variable across populations, with prevalence in studies ranging from 7% to 58%.[80–82] The ARIC cohort and others have demonstrated a close trend between the degree of hypertension and likelihood of albuminuria, surprisingly even at high-normal levels of BP.[83]

Albuminuria is well demonstrated as a predictor of incident renal disease, progression of CKD, and end-stage renal disease (ESRD) in the general and diabetic populations, even being found to be more predictive of future renal deterioration than decreased renal function.[84] Studies specific to hypertensive patients demonstrated higher prevalence of CKD and greater acceleration in loss of kidney function in hypertensive patients with albuminuria.[85] Hypertensive patients in the Microalbuminuria: A Genoa Investigation on Complications (MAGIC) study had sevenfold higher incidence of chronic renal insufficiency if microalbuminuria was present at baseline.[86]

As a secondary marker for systemic endothelial dysfunction, albuminuria is also predictive of target organ events outside the kidney. Albuminuria correlates with the degree of atherosclerosis in high-risk populations and has been proposed as a surrogate for arterial stiffness. Robust general population data also associate the degree and progression of albuminuria with LVH and concentric hypertrophy, presence and progression of carotid plaques, and cardiovascular events.[87–89] Albuminuria is well established as an independent predictor of all-cause mortality to a degree that may be more predictive than BP control.[90,91] In hypertensive patients, microalbuminuria is an independent risk predictor for major cardiovascular events and cardiovascular mortality.[92,93] Macroalbuminuria was found in a metaanalysis to be associated with a 2.3-fold risk of all-cause mortality.[85]

Early detection of microalbuminuria may signal reversible vascular dysfunction before overt end organ failure. Currently the National Kidney Foundation Guidelines recommend screening diabetic patients for albuminuria yearly. The United States Preventative Services Task Force (USPSTF) has so far concluded that there is insignificant evidence to support routine urinary albumin screening in asymptomatic adults.[94,95] However, in a trial implementing urinary albumin screening in a general population of >40,000 patients, baseline microalbuminuria with a cutoff of 20 mg/L had 58% sensitivity and 92% specificity at predicting the need for renal replacement therapy (RRT) within 9 years; nearly 40% of those patients had no prior diagnosis of renal dysfunction.[96]

There is also evidence that reductions in urinary albumin excretion with BP pharmacotherapy may be associated with improved prognosis independent of the BP-lowering effects of these therapies alone, through incompletely understood mechanisms. In a metaanalysis, each 30% reduction in albuminuria during antihypertensive drug therapy decreased risk of ESRD by 24%, independent of BP.[97]

Given these findings, there is interest in albuminuria as a therapeutic target. If such practice is implemented, thresholds for normal values may require adjustment, given that significant increase in morbidity had been demonstrated using cutoff values as low as 5 μg/min (equal to 7.2 mg/24 h).[87,90,98]

Multimarker Risk Stratification Panels

Many of these markers may have additive and/or multiplicative discrimination in combination for predicting morbidity associated with hypertension. Therefore a worthy goal is to develop a multimarker panel for risk stratification and potentially also to establish therapeutic targets. One retrospective analysis of hypertensive patients found that a four-marker panel of pro-BNP, transforming growth factor beta (TGF-β), CT-1, and cystatin C was most predictive of HF presence.[52] In a study comprised of the MESA and Dallas Heart Study cohorts, cardiovascular risk prediction using LVH by ECG, coronary artery calcium, NT-proBNP, hs-troponin, and hsCRP was well correlated with global composite cardiovascular outcome over 10 years, with increasing predictive value for each abnormal component. The analyses adjusted for hypertension status, validating this multimarker panel for patients with and without hypertension.[99] Based on the aforementioned findings, the most powerful predictive tools will likely use the compounded prognostic value of multiple markers representing diverse pathologic processes.

USING BIOMARKERS TO PERSONALIZE ANTIHYPERTENSIVE THERAPY

Hypertension is a diverse disease that invites individualized therapy. Opportunities to customize therapy are in the management of treatment-resistant hypertension, the choice of intensity of BP therapy (e.g., to a goal of 140 mmHg vs. 120 mmHg SBP), and the choice of drug class, particularly for patients with comorbidities that warrant special consideration for targeted benefits or risk of harm from antihypertensive therapy. It

may be that future guidelines delineate appropriate antihypertensive therapy options in the setting of various biomarkers of subclinical target organ dysfunction, aiming to prevent further damage. In addition, there is a relatively new field of thought surrounding "hypertension phenotypes," or the concept that, in certain individuals, one physiologic driver of hypertension dominates over the others, and therapy targeting this mechanism will be most efficacious. Conversely, treating with empiric antihypertensive drugs that do not counteract the dominant mechanism may lead to suspicion of nonadherence or to inappropriate labels of treatment-resistant hypertension. This section will discuss evidence surrounding the identification of these phenotypes and will include special attention to cases of true resistant and refractory hypertension.

Using Biomarkers to Select Therapeutic Targets for Antihypertensive Therapies

Primary physiologic targets for antihypertensive therapy are volume overload, vasoconstriction, RAAS overactivation, decreased vascular compliance, and hyperdynamic cardiac state. The strongest data for targeted therapy relate to RAAS overactivation.

Targeted therapy: RAAS system

RAAS-blocking agents and diuretics are first-line antihypertensive therapies. In a landmark article, Laragh, et al. proposed two primary phenotypes driving relative patient response to these classes of agents (Fig. 3.5). In the first phenotype the primary driver of hypertension is inappropriate RAAS activation relative to total body sodium and water content ("R" phenotype), making this an ideal candidate for RAAS blockade. The second is an individual with volume overload due to inappropriate renal salt handling and/or excess salt ingestion in whom renin pathway signaling is appropriately suppressed by negative feedback ("V" phenotype). This patient in theory would have little response to RAAS blockade and require diuresis to overcome the already overwhelmed compensatory mechanisms.[100] This theory has been subjected to trials with mixed results. In Laragh's 2011 trial, newly diagnosed hypertensive patients were divided by plasma renin level into R (elevated renin) and V (suppressed renin) phenotypes; patients within each group were then randomized into anti-RAAS therapy or diuretic therapy. Those with suppressed renin levels demonstrated a more frequent paradoxical pressor response to anti-RAAS therapy, and lowest BPs were achieved in patients receiving phenotype-matched therapy.[101] In another trial, patients had better BP outcomes when randomized to renin-guided

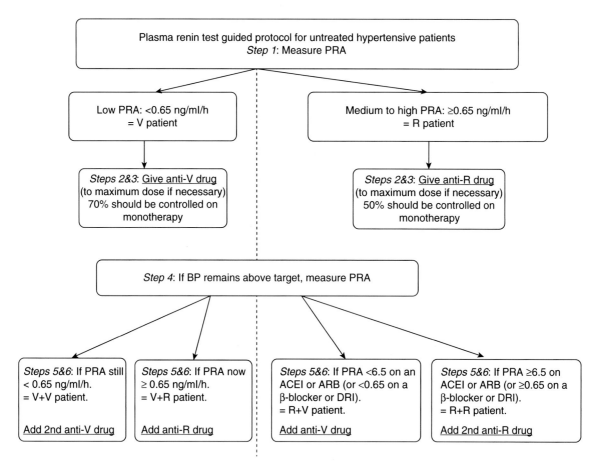

FIG. 3.5 Proposed renin-guided therapy for hypertensive patients. (From Laragh JH, Sealey JE. The plasma renin test reveals the contribution of body sodium-volume content (V) and renin-angiotensin (R) vasoconstriction to long-term blood pressure. *Am J Hypertens.* 2011;24(11):1164–1180; with permission.)

therapy than to nonalgorithmic specialist hypertension management.[102] A longstanding related theory held that a subset of patients with inherent paradoxical renin response may have excessive reactive renin secretion in response to RAAS blockade, called "Ang II/aldosterone escape." This was refuted in a trial for renin blocker aliskiren in which response was most marked, in fact, in those with highest baseline renin.[103]

However, other studies have failed to demonstrate a significant association between RAAS pathway levels and response to RAAS blockade.[104,105] One author suggested that given marginal benefit derived even in a homogenous cohort, determining cutoff renin levels generalizable to the population would be extremely difficult; clearly further validation is necessary before routine measurement of renin levels for this purpose is put into general practice.[104] A more targeted potential benefit of this approach is in the treatment of patients

not responsive to initial empiric RAAS blockade. For example, reanalysis of aliskiren trials has demonstrated that BP is insufficiently reduced in those with low baseline renin or in those in whom renin levels do not decrease in response to therapy.[106] In a small cohort study, patients with treatment-resistant hypertension and low renin on serology were taken off of RAAS blockers in favor of alternative agents. When compared with controls, in whom aldosterone antagonist agents were added empirically, those on renin-guided therapy were on fewer total medications with similar BP outcomes.[102,107] On-therapy renin levels clearly must be interpreted in the context of drug mechanism; for example, those on direct renin inhibitors exhibit low PRA but reactive elevation in PRC due to negative feedback. Angiotensin-converting enzyme inhibitors (ACEs) and angiotensin II receptor blockers (ARBs) moderately increase renin levels, and beta blocker therapy suppresses renin release.[108,109] Beta blockers have been demonstrated to have greater antihypertensive effect in high-renin patients than diuretics, offering a second-line option for those with contraindication or intolerance to direct RAAS blockade.[110] Given high variability of baseline and on-treatment renin levels across populations, further trials with clinical endpoints are needed to validate renin-guided therapy.

A newer target for identifying RAAS overactivity is urinary angiotensinogen, which is more specific than plasma levels for intrarenal RAAS activation. Urinary angiotensin is elevated disproportionately in diabetic patients, making interpretation difficult in this group. Urinary angiotensinogen is higher in hypertensive patients, decreases in response to therapy, and is correlated with salt sensitivity of blood pressure.[111,112]

There is robust evidence that renal response to sodium load varies widely. Salt-sensitive patients are those in whom BP increases with sodium load and responds to sodium restriction. The prevailing theory is that this is due to inappropriately low sodium clearance, with the relationship curve between arterial pressure and sodium clearance chronically shifted to the right, thus requiring higher BP to excrete sodium.[113] The first mechanism implicated in this process is AT-1-triggered activation of tubular

sodium channels in the subclinical hyperaldosterone state represented by many essential hypertensives, particularly in the setting of obesity.[113] Biomarkers identified as potentially more specific indicators of salt-sensitive state are 24-hour urinary sodium and ET-1.[114,115] Additionally, there is evidence for Ang II-mediated but aldosterone-independent mineralocorticoid receptor activation, likely via inflammation and/or production of ROS.[116] Those with this pattern have augmented BP response when statins are added to antihypertensive therapy, indicating a role for inflammatory marker analysis in salt-sensitive patients.[117] Finally, sympathetic overactivity (often isolated to the kidneys) leads to salt sensitivity via β-1-mediated renin production and α-1 direct activity on the renal tubules.[118] Evidence of hyperactive sympathetic drive may identify candidates for renal denervation [described further below].

Targeted therapy: inflammatory states
There is great interest in identifying hypertensive patients with overactivation of the inflammatory cascade, with the goal of targeted therapy via traditional antihypertensive agents as well as nontraditional drugs with novel mechanisms (Fig. 3.6).

RAAS inhibition has BP-mediated and non-BP–mediated antiinflammatory properties, due in part to

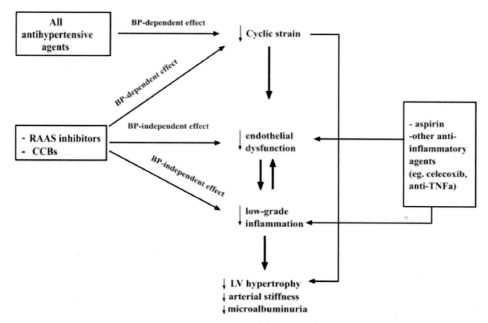

FIG. 3.6 Blood pressure–dependent or blood pressure–independent antiinflammatory effects of antihypertensive and purely antiinflammatory agents. (From Pietri P, Vlachopoulos C, Tousoulis D. Inflammation and Arterial Hypertension: From Pathophysiological Links to Risk Prediction. *Curr Med Chem.* 2015;22(23):2754–2761; with permission.)

suppressed renal vascular adhesion molecule expression and macrophage infiltration. In the Valsartan-Managing Blood Pressure Aggressively and Evaluating Reductions in hs-CRP (Val-MARC) trial, randomization to valsartan versus valsartan-hydrochlorathiazide (HCTZ) resulted in greater BP reduction in the combination arm, but greater decrease in hsCRP in the valsartan arm, supporting the BP-independent antiinflammatory properties of ARBs.[119] Thiazide diuretics have been demonstrated previously to promote inflammation. Combination therapy with amlodipine and RAAS blockade has established superiority over HCTZ in decreasing markers of inflammation and in preventing cardiovascular morbidity and mortality independent of BP effects.[120] The antiinflammatory mechanism for calcium channel blockers (CCBs) involves anti-polymorphonuclear leukocyte (PML) priming and antioxidant properties.[121] Therefore some degree of therapeutic benefit derived from RAAS inhibitors and CCBs in preventing target organ damage may be via antiinflammatory properties.

Serum CRP decreases in response to RAAS-blocking, CCB, and beta blocker agents.[121-123] TNF-α and IL-6 respond to ARBs.[122] Intracellular Adhesion Molecule 1 (ICAM-1) decreases in response to both ACE and ARB therapies and fibrinogen in response to ACE inhibition but not ARB.[124] PAI-1 decreases with ACE therapy.[125] Synchronously, patients with elevated CRP have greater BP-lowering response to RAAS blockade than those with normal CRP.[126] Before using inflammatory markers in choice of therapy or as a therapeutic target, it will be most important to demonstrate that antiinflammatory effects of antihypertensive agents correlate with improved clinical outcomes. In a mixed hypertensive and normotensive post-CVA population, ACE therapy resulted in 2.6-fold lower CRP level than other BP agents, which notably was accompanied by 60% decrease in risk of future cardiovascular events, independent of BP changes.[127] There is opportunity for similar studies correlating improved markers of inflammation with decreased incidence of target organ events in hypertensive patients.

Another consideration is the use of inflammatory markers to identify hypertensive patients who may benefit from targeted antiinflammatory drugs to prevent downstream damage. Statins in combination with antihypertensive therapy improve markers of inflammation and in turn diminish cardiovascular event rate.[128] More recently, IL-1β monoclonal antibody therapy had similar favorable outcomes in a high-risk population.[129] The potential next step is investigation into relative clinical outcomes of antiinflammatory therapy in hypertensive patients with elevated inflammatory biomarkers compared with those with normal inflammatory markers.

Targeted therapy: oxidative stress

Another potential target for therapy among hypertensive adults outside of blood pressure itself is oxidative stress. In those with elevated uric acid, an attractive adjunct to traditional antihypertensive therapy are XO inhibitors. These agents (allopurinol, febuxostat, and/or probenecid) have demonstrated BP-lowering effects, diminished RAAS activation, improved vascular resistance, slowed progression of CKD, and resolution of prehypertension (in adolescents).[130-133] However, recent randomized controlled trials failed to demonstrate change in the degree of brachial artery vasodilation, antihypertensive effect, or significant alterations in RAAS in response to urate-lowering effect of XO inhibitors, inviting further study to identify the level of uric acid elevation at which clinical benefit occurs.[134,135] Of note, a recent trial also showed that while it was noninferior to allopurinol for CVD outcomes, febuxostat increased CV and all-cause death.[136]

Biomarker Use in Resistant and Refractory Hypertension

Resistant hypertension is defined as BP that remains above goal despite the use of three antihypertensive medications from different classes at optimal dose amounts. One of these should be a diuretic. Resistance is present in 10%–20% of hypertensive patients, but prevalence in those with concurrent CKD approaches 35%–40%.[137] Resistant hypertension confers risk of vascular comorbidities and mortality which exceeds that in the general hypertensive population and is exaggerated further in those with concurrent CKD. The following section will highlight considerations in which biomarkers may be useful in the care of patients with resistant hypertension.

Biomarkers in Pseudoresistance

Pseudoresistance is hypertension meeting criteria for resistant hypertension; however, medication nonadherence or white coat hypertension is responsible. At present, urinary levels of 40 of the most common drugs from nearly all classes of antihypertensive agents (with the exception of nitrates) may be identified via chromatography-mass spectrophotometry with nondetection generally set at levels consistent with four half-lives of the drug.[138] Serum or urine testing for antihypertensive medications has demonstrated nonadherence rates between 25% and 70%, and 10%–35% have complete lack of detectable antihypertensive drug levels.[138-140] Although this testing is available in clinical practice, the technology is costly. Given the high prevalence of nonadherence, there is a valid argument for

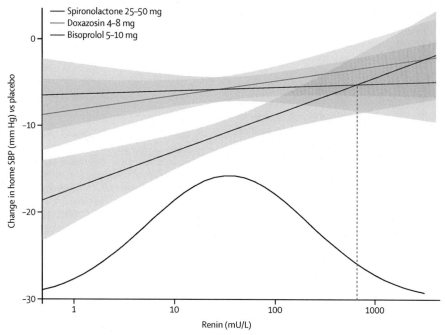

FIG. 3.7 Blood pressure response to spironolactone in relation to plasma renin. (From Williams B, MacDonald TM, Morant S, et al. Spironolactone versus placebo, bisoprolol, and doxazosin to determine the optimal treatment for drug-resistant hypertension (PATHWAY-2): a randomised, double-blind, crossover trial. *Lancet.* 2015;386(10008):2059–2068; with permission.)

the cost-effectiveness of this strategy compared with the compounded cost of multidrug regimens, progression to invasive antihypertensive therapy, and downstream expenditures related to target organ failure and events. In a recent study, patients found by serum or urine drug levels to be nonadherent received in-office physician counseling. At follow-up, ratio of prescribed drugs to detected drugs tripled with a responding decrease in SBP by mean 19.5 mmHg and a linear trend between adherence ratio and change in BP.[141]

For patients on RAAS-blocking agents, urinary renin and angiotensinogen, when initially elevated, demonstrate a predictable decrease with the initiation of therapy, making these tests potentially useful in analysis of patient adherence.[142]

Biomarkers in the evaluation and treatment of resistant hypertension

The major driver behind true resistant hypertension seems to be fluid retention, although there is likely a multifactorial component. Trials have identified a hyperaldosterone state with suppressed plasma renin to be prevalent in those with resistant hypertension, suggesting sodium retention as the primary driver and

aldosterone receptors as a key therapeutic target.[143] There is significant evidence supporting the use of spironolactone as the add-on fourth agent of choice in cases of resistant hypertension. This was further supported in the Pathway-2 cohort by a marked inverse correlation between renin level and degree of BP reduction by spironolactone (Fig. 3.7). Thiazide diuretics are also well supported as an adjunct to therapy, though these have generally already been prescribed. It should be noted that patients in the Pathway-2 study with the highest renin levels actually had greater response to beta blocker (which has renin-blocking activity), a finding which lends support to the potential benefit of checking renin levels in patients with difficult-to-treat hypertension.

Refractory hypertension

5%–10% of patients referred to hypertension clinics are diagnosed with refractory hypertension, and this population has a diminished response to spironolactone therapy. It has recently been suggested that sympathetic overactivation is the driving mechanism for hypertension in this group. Renal denervation (ablation of the autonomic nerve fibers along the renal artery) may provide benefit, but outcomes of retrospective case series and sham-controlled trials are mixed.[144–147] Carotid baroreflex activation therapy, another invasive antisympathetic therapy, has completed phase III clinical trials but is yet to reach mainstream clinical practice. Biomarkers specific to sympathetic overactivity may improve selection of candidates for both procedures. For example, brain-derived neurotrophic factor, a neuronal growth factor that regulates neurotransmitter production, is transiently downregulated immediately after successful renal denervation, establishing this as a potential preprocedural biomarker for identifying sympathetic drive in those hypertensive patients who may benefit most from antisympathetic therapy.[148]

Practical Considerations in Biomarker-Driven Therapy

Major society guidelines recommend that for most patients, drug class selection remains at the discretion of the clinician. Comorbid conditions such as HF with reduced ejection fraction (HFrEF), chronic renal disease, and post-MI state can guide therapy selection based on strong indications for ACE, ARB, angiotensin receptor-neprilysin inhibitor (ARNI), and/or beta blockade in these conditions. There is sufficient evidence to conclude that those with known high renin levels should be treated with ACE or ARB as first line, but not enough to support routine renin testing. Therefore the clinical challenge of treating hypertension, particularly in resistant or refractory cases, may in the future become less onerous and more personalized using a biomarker-guided treatment strategy. Future clinical trials are necessary to confirm this provocative hypothesis.

CONCLUSION

At present, BP itself is the predominant "biomarker" for the diagnosis, prognostication, and monitoring of hypertension. Novel blood-based biomarkers representing diverse mechanisms and consequences of hypertension are now known to be predictive of incident hypertension and/or target organ damage. We believe that further development of multimarker panels may improve risk stratification in healthy patients and newly diagnosed hypertensives. When alternative reasons are ruled out, the possibility that abnormal levels of troponin, NT-proBNP, inflammatory markers, hyperuricemia, and albuminuria in particular are representative of subclinical target organ damage in hypertensive patients should be carefully entertained. There is great opportunity to identify dominant RAAS activation, fluid overload, or sympathetic activity as phenotypic subclasses in hypertensive patients. The potential to tailor therapy to biomarker response invites further studies that may shape future guidelines.

REFERENCES

1. Rose G. Sick individuals and sick populations. *Int J Epidemiol*. 1985;14(1):32–38. https://doi.org/10.1093/ije/14.1.32.
2. Roberts J, Maurer K. Blood Pressure of Persons 6–74 Years of Age in the United States. National Center for Health Statistics. *Vital Health Stat*. 1976;1.
3. Tirosh A, Afek A, Rudich A, et al. Progression of normotensive adolescents to hypertensive adults: a study of 26,980 teenagers. *Hypertension*. 2010;56(2):203–209. https://doi.org/10.1161/HYPERTENSIONAHA.109.146415.
4. Allen NB, Siddique J, Wilkins JT, et al. Blood pressure trajectories in early adulthood and subclinical atherosclerosis in middle age. *JAMA*. 2014;311(5):490–497. https://doi.org/10.1001/jama.2013.285122.
5. Banegas JR, Ruilope LM, de la Sierra A, et al. Relationship between clinic and ambulatory blood-pressure measurements and mortality. *N Engl J Med*. 2018;378(16):1509–1520. https://doi.org/10.1056/NEJMoa1712231.
6. Newton-Cheh C, Guo CY, Gona P, et al. Clinical and genetic correlates of aldosterone-to-renin ratio and relations to blood pressure in a community sample. *Hypertension*. 2007;49(4):846–856. https://doi.org/10.1161/01.HYP.0000258554.87444.91.
7. Brown JM, Robinson-Cohen C, Luque-Fernandez MA, et al. The Spectrum of subclinical primary aldosteronism and incident hypertension: a cohort study. *Ann Intern Med*. 2017. https://doi.org/10.7326/M17-0882.
8. van Ballegooijen AJ, Kestenbaum B, Sachs MC, et al. Association of 25-hydroxyvitamin D and parathyroid hormone with incident hypertension: MESA (Multi-Ethnic Study of Atherosclerosis). *J Am Coll Cardiol*. 2014;63(12):1214–1222. https://doi.org/10.1016/j.jacc.2014.01.012.
9. Yao L, Folsom AR, Pankow JS, et al. Parathyroid hormone and the risk of incident hypertension. *J Hypertens*. 2016;34(2):196–203. https://doi.org/10.1097/HJH.0000000000000794.
10. Kunutsor SK, Apekey TA, Steur M. Vitamin D and risk of future hypertension: meta-analysis of 283,537 participants. *Eur J Epidemiol*. 2013;28(3):205–221. https://doi.org/10.1007/s10654-013-9790-2.
11. Sugden JA, Davies JI, Witham MD, Morris AD, Struthers AD. Vitamin D improves endothelial function in patients with Type 2 diabetes mellitus and low vitamin D levels. *Diabet Med*. 2008;25(3):320–325. https://doi.org/10.1111/j.1464-5491.2007.02360.x.
12. Sanchez OA, Jacobs DR, Bahrami H, et al. Increasing aminoterminal-pro-B-type natriuretic peptide precedes the development of arterial hypertension: the multiethnic study of atherosclerosis. *J Hypertens*. 2015;33(5):966–974. https://doi.org/10.1097/HJH.0000000000000500.

13. Bower JK, Lazo M, Matsushita K, et al. N-terminal pro-brain natriuretic peptide (NT-proBNP) and risk of hypertension in the atherosclerosis risk in communities (ARIC) study. *Am J Hypertens*. 2015;28(10):1262–1266. https://doi.org/10.1093/ajh/hpv026.

14. McEvoy JW, Chen Y, Nambi V, et al. High-sensitivity cardiac troponin T and risk of hypertension. *Circulation*. 2015;132(9):825–833. https://doi.org/10.1161/CIRCU-LATIONAHA.114.014364.

15. Ho JE, Larson MG, Ghorbani A, et al. Soluble ST2 predicts elevated SBP in the community. *J Hypertens*. 2013;31(7):1431–1436; discussion 1436. https://doi.org/10.1097/HJH.0b013e3283611bdf.

16. Fox ER, Musani SK, Singh P, et al. Association of plasma B-type natriuretic peptide concentrations with longitudinal blood pressure tracking in African Americans: findings from the Jackson Heart Study. *Hypertension*. 2013;61(1):48–54. https://doi.org/10.1161/HYPERTEN-SIONAHA.112.197657.

17. Freitag MH, Larson MG, Levy D, et al. Plasma brain natriuretic peptide levels and blood pressure tracking in the Framingham Heart Study. *Hypertension*. 2003;41(4):978–983. https://doi.org/10.1161/01.HYP.0000061116.20490.8D.

18. Hage FG, Oparil S, Xing D, Chen YF, McCrory MA, Szalai AJ. C-reactive protein-mediated vascular injury requires complement. *Arter Thromb Vasc Biol*. 2010;30(6):1189–1195. https://doi.org/10.1161/ATVBAHA.110.205377.

19. Lakoski SG, Herrington DM, Siscovick DM, Hulley SB. C-reactive protein concentration and incident hypertension in young adults: the CARDIA study. *Arch Intern Med*. 2006;166(3):345–349. https://doi.org/10.1001/archinte.166.3.345.

20. Sesso HD, Jiménez MC, Wang L, Ridker PM, Buring JE, Gaziano JM. Plasma inflammatory markers and the risk of developing hypertension in men. *J Am Heart Assoc*. 2015;4(9):e001802. https://doi.org/10.1161/JAHA.115.001802.

21. Lakoski SG, Cushman M, Siscovick DS, et al. The relationship between inflammation, obesity and risk for hypertension in the Multi-Ethnic Study of Atherosclerosis (MESA). *J Hum Hypertens*. 2011;25(2):73–79. https://doi.org/10.1038/jhh.2010.91.

22. Cheung BM, Ong KL, Tso AW, et al. C-reactive protein as a predictor of hypertension in the Hong Kong cardiovascular risk factor prevalence study (CRISPS) cohort. *J Hum Hypertens*. 2012;26(2):108–116. https://doi.org/10.1038/jhh.2010.125.

23. Sesso HD, Buring JE, Rifai N, Blake GJ, Gaziano JM, Ridker PM. C-reactive protein and the risk of developing hypertension. *JAMA*. 2003;290(22):2945–2951. https://doi.org/10.1001/jama.290.22.2945.

24. Shin JY, Lee HR, Shim JY. Significance of high-normal serum uric acid level as a risk factor for arterial stiffness in healthy Korean men. *Vasc Med*. 2012;17(1):37–43. https://doi.org/10.1177/1358863X11434197.

25. Leiba A, Vinker S, Dinour D, Holtzman EJ, Shani M. Uric acid levels within the normal range predict increased risk of hypertension: a cohort study. *J Am Soc Hypertens*. 2015;9(8):600–609. https://doi.org/10.1016/j.jash.2015.05.010.

26. Sun HL, Pei D, Lue KH, Chen YL. Uric acid levels can predict metabolic syndrome and hypertension in adolescents: a 10-year longitudinal study. *PLoS One*. 2015;10(11):e0143786. https://doi.org/10.1371/journal.pone.0143786.

27. Mellen PB, Bleyer AJ, Erlinger TP, et al. Serum uric acid predicts incident hypertension in a biethnic cohort: the atherosclerosis risk in communities study. *Hypertension*. 2006;48(6):1037–1042. https://doi.org/10.1161/01.HYP.0000249768.26560.66.

28. Mazzali M, Hughes J, Kim YG, et al. Elevated uric acid increases blood pressure in the rat by a novel crystal-independent mechanism. *Hypertension*. 2001;38(5):1101–1106. https://www.ncbi.nlm.nih.gov/pubmed/11711505.

29. Peng H, Yeh F, de Simone G, et al. Relationship between plasma plasminogen activator inhibitor-1 and hypertension in American Indians: findings from the Strong Heart Study. *J Hypertens*. 2017;35(9):1787–1793. https://doi.org/10.1097/HJH.0000000000001375.

30. Ingelsson E, Pencina MJ, Tofler GH, et al. Multimarker approach to evaluate the incidence of the metabolic syndrome and longitudinal changes in metabolic risk factors: the Framingham Offspring Study. *Circulation*. 2007;116(9):984–992. https://doi.org/10.1161/CIRCU-LATIONAHA.107.708537.

31. Wang TJ, Gona P, Larson MG, et al. Multiple biomarkers and the risk of incident hypertension. *Hypertension*. 2007;49(3):432–438. https://doi.org/10.1161/01.HYP.0000256956.61872.aa.

32. Park SK, Moon SY, Oh CM, Ryoo JH, Park MS. High normal urine albumin-to-creatinine ratio predicts development of hypertension in Korean men. *Circ J*. 2014;78(3):656–661. https://www.ncbi.nlm.nih.gov/pubmed/24334637.

33. Wang TJ, Evans JC, Meigs JB, et al. Low-grade albuminuria and the risks of hypertension and blood pressure progression. *Circulation*. 2005;111(11):1370–1376. https://doi.org/10.1161/01.CIR.0000158434.69180.2D.

34. Forman JP, Fisher ND, Schopick EL, Curhan GC. Higher levels of albuminuria within the normal range predict incident hypertension. *J Am Soc Nephrol*. 2008;19(10):1983–1988. https://doi.org/10.1681/ASN.2008010038.

35. Huang M, Matsushita K, Sang Y, Ballew SH, Astor BC, Coresh J. Association of kidney function and albuminuria with prevalent and incident hypertension: the Atherosclerosis Risk in Communities (ARIC) study. *Am J Kidney Dis*. 2015;65(1):58–66. https://doi.org/10.1053/j.ajkd.2014.06.025.

36. Lieb W, Larson MG, Benjamin EJ, et al. Multimarker approach to evaluate correlates of vascular stiffness: the Framingham Heart Study. *Circulation*. 2009;119(1):37–43. https://doi.org/10.1161/CIRCULATIONAHA.108.816108.

37. Paynter NP, Cook NR, Everett BM, Sesso HD, Buring JE, Ridker PM. Prediction of incident hypertension risk in women with currently normal blood pressure. *Am J Med.* 2009;122(5):464–471. https://doi.org/10.1016/j.amjmed.2008.10.034.

38. McEvoy JW, Chen Y, Rawlings A, et al. Diastolic blood pressure, subclinical myocardial damage, and cardiac events: implications for blood pressure control. *J Am Coll Cardiol.* 2016;68(16):1713–1722. https://doi.org/10.1016/j.jacc.2016.07.754.

39. Velagaleti RS, Gona P, Levy D, et al. Relations of biomarkers representing distinct biological pathways to left ventricular geometry. *Circulation.* 2008;118(22):2252–2258. https://doi.org/10.1161/CIRCULATIONAHA.108.817411. 5pp. following 2258.

40. Campbell DJ, Woodward M, Chalmers JP, et al. Prediction of myocardial infarction by N-terminal-pro-B-type natriuretic peptide, C-reactive protein, and renin in subjects with cerebrovascular disease. *Circulation.* 2005;112(1):110–116. https://doi.org/10.1161/CIRCULATIONAHA.104.525527.

41. Parikh NI, Gona P, Larson MG, et al. Plasma renin and risk of cardiovascular disease and mortality: the Framingham Heart Study. *Eur Heart J.* 2007;28(21):2644–2652. https://doi.org/10.1093/eurheartj/ehm399.

42. Gonzalez MC, Cohen HW, Sealey JE, Laragh JH, Alderman MH. Enduring direct association of baseline plasma renin activity with all-cause and cardiovascular mortality in hypertensive patients. *Am J Hypertens.* 2011;24(11):1181–1186. https://doi.org/10.1038/ajh.2011.172.

43. Kobori H, Urushihara M. Augmented intrarenal and urinary angiotensinogen in hypertension and chronic kidney disease. *Pflugers Arch.* 2013;465(1):3–12. https://doi.org/10.1007/s00424-012-1143-6.

44. Saito T, Urushihara M, Kotani Y, Kagami S, Kobori H. Increased urinary angiotensinogen is precedent to increased urinary albumin in patients with type 1 diabetes. *Am J Med Sci.* 2009;338(6):478–480. https://doi.org/10.1097/MAJ.0b013e3181b90c25.

45. Phelan D, Watson C, Martos R, et al. Modest elevation in BNP in asymptomatic hypertensive patients reflects subclinical cardiac remodeling, inflammation and extracellular matrix changes. *PLoS One.* 2012;7(11). https://doi.org/10.1371/journal.pone.0049259.

46. Huang Y, Song Y, Mai W, et al. Association of N-terminal pro brain natriuretic peptide and impaired aortic elastic property in hypertensive patients. *Clin Chim Acta.* 2011;412(23–24):2272–2276. https://doi.org/10.1016/j.cca.2011.08.022.

47. Kaypakli O, Gür M, Gözükara MY, et al. Association between high-sensitivity troponin T, left ventricular hypertrophy, and myocardial performance index. *Herz.* 2015;40(7):1004–1010. https://doi.org/10.1007/s00059-015-4322-3.

48. Elbasan Z, Gür M, Sahin DY, et al. N-terminal pro-brain natriuretic peptide levels and abnormal geometric patterns of left ventricle in untreated hypertensive patients. *Clin Exp Hypertens.* 2014;36(3):153–158. https://doi.org/10.3109/10641963.2013.804538.

49. Uçar H, Gür M, Kivrak A, et al. High-sensitivity cardiac troponin T levels in newly diagnosed hypertensive patients with different left ventricle geometry. *Blood Press.* 2014;23(4):240–247. https://doi.org/10.3109/08037051.2013.840429.

50. Mueller T, Gegenhuber A, Dieplinger B, Poelz W, Haltmayer M. Capability of B-type natriuretic peptide (BNP) and amino-terminal proBNP as indicators of cardiac structural disease in asymptomatic patients with systemic arterial hypertension. *Clin Chem.* 2005;51(12):2245–2251. https://doi.org/10.1373/clinchem.2005.056648.

51. Conen D, Zeller A, Pfisterer M, Martina B. Usefulness of B-type natriuretic peptide and C-reactive protein in predicting the presence or absence of left ventricular hypertrophy in patients with systemic hypertension. *Am J Cardiol.* 2006;97(2):249–252. https://doi.org/10.1016/j.amjcard.2005.08.028.

52. Bielecka-Dabrowa A, Michalska-Kasiczak M, Gluba A, et al. Biomarkers and echocardiographic predictors of myocardial dysfunction in patients with hypertension. *Sci Rep.* 2015;5:8916. https://doi.org/10.1038/srep08916.

53. Ceyhan C, Unal S, Yenisey C, Tekten T, Ceyhan FB. The role of N terminal pro-brain natriuretic peptide in the evaluation of left ventricular diastolic dysfunction: correlation with echocardiographic indexes in hypertensive patients. *Int J Cardiovasc Imaging.* 2008;24(3):253–259. https://doi.org/10.1007/s10554-007-9256-2.

54. Okuyama R, Ishii J, Takahashi H, et al. Combination of high-sensitivity troponin I and N-terminal pro-B-type natriuretic peptide predicts future hospital admission for heart failure in high-risk hypertensive patients with preserved left ventricular ejection fraction. *Heart Vessel.* 2017;32(7):880–892. https://doi.org/10.1007/s00380-017-0948-9.

55. Setsuta K, Kitahara Y, Arae M, Ohbayashi T, Seino Y, Mizuno K. Elevated cardiac troponin T predicts adverse outcomes in hypertensive patients. *Int Heart J.* 2011;52(3):164–169. https://www.ncbi.nlm.nih.gov/pubmed/21646739.

56. Olsen MH, Wachtell K, Tuxen C, et al. N-terminal pro-brain natriuretic peptide predicts cardiovascular events in patients with hypertension and left ventricular hypertrophy: a LIFE study. *J Hypertens.* 2004;22(8):1597–1604. https://www.ncbi.nlm.nih.gov/pubmed/15257184.

57. Pokharel Y, Sun W, de Lemos JA, et al. High-sensitivity troponin T and cardiovascular events in systolic blood pressure Categories: Atherosclerosis Risk in Communities Study. *Hypertension.* 2015;65(1):78–84. https://doi.org/10.1161/HYPERTENSIONAHA.114.04206.

58. McEvoy JW, Martin SS, Dardari ZA, et al. Coronary artery calcium to guide a personalized risk-based approach to initiation and intensification of antihypertensive therapy. *Circulation.* 2017;135(2):153–165. https://doi.org/10.1161/CIRCULATIONAHA.116.025471.

59. Wong HK, Cheung TT, Cheung BM. Adrenomedullin and cardiovascular diseases. *JRSM Cardiovasc Dis.* 2012;1(5). https://doi.org/10.1258/cvd.2012.012003.

60. Al-Omari MA, Khaleghi M, Mosley TH, et al. Mid-regional pro-adrenomedullin is associated with pulse pressure, left ventricular mass, and albuminuria in African Americans with hypertension. *Am J Hypertens.* 2009;22(8):860–866. https://doi.org/10.1038/ajh.2009.82.

61. Xue Y, Taub P, Iqbal N, Fard A, Clopton P, Maisel A. Mid-region pro-adrenomedullin adds predictive value to clinical predictors and Framingham risk score for long-term mortality in stable outpatients with heart failure. *Eur J Heart Fail.* 2013;15(12):1343–1349. https://doi.org/10.1093/eurjhf/hft116.

62. Wild PS, Schnabel RB, Lubos E, et al. Midregional proadrenomedullin for prediction of cardiovascular events in coronary artery disease: results from the AtheroGene study. *Clin Chem.* 2012;58(1):226–236. https://doi.org/10.1373/clinchem.2010.157842.

63. Ojji DB, Opie LH, Lecour S, Lacerda L, Adeyemi O, Sliwa K. Relationship between left ventricular geometry and soluble ST2 in a cohort of hypertensive patients. *J Clin Hypertens.* 2013;15(12):899–904. https://doi.org/10.1111/jch.12205.

64. López B, González A, Lasarte JJ, et al. Is plasma cardiotrophin-1 a marker of hypertensive heart disease? *J Hypertens.* 2005;23(3):625–632. https://www.ncbi.nlm.nih.gov/pubmed/15716706.

65. Wang YC, Yu CC, Chiu FC, et al. Soluble ST2 as a biomarker for detecting stable heart failure with a normal ejection fraction in hypertensive patients. *J Card Fail.* 2013;19(3):163–168. https://doi.org/10.1016/j.cardfail.2013.01.010.

66. López B, González A, Querejeta R, Barba J, Díez J. Association of plasma cardiotrophin-1 with stage C heart failure in hypertensive patients: potential diagnostic implications. *J Hypertens.* 2009;27(2):418–424. https://doi.org/10.1097/HJH.0b013e32831ac981.

67. Mahmud A, Feely J. Arterial stiffness is related to systemic inflammation in essential hypertension. *Hypertension.* 2005;46(5):1118–1122. https://doi.org/10.1161/01.HYP.0000185463.27209.b0.

68. Amer MS, Elawam AE, Khater MS, Omar OH, Mabrouk RA, Taha HM. Association of high-sensitivity C-reactive protein with carotid artery intima-media thickness in hypertensive older adults. *J Am Soc Hypertens.* 2011;5(5):395–400. https://doi.org/10.1016/j.jash.2011.03.004.

69. Hashimoto H, Kitagawa K, Hougaku H, Etani H, Hori M. Relationship between C-reactive protein and progression of early carotid atherosclerosis in hypertensive subjects. *Stroke.* 2004;35(7):1625–1630. https://doi.org/10.1161/01.STR.0000130422.89335.81.

70. Kaptoge S, Di Angelantonio E, Lowe G, et al. C-reactive protein concentration and risk of coronary heart disease, stroke, and mortality: an individual participant meta-analysis. *Lancet.* 2010;375(9709):132–140. https://doi.org/10.1016/S0140-6736(09)61717-7.

71. Iwashima Y, Horio T, Kamide K, Rakugi H, Ogihara T, Kawano Y. C-reactive protein, left ventricular mass index, and risk of cardiovascular disease in essential hypertension. *Hypertens Res.* 2007;30(12):1177–1185. https://doi.org/10.1291/hypres.30.1177.

72. Pietri P, Vyssoulis G, Vlachopoulos C, et al. Relationship between low-grade inflammation and arterial stiffness in patients with essential hypertension. *J Hypertens.* 2006;24(11):2231–2238. https://doi.org/10.1097/01.hjh.0000249701.49854.21.

73. Zhang W, Wang W, Yu H, et al. Interleukin 6 underlies angiotensin II-induced hypertension and chronic renal damage. *Hypertension.* 2012;59(1):136–144. https://doi.org/10.1161/HYPERTENSIONAHA.111.173328.

74. Mehaffey E, Majid DSA. Tumor necrosis factor-α, kidney function, and hypertension. *Am J Physiol Ren Physiol.* 2017;313(4):F1005–F1008. https://doi.org/10.1152/ajprenal.00535.2016.

75. Kaptoge S, Seshasai SRK, Gao P, et al. Inflammatory cytokines and risk of coronary heart disease: new prospective study and updated meta-analysis. *Eur Heart J.* 2014;35:578–589. https://doi.org/10.1093/eurheartj/eht367.

76. Shankar A, Sun L, Klein BE, et al. Markers of inflammation predict the long-term risk of developing chronic kidney disease: a population-based cohort study. *Kidney Int.* 2011;80(11):1231–1238. https://doi.org/10.1038/ki.2011.283.

77. Verdecchia P, Schillaci G, Reboldi G, Santeusanio F, Porcellati C, Brunetti P. Relation between serum uric acid and risk of cardiovascular disease in essential hypertension. The PIUMA study. *Hypertension.* 2000;36(6):1072–1078. https://www.ncbi.nlm.nih.gov/pubmed/11116127.

78. Lip GY, Beevers M, Beevers DG. Serum urate is associated with baseline renal dysfunction but not survival or deterioration in renal function in malignant phase hypertension. *J Hypertens.* 2000;18(1):97–101. https://www.ncbi.nlm.nih.gov/pubmed/10678549.

79. Deckert T, Feldt-Rasmussen B, Borch-Johnsen K, Jensen T, Kofoed-Enevoldsen A. Albuminuria reflects widespread vascular damage. The Steno hypothesis. *Diabetologia.* 1989;32(4):219–226. https://www.ncbi.nlm.nih.gov/pubmed/2668076.

80. Böhm M, Thoenes M, Danchin N, Bramlage P, La Puerta P, Volpe M. Association of cardiovascular risk factors with microalbuminuria in hypertensive individuals: the i-SEARCH global study. *J Hypertens.* 2007;25(11):2317–2324. https://doi.org/10.1097/HJH.0b013e3282ef1c5f.

81. Bigazzi R, Bianchi S, Campese VM, Baldari G. Prevalence of microalbuminuria in a large population of patients with mild to moderate essential hypertension. *Nephron.* 1992;61(1):94–97. https://www.ncbi.nlm.nih.gov/pubmed/1528348.

82. Pontremoli R, Sofia A, Ravera M, et al. Prevalence and clinical correlates of microalbuminuria in essential hypertension: the MAGIC Study. Microalbuminuria: a Genoa Investigation on Complications. *Hypertension.* 1997;30(5):1135–1143. https://www.ncbi.nlm.nih.gov/pubmed/9369267.

83. Hsu CC, Brancati FL, Astor BC, et al. Blood pressure, atherosclerosis, and albuminuria in 10,113 participants in the atherosclerosis risk in communities study. *J Hypertens.* 2009;27(2):397–409. https://www.ncbi.nlm.nih.gov/pubmed/19226709.

84. Halbesma N, Kuiken DS, Brantsma AH, et al. Macroalbuminuria is a better risk marker than low estimated GFR to identify individuals at risk for accelerated GFR loss in population screening. *J Am Soc Nephrol.* 2006;17(9):2582–2590. https://doi.org/10.1681/ASN.2005121352.

85. Mahmoodi BK, Matsushita K, Woodward M, et al. Associations of kidney disease measures with mortality and end-stage renal disease in individuals with and without hypertension: a meta-analysis. *Lancet.* 2012;380(9854):1649–1661. https://doi.org/10.1016/S0140-6736(12)61272-0.

86. Viazzi F, Leoncini G, Conti N, et al. Microalbuminuria is a predictor of chronic renal insufficiency in patients without diabetes and with hypertension: the MAGIC study. *Clin J Am Soc Nephrol.* 2010;5(6):1099–1106. https://doi.org/10.2215/CJN.07271009.

87. Palatini P, Graniero GR, Canali C, et al. Relationship between albumin excretion rate, ambulatory blood pressure and left ventricular hypertrophy in mild hypertension. *J Hypertens.* 1995;13(12 Pt 2):1796–1800. https://www.ncbi.nlm.nih.gov/pubmed/8903654.

88. Jørgensen L, Jenssen T, Johnsen SH, et al. Albuminuria as risk factor for initiation and progression of carotid atherosclerosis in non-diabetic persons: the Tromsø Study. *Eur Heart J.* 2007;28(3):363–369. https://doi.org/10.1093/eurheartj/ehl394.

89. Astor BC, Hallan SI, Miller ER, Yeung E, Coresh J. Glomerular filtration rate, albuminuria, and risk of cardiovascular and all-cause mortality in the US population. *Am J Epidemiol.* 2008;167(10):1226–1234. https://doi.org/10.1093/aje/kwn033.

90. Matsushita K, van der Velde M, Astor BC, et al. Association of estimated glomerular filtration rate and albuminuria with all-cause and cardiovascular mortality in general population cohorts: a collaborative meta-analysis. *Lancet.* 2010;375(9731):2073–2081. https://doi.org/10.1016/S0140-6736(10)60674-5.

91. Gerstein HC, Mann JF, Yi Q, et al. Albuminuria and risk of cardiovascular events, death, and heart failure in diabetic and nondiabetic individuals. *JAMA.* 2001;286(4):421–426. http://www.ncbi.nlm.nih.gov/pubmed/11466120.

92. Bigazzi R, Bianchi S, Baldari D, Campese VM. Microalbuminuria predicts cardiovascular events and renal insufficiency in patients with essential hypertension. *J Hypertens.* 1998;16(9):1325–1333. https://www.ncbi.nlm.nih.gov/pubmed/9746120.

93. Pascual JM, Rodilla E, Costa JA, Garcia-Escrich M, Gonzalez C, Redon J. Prognostic value of microalbuminuria during antihypertensive treatment in essential hypertension. *Hypertension.* 2014;64(6):1228–1234. https://doi.org/10.1161/HYPERTENSIONAHA.114.04273.

94. National Kidney Foundation. KDOQI clinical practice guideline for diabetes and CKD: 2012 update. *Am J Kidney Dis.* 2012;60(5):850–886. https://doi.org/10.1053/j.ajkd.2012.07.005.

95. Moyer VA. Force USPST. Screening for chronic kidney disease: U.S. Preventive Services Task Force recommendation statement. *Ann Intern Med.* 2012;157(8):567–570. https://doi.org/10.7326/0003-4819-157-8-201210160-00533.

96. van der Velde M, Halbesma N, de Charro FT, et al. Screening for albuminuria identifies individuals at increased renal risk. *J Am Soc Nephrol.* 2009;20(4):852–862. https://doi.org/10.1681/ASN.2008060655.

97. Heerspink HJ, Kröpelin TF, Hoekman J, de Zeeuw D. Consortium RA as SE (REASSURE). Drug-induced reduction in albuminuria is associated with subsequent renoprotection: a meta-analysis. *J Am Soc Nephrol.* 2015;26(8):2055–2064. https://doi.org/10.1681/ASN.2014070688.

98. Klausen KP, Parving HH, Scharling H, Jensen JS. The association between metabolic syndrome, microalbuminuria and impaired renal function in the general population: impact on cardiovascular disease and mortality. *J Intern Med.* 2007;262(4):470–478. https://doi.org/10.1111/j.1365-2796.2007.01839.x.

99. de Lemos JA, Ayers CR, Levine B, et al. Multimodality strategy for cardiovascular risk assessment: performance in 2 population-based cohorts. *Circulation.* 2017;135(22):2119–2132. https://doi.org/10.1161/CIRCULATIONAHA.117.027272.

100. Laragh JH, Sealey JE. The plasma renin test reveals the contribution of body sodium-volume content (V) and renin-angiotensin (R) vasoconstriction to long-term blood pressure. *Am J Hypertens.* 2011;24(11):1164–1180. https://doi.org/10.1038/ajh.2011.171.

101. Alderman MH, Cohen HW, Sealey JE, Laragh JH. Pressor responses to antihypertensive drug types. *Am J Hypertens.* 2010;23(9):1031–1037. https://doi.org/10.1038/ajh.2010.114.

102. Egan BM, Basile JN, Rehman SU, et al. Plasma Renin test-guided drug treatment algorithm for correcting patients with treated but uncontrolled hypertension: a randomized controlled trial. *Am J Hypertens.* 2009;22(7):792–801. https://doi.org/10.1038/ajh.2009.63.

103. Stanton AV, Dicker P, O'Brien ET. Aliskiren monotherapy results in the greatest and the least blood pressure lowering in patients with high- and low-baseline PRA levels, respectively. *Am J Hypertens.* 2009;22(9):954–957. https://doi.org/10.1038/ajh.2009.114.

104. Schilders JE, Wu H, Boomsma F, van den Meiracker AH, Danser AH. Renin-angiotensin system phenotyping as a guidance toward personalized medicine for ACE inhibitors: can the response to ACE inhibition be predicted on the basis of plasma renin or ACE? *Cardiovasc Drugs Ther.* 2014;28(4):335–345. https://doi.org/10.1007/s10557-014-6537-6.

105. Jansen PM, Frenkel WJ, van den Born BJ, et al. Determinants of blood pressure reduction by eplerenone in uncontrolled hypertension. *J Hypertens.* 2013;31(2):404–413. https://doi.org/10.1097/HJH.0b013e32835b71d6.

106. Sealey JE, Laragh JH. Aliskiren fails to lower blood pressure in patients who have either low PRA levels or whose PRA falls insufficiently or reactively rises. *Am J Hypertens.* 2009;22(1):112–121. https://doi.org/10.1038/ajh.2008.275.

107. Egan BM, Laken MA, Sutherland SE, et al. Aldosterone antagonists or renin-guided therapy for treatment-resistant hypertension: a comparative effectiveness pilot study in primary care. *Am J Hypertens.* 2016;29(8):976–983. https://doi.org/10.1093/ajh/hpw016.

108. Seifarth C, Trenkel S, Schobel H, Hahn EG, Hensen J. Influence of antihypertensive medication on aldosterone and renin concentration in the differential diagnosis of essential hypertension and primary aldosteronism. *Clin Endocrinol.* 2002;57(4):457–465. https://www.ncbi.nlm.nih.gov/pubmed/12354127.

109. Nussberger J, Gradman AH, Schmieder RE, Lins RL, Chiang Y, Prescott MF. Plasma renin and the antihypertensive effect of the orally active renin inhibitor aliskiren in clinical hypertension. *Int J Clin Pract.* 2007;61(9):1461–1468. https://doi.org/10.1111/j.1742-1241.2007.01473.x.

110. Turner ST, Schwartz GL, Chapman AB, et al. Plasma renin activity predicts blood pressure responses to beta-blocker and thiazide diuretic as monotherapy and add-on therapy for hypertension. *Am J Hypertens.* 2010;23(9):1014–1022. https://doi.org/10.1038/ajh.2010.98.

111. Kobori H, Urushihara M, Xu JH, Berenson GS, Navar LG. Urinary angiotensinogen is correlated with blood pressure in men (Bogalusa Heart Study). *J Hypertens.* 2010;28(7):1422–1428. https://doi.org/10.1097/HJH.0b013e3283392673.

112. Rebholz CM, Chen J, Zhao Q, et al. Urine angiotensinogen and salt-sensitivity and potassium-sensitivity of blood pressure. *J Hypertens.* 2015;33(7):1394–1400. https://doi.org/10.1097/HJH.0000000000000564.

113. Ando K, Fujita T. Pathophysiology of salt sensitivity hypertension. *Ann Med.* 2012;44(suppl 1):S119–S126. https://doi.org/10.3109/07853890.2012.671538.

114. Ghazi L, Dudenbostel T, Lin CP, Oparil S, Calhoun DA. Urinary sodium excretion predicts blood pressure response to spironolactone in patients with resistant hypertension independent of aldosterone status. *J Hypertens.* 2016;34(5):1005–1010. https://doi.org/10.1097/HJH.0000000000000870.

115. Ergul A. Hypertension in black patients: an emerging role of the endothelin system in salt-sensitive hypertension. *Hypertension.* 2000;36(1):62–67. https://www.ncbi.nlm.nih.gov/pubmed/10904013.

116. Ghazi L, Drawz P. Advances in understanding the renin-angiotensin-aldosterone system (RAAS) in blood pressure control and recent pivotal trials of RAAS blockade in heart failure and diabetic nephropathy. *F1000Res.* 2017;6. https://doi.org/10.12688/f1000research.9692.1.

117. Zhou MS, Tian R, Jaimes EA, Raij L. Combination therapy of amlodipine and atorvastatin has more beneficial vascular effects than monotherapy in salt-sensitive hypertension. *Am J Hypertens.* 2014;27(6):873–880. https://doi.org/10.1093/ajh/hpt272.

118. Fujita T. Aldosterone in salt-sensitive hypertension and metabolic syndrome. *J Mol Med.* 2008;86(6):729–734. https://doi.org/10.1007/s00109-008-0343-1.

119. Ridker PM, Danielson E, Rifai N, Glynn RJ, Investigators V-M. Valsartan, blood pressure reduction, and C-reactive protein: primary report of the Val-MARC trial. *Hypertension.* 2006;48(1):73–79. https://doi.org/10.1161/01.HYP.0000226046.58883.32.

120. Martinez-Martin FJ, Rodriguez-Rosas H, Peiro-Martinez I, Soriano-Perera P, Pedrianes-Martin P, Comi-Diaz C. Olmesartan/amlodipine vs olmesartan/hydrochlorothiazide in hypertensive patients with metabolic syndrome: the OLAS study. *J Hum Hypertens.* 2011;25(6):346–353. https://doi.org/10.1038/jhh.2010.104.

121. Farah R, Khamisy-Farah R, Shurtz-Swirski R. Calcium channel blocker effect on insulin resistance and inflammatory markers in essential hypertension patients. *Int Angiol.* 2013;32(1):85–93. https://www.ncbi.nlm.nih.gov/pubmed/23435396.

122. Fliser D, Buchholz K, Haller H. Investigators ET on O and P in I and A (EUTOPIA). Antiinflammatory effects of angiotensin II subtype 1 receptor blockade in hypertensive patients with microinflammation. *Circulation.* 2004;110(9):1103–1107. https://doi.org/10.1161/01.CIR.0000140265.21608.8E.

123. Palmas W, Ma S, Psaty B, Goff DC, Darwin C, Barr RG. Antihypertensive medications and C-reactive protein in the multi-ethnic study of atherosclerosis. *Am J Hypertens.* 2007;20(3):233–241. https://doi.org/10.1016/j.amjhyper.2006.08.006.

124. Fogari R, Zoppi A, Lazzari P, et al. ACE inhibition but not angiotensin II antagonism reduces plasma fibrinogen and insulin resistance in overweight hypertensive patients. *J Cardiovasc Pharmacol.* 1998;32(4):616–620. https://doi.org/.

125. Erdem Y, Usalan C, Haznedaroğlu IC, et al. Effects of angiotensin converting enzyme and angiotensin II receptor inhibition on impaired fibrinolysis in systemic hypertension. *Am J Hypertens.* 1999;12(11 Pt 1):1071–1076. https://www.ncbi.nlm.nih.gov/pubmed/10604482.

126. Schrover IM, Dorresteijn JAN, Smits JE, Danser AHJ, Visseren FLJ, Spiering W. Identifying treatment response to antihypertensives in patients with obesity-related hypertension. *Clin Hypertens.* 2017;23:20. https://doi.org/10.1186/s40885-017-0077-x.

127. Di Napoli M, Papa F. Angiotensin-converting enzyme inhibitor use is associated with reduced plasma concentration of C-reactive protein in patients with first-ever ischemic stroke. *Stroke.* 2003;34(12):2922–2929. https://doi.org/10.1161/01.STR.0000099124.84425.BB.

128. Ridker PM, Danielson E, Fonseca FA, et al. Reduction in C-reactive protein and LDL cholesterol and cardiovascular event rates after initiation of rosuvastatin: a prospective study of the JUPITER trial. *Lancet.* 2009;373(9670):1175–1182. https://doi.org/10.1016/S0140-6736(09)60447-5.

129. Ridker PM, Everett BM, Thuren T, et al. Antiinflammatory therapy with canakinumab for atherosclerotic disease. *N Engl J Med.* 2017;377(12):1119–1131. https://doi.org/10.1056/NEJMoa1707914.

130. Agarwal V, Hans N, Messerli FH. Effect of allopurinol on blood pressure: a systematic review and meta-analysis. *J Clin Hypertens.* 2013;15(6):435–442. https://doi.org/10.1111/j.1751-7176.2012.00701.x.

131. Tani S, Nagao K, Hirayama A. Effect of febuxostat, a xanthine oxidase inhibitor, on cardiovascular risk in hyperuricemic patients with hypertension: a prospective, open-label, pilot study. *Clin Drug Investig.* 2015;35(12):823–831. https://doi.org/10.1007/s40261-015-0349-8.

132. Soletsky B, Feig DI. Uric acid reduction rectifies prehypertension in obese adolescents. *Hypertens (Dallas, Tex 1979).* 2012;60(5):1148–1156. https://doi.org/10.1161/HYPERTENSIONAHA.112.196980.

133. Kohagura K, Tana T, Higa A, et al. Effects of xanthine oxidase inhibitors on renal function and blood pressure in hypertensive patients with hyperuricemia. *Hypertens Res.* 2016;39(8):593–597. https://doi.org/10.1038/hr.2016.37.

134. Borgi L, McMullan C, Wohlhueter A, Curhan GC, Fisher ND, Forman JP. Effect of uric acid-lowering agents on endothelial function: a randomized, double-blind, placebo-controlled trial. *Hypertension.* 2017;69(2):243–248. https://doi.org/10.1161/HYPERTENSIONAHA.116.08488.

135. McMullan CJ, Borgi L, Fisher N, Curhan G, Forman J. Effect of uric acid lowering on renin-angiotensin-system activation and ambulatory BP: a randomized controlled trial. *Clin J Am Soc Nephrol.* 2017;12(5):807–816. https://doi.org/10.2215/CJN.10771016.

136. White WB, Saag KG, Becker MA, et al. Cardiovascular safety of febuxostat or allopurinol in patients with Gout. *N Engl J Med.* 2018;378(13):1200–1210. https://www-ncbi-nlm-nih-gov.ezp.welch.jhmi.edu/pubmed/?term=N+Engl+J+Med+2018%3B+378%3A1200-1210.

137. Thomas G, Xie D, Chen HY, et al. Prevalence and prognostic significance of apparent treatment resistant hypertension in chronic kidney disease: report from the chronic renal insufficiency cohort study. *Hypertension.* 2016;67(2):387–396. https://doi.org/10.1161/HYPERTENSIONAHA.115.06487.

138. Tomaszewski M, White C, Patel P, et al. High rates of non-adherence to antihypertensive treatment revealed by high-performance liquid chromatography-tandem mass spectrometry (HP LC-MS/MS) urine analysis. *Heart.* 2014;100(11):855–861. https://doi.org/10.1136/heartjnl-2013-305063.

139. Strauch B, Petrák O, Zelinka T, et al. Precise assessment of noncompliance with the antihypertensive therapy in patients with resistant hypertension using toxicological serum analysis. *J Hypertens.* 2013;31(12):2455–2461. https://doi.org/10.1097/HJH.0b013e3283652c61.

140. Ceral J, Habrdova V, Vorisek V, Bima M, Pelouch R, Solar M. Difficult-to-control arterial hypertension or uncooperative patients? The assessment of serum antihypertensive drug levels to differentiate non-responsiveness from non-adherence to recommended therapy. *Hypertens Res.* 2011;34(1):87–90. https://doi.org/10.1038/hr.2010.183.

141. Gupta P, Patel P, Štrauch B, et al. Biochemical screening for nonadherence is associated with blood pressure reduction and Improvement in adherence. *Hypertension.* 2017;70(5):1042–1048. https://doi.org/10.1161/HYPERTENSIONAHA.117.09631.

142. van den Heuvel M, Batenburg WW, Jainandunsing S, et al. Urinary renin, but not angiotensinogen or aldosterone, reflects the renal renin-angiotensin-aldosterone system activity and the efficacy of renin-angiotensin-aldosterone system blockade in the kidney. *J Hypertens.* 2011;29(11):2147–2155. https://doi.org/10.1097/HJH.0b013e32834bbcbf.

143. Gaddam KK, Nishizaka MK, Pratt-Ubunama MN, et al. Characterization of resistant hypertension: association between resistant hypertension, aldosterone, and persistent intravascular volume expansion. *Arch Intern Med.* 2008;168(11):1159–1164. https://doi.org/10.1001/archinte.168.11.1159.

144. Esler MD, Krum H, Sobotka PA, et al. Renal sympathetic denervation in patients with treatment-resistant hypertension (The Symplicity HTN-2 Trial): a randomised controlled trial. *Lancet.* 2010;376(9756):1903–1909. https://doi.org/10.1016/S0140-6736(10)62039-9.

145. Bhatt DL, Kandzari DE, O'Neill WW, et al. A controlled trial of renal denervation for resistant hypertension. *N Engl J Med.* 2014;370(15):1393–1401. https://doi.org/10.1056/NEJMoa1402670.

146. Azizi M, Sapoval M, Gosse P, et al. Optimum and stepped care standardised antihypertensive treatment with or without renal denervation for resistant hypertension (DENERHTN): a multicentre, open-label, randomised controlled trial. *Lancet.* 2015;385(9981):1957–1965. https://doi.org/10.1016/S0140-6736(14)61942-5.

147. Townsend RR, Mahfoud F, Kandzari DE, et al. Catheter-based renal denervation in patients with uncontrolled hypertension in the absence of antihypertensive medications (SPYRAL HTN-OFF MED): a randomised, sham-controlled, proof-of-concept trial. *Lancet.* 2017;390(10108):2160–2170. https://doi.org/10.1016/S0140-6736(17)32281-X.

148. Dörr O, Liebetrau C, Möllmann H, et al. Brain-derived neurotrophic factor as a marker for immediate assessment of the success of renal sympathetic denervation. *J Am Coll Cardiol.* 2015;65(11):1151–1153. https://doi.org/10.1016/j.jacc.2014.11.071.

CHAPTER 4

Diabetes: Key Markers of Injury and Prognosis

IAN J. NEELAND, MD • KERSHAW V. PATEL, MD

DIABETES MELLITUS—A DISEASE DEFINED BY BIOMARKERS

Diabetes mellitus (DM) is a global epidemic that encompasses multiple disorders related to altered metabolic homeostasis of glucose and related systems. Although diabetes can manifest as an autoimmune disease of pancreatic islet cells (the primary mechanism in type 1 diabetes), gestational diabetes, or secondary to medications, the vast majority (90%–95%) of individuals suffering with diabetes have type 2 diabetes mellitus (T2DM). Insulin resistance and other abnormalities seen in the metabolic syndrome are typically found in T2DM. The burden of diabetes is growing globally with a worldwide estimated prevalence of 2.8% in 2000 expected to increase to 4.4% by 2030.[1] In the United States (US) alone, diabetes was responsible for more than 70,000 deaths and was the seventh leading cause of death in 2014.[2] The economic burden of diabetes in the US is also significant. In 2002 the estimated cost of diabetes was $132 billion.[3]

The hallmark of diabetes is elevation in blood glucose levels with or without insulin resistance in skeletal muscle and liver. The definition of diabetes has evolved over the last 40 years. In 1979 the National Diabetes Data Group used distributions of serum glucose levels to define threshold values.[4] Diabetes was diagnosed by symptoms, fasting plasma glucose cutoff of greater than or equal to 140 mg/dL, or a 2-h plasma glucose greater than or equal to 200 mg/dL after a 75-g oral glucose load (glucose tolerance test). In 1997 the Expert Committee on the Diagnosis and Classification of Diabetes Mellitus shifted the diagnostic criteria focus to thresholds based on levels at which long-term microvascular complications (retinopathy and nephropathy) were seen.[5] Although plasma glucose levels seen in the population have a wide distribution, there is a threshold at which patients are more likely to develop microvascular diseases. For example, among Pima Indian residents in Arizona, a higher incidence of retinopathy and nephropathy were found at specific fasting plasma

glucose and 2-h plasma glucose levels.[6] The Expert Committee also revised the diagnostic criteria so that the various tests reflected equivalent levels of hyperglycemia and microvascular risk. The fasting plasma glucose cutoff for diagnosing diabetes was later lowered to a level ≥126 mg/dL, and this test was preferred over the oral glucose tolerance test because glucose tolerance testing is less convenient, more costly, less reproducible, and may not be physiologic.

In 2008 the International Diabetes Foundation, European Association for the Study of Diabetes, and the American Diabetes Association harmonized new methods for diagnosing diabetes.[7] Glycated hemoglobin (Hb A1c) was incorporated in the definition as it reflects long-term exposure to serum glucose, and Hb A1c thresholds are associated with complications of diabetes. Contemporary guidelines include an Hb A1c threshold greater than or equal to 6.5% confirmed with repeat testing as part of the diagnosis for diabetes[8] (Table 4.1). Thresholds for diagnosing diabetes therefore have shifted over time from a population distribution approach to biomarkers reflecting long-term exposure and risk for clinical outcomes. An important limitation to the current diagnostic criteria, however, is that the glycemic thresholds reflect risk for developing microvascular diseases but not necessarily macrovascular complications. Differential exposure to elevated plasma glucose levels is one proposed mechanism for the variation in microvascular and macrovascular complications seen with diabetes as tissues in the kidney, retina, and vascular endothelium are exposed to high glucose levels in an insulin-independent manner, in contrast to striated muscle, such as cardiac myocytes, which requires insulin-dependent glucose transport resulting in lower exposure to hyperglycemia.[9] Because studies have not shown that improved glycemic control in diabetes impacts macrovascular disease (cardiovascular death, coronary heart disease, and stroke), there is a need for blood-based biomarkers for cardiovascular injury and prognosis that can aid the clinician in risk

Biomarkers in Cardiovascular Disease. https://doi.org/10.1016/B978-0-323-54835-9.00004-1

TABLE 4.1
Current Diagnostic Criteria for Diabetes Mellitus

Biomarker	Criterion for Diagnosis
Fasting plasma glucose	≥126 mg/dL[a]
Random plasma glucose	≥200 mg/dL with classic symptoms of hyperglycemia or hyperglycemic crisis
Two-hour plasma glucose	≥200 mg/dL during an OGTT[b]
Hemoglobin A1c	≥126 mg/dL[c]

[a]Fasting is defined as no caloric intake for at least 8h before testing.
[b]OGTT = oral glucose tolerance test; equivalent glucose load of 75-g anhydrous glucose dissolved in water.
[c]Using a certified and standardized laboratory test.
Initial test should be confirmed with repeat testing in the absence of unequivocal hyperglycemia.
Data from American Diabetes Association. Diagnosis and classification of diabetes mellitus. *Diabetes Care.* January 2014;37(Suppl. 1):S81–S90.

stratification, primary and secondary prevention, initiation of therapy, monitoring treatment efficacy, and determining long-term prognosis.

BIOMARKERS OF GLYCEMIC CONTROL— MICROVASCULAR DISEASE

Current evidence supports a direct relationship between glycemic control (vis-à-vis clinical thresholds of plasma glucose and Hb A1c) and progression of microvascular disease, including nephropathy, retinopathy, and neuropathy.[9] The UK Prospective Diabetes Study (UKPDS) 33 trial established that intensive glycemic control in patients with T2DM reduces the risk of microvascular complications.[10] In this trial, 3,867 patients with T2DM were randomized to intensive treatment with antihyperglycemic medications or conventional treatment. The median Hb A1c level in the intensive group was 7% compared with 7.9% in the conventional treatment arm over the 10-year study period. The risk for any diabetes end point (sudden death, death from hyperglycemia or hypoglycemia, fatal or nonfatal myocardial infarction, angina, heart failure, stroke, renal failure, and others) was 12% lower in the intensive treatment group than that in the conventional treatment group, driven mostly by a 25% risk reduction in microvascular events. UKPDS 33 did not demonstrate any significant difference in myocardial infarction or mortality between the intensive and conservative treatment groups. The Diabetes Control and Complications Trial (DCCT) also showed

that intensive glycemic control using at least three daily insulin injections or an insulin pump and frequent blood glucose monitoring reduced the incidence and progression of retinopathy and other microvascular complications in a trial of 1,441 patients with type 1 diabetes mellitus (T1DM).[11] The mean ± standard deviation (SD) blood glucose achieved was 155 ± 30 mg/dL in the intensive therapy group compared with 231 ± 55 mg/dL in the conventional therapy group. During 6 years of follow-up, the relative risk (RR) of retinopathy was reduced by 63% (95% confidence interval [CI], 52% to 71%), risk of nephropathy (microalbuminuria, defined by urinary albumin exertion ≥ 40 mg/day) was reduced by 39% (95% CI, 21%–42%), and risk of neuropathy was reduced by 60% (95% CI, 38%–74%) in the intensive therapy group compared with those in the conventional group.[11] Similar outcomes were seen in the Action to Control Cardiovascular Risk in Diabetes (ACCORD) trial in which 10,251 participants with T2DM at high risk for cardiovascular disease were randomized to receive either intensive or standard treatment for glycemic control using a target Hb A1c level of <6.0% or 7.0%–7.9%, respectively.[12,13] A subgroup of these patients (n = 2,856) were evaluated at 4 years of follow-up for progression of diabetic retinopathy.[14] In ACCORD trial, median Hb A1c levels were 6.4% among participants receiving intensive therapy compared with 7.5% among those receiving standard therapy. Targeting a lower Hb A1c level significantly decreased the odds of diabetic retinopathy progression (adjusted odds ratio [OR], 0.67; 95% CI, 0.51 to 0.87). In the Action in Diabetes and Vascular Disease: Preterax and Diamicron Modified Release Controlled Evaluation (ADVANCE) trial, 11,140 patients with T2DM were randomly assigned to standard or intensive glucose control. Patients randomized to the intensive glucose control group received the sulfonylurea gliclazide and other glucose-lowering medications to reach a goal Hb A1c value of ≤6.5%.[15] The intensive glucose control group achieved a lower mean Hb A1c than the standard glucose control group after a median of 5 years of follow-up (6.5% vs. 7.3%, respectively). Intensive glucose control led to a lower incidence of combined microvascular and macrovascular events than standard glucose control (18.1% vs. 20.0%; hazard ratio [HR], 0.90; 95% CI, 0.82 to 0.98), driven by the reduction in major microvascular events (9.4% vs. 10.9%; HR, 0.86; 95% CI, 0.77 to 0.97). The reduction in microvascular events was mostly related to the reduction in the incidence of nephropathy, not retinopathy. A recent systematic review and meta-analysis that includes the above mentioned three trials and a total of 28,614 study

TABLE 4.2
Relative Risk Estimates for Microvascular Events in Major Clinical Trials of Intensive Versus Conventional Glucose Control

Cardiovascular Event	Intensive (n)	Conventional (n)	Risk Ratio (95% CI)
Composite microvascular outcome	1,331/13,770	1,312/11,830	0.88 (0.79–0.97)
Retinopathy	740/6,175	660/4,618	0.80 (0.67–0.94)
Nephropathy	3,402/14,675	3,497/13,094	0.83 (0.64–1.06)

Data from Hemmingsen B, et al. Intensive glycemic control for patients with type 2 diabetes: systematic review with meta-analysis and trial sequential analysis of randomised clinical trials. *BMJ*. 2011;343:d6898. https://doi.org/10.1136/bmj.d6898.

TABLE 4.3
Relative Risk Estimates for Cardiovascular Disease Events in Major Clinical Trials of Intensive Versus Conventional Glucose Control

Cardiovascular Event	Intensive (n)	Conventional (n)	Relative Risk (95% CI)
Cardiovascular disease	1,643/14,662	1,456/13,140	0.90 (0.83–0.98)
Coronary heart disease	1,106/14,662	1,003/13,140	0.89 (0.81–0.96)
Stroke	502/14,662	432/13,140	0.98 (0.86–1.11)
Congestive heart failure	539/14,662	490/13,140	1.01 (0.89–1.14)
Cardiovascular mortality	729/14,662	595/13,140	0.97 (0.76–1.24)
All-cause mortality	1,396/14,662	1,133/13,140	0.98 (0.84–1.15)

Data from Kelly TN, et al. Systematic Review: Glucose Control and Cardiovascular Disease in Type 2 Diabetes. *Ann Intern Med*. 2009;130:394–403.

participants confirmed that intensive glycemic control led to a reduction in microvascular events compared with conventional glycemic control[16] (Table 4.2).

BIOMARKERS OF GLYCEMIC CONTROL—MACROVASCULAR DISEASE

Despite reductions in microvascular complications with intensive glycemic control in patients with diabetes, trials of glucose-lowering interventions using clinical targets of blood glucose and Hb A1c levels have not consistently shown a reduction in macrovascular complications. Macrovascular refers to cardiovascular death, coronary heart disease, and stroke; heart failure is not generally included as an outcome. In the ADVANCE trial, intensive glucose control did not significantly lower the composite outcome of macrovascular events, including cardiovascular death, nonfatal myocardial infarction, or nonfatal stroke.[15] In the ACCORD trial, intensive therapy with goal Hb A1c of <6.0% was terminated due to higher mortality seen in this group relative to standard therapy with goal Hb A1c ranging 7%–7.9%. Before terminating the intensive therapy

strategy because of higher all-cause mortality, the two groups did not differ significantly in the composite primary outcome of cardiovascular death, nonfatal myocardial infarction, or nonfatal stroke.[13] In a systematic review and meta-analysis of 5 trials involving 27,802 study participants comparing intensive versus conventional glucose control, summary analyses showed a small reduction in cardiovascular disease with intensive glucose control (RR, 0.90; 95% CI, 0.83–0.98) but not cardiovascular or all-cause death[17] (Table 4.3).

Additional evidence arguing against hyperglycemia as an important modifiable biomarker for macrovascular disease comes from trials examining the sodium glucose cotransporter 2 inhibitors (SGLT2i) and glucagon-like peptide 1 analogues (GLP1a). Empagliflozin and canagliflozin are SGLT2i that block glucose reabsorption in the proximal tubule of the nephron and were studied in two large cardiovascular outcomes trials. In Empagliflozin Cardiovascular Outcome Event Trial in Type 2 Diabetes Mellitus Patients (EMPA-REG OUTCOME), 7,020 patients with diabetes and established cardiovascular disease were randomly assigned treatment with empagliflozin or placebo on a background

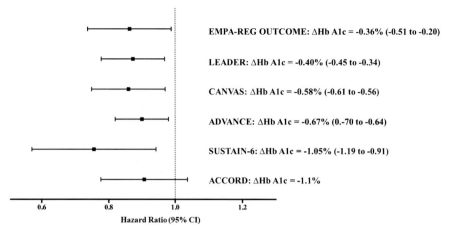

FIG. 4.1 Change in glycemic control and study outcomes in clinical trials. Placebo-adjusted mean change (95% confidence interval) in glycated hemoglobin (Hb A1c) and corresponding hazard ratio (95% confidence interval) of study outcome for intervention versus control group in clinical trials. (Data from individual trial reporting as referenced in the text.)

of standard of care therapies.[18] In the intention-to-treat analysis the adjusted mean difference in Hb A1c between the empagliflozin 25-mg and placebo groups was approximately –0.36% at week 206. Despite relatively small improvements in glucose control, the composite risk of death from cardiovascular causes, nonfatal myocardial infarction, or nonfatal stroke was 14% lower with empagliflozin treatment, with a 38% relative risk reduction in cardiovascular death. In Canagliflozin Cardiovascular Assessment Study (CANVAS), 10,142 patients with diabetes and high cardiovascular risk were randomized to receive either canagliflozin or placebo.[19] The mean difference in glycated hemoglobin between the two groups was –0.58%, and the canagliflozin group had a 14% lower rate of the composite outcome of death from cardiovascular causes, nonfatal myocardial infarction, or nonfatal stroke than the placebo group. Liraglutide and semaglutide are GLP1a that stimulate insulin secretion and have extrapancreatic tissue affects and were studied in large cardiovascular outcomes trials. The Liraglutide Effect and Action in Diabetes: Evaluation of Cardiovascular Outcome Results (LEADER) trial randomized patients with diabetes and high cardiovascular risk to either liraglutide or placebo.[20] Study participants receiving liraglutide had a 0.4% reduction in glycated hemoglobin at 36 months and a 13% reduction in the composite outcome of death from cardiovascular causes, nonfatal myocardial infarction, or nonfatal stroke. In SUSTAIN-6 trial, patients with diabetes and increased cardiovascular risk were randomized to receive either semaglutide or placebo.[21] At 104 weeks, the mean difference in

Hb A1c between the semaglutide 1.0-mg and placebo groups was –1.05%. The semaglutide group showed a 26% risk reduction in the composite outcome of cardiovascular death, nonfatal myocardial infarction, or nonfatal stroke. Taken together, the relatively less Hb A1c lowering and the magnitude of cardiovascular effects suggests that it is unlikely that the cardiovascular benefits of SGLT2i and GLP1a are primarily due to their glucose-lowering effect and that other factors are likely contributing to these positive outcomes[22] (Fig. 4.1).

NONGLYCEMIC BIOMARKERS OF CARDIOVASCULAR RISK AND PROGNOSIS

Although trials have clearly demonstrated that glycemic control, measured by serum glucose and Hb A1c, estimates risk for microvascular complications in patients with diabetes, average glucose exposure explained only about 11% of the variation in retinopathy risk for the entire study population in DCCT, suggesting that additional factors unrelated to blood glucose levels may contribute to microvascular risk.[23] Furthermore, many nonglycemic serum-based biomarkers in diabetes may contribute to cardiovascular risk stratification and prognostication.

Lipids

Evidence suggests that lipid levels are important biomarkers in the pathogenesis of diabetic vascular complications.[24] Abnormal blood lipid levels are common in patients with diabetes, especially in those with T2DM. Elevated levels of triglycerides and low levels

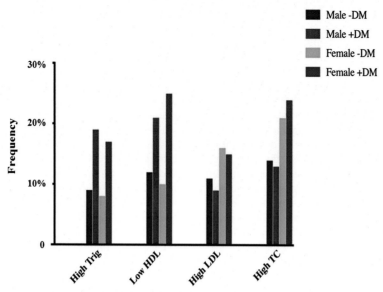

FIG. 4.2 Frequency of dyslipidemia in patients with diabetes mellitus. High is defined by values >90th percentile of the US population. Low is defined by values <10th percentile in the US population. *DM*, diabetes mellitus; *HDL*, high-density lipoprotein cholesterol; *LDL*, low-density lipoprotein cholesterol; *TC*, total cholesterol; *Trig*, triglycerides. (Data from Mooradian AD. Dyslipidemia in type 2 diabetes mellitus. *Nat Clin Pract Endocrinol Metab.* 2009;5(3):150-9.)

of high-density lipoprotein (HDL) cholesterol are two of the most common abnormalities and are thought to contribute to elevated risk for cardiovascular disease (Fig. 4.2).[25] Current guidelines from the American Diabetes Association recommend a screening lipid profile at the time of first diagnosis and periodically thereafter.[26] Statin therapy is an important treatment consideration in any patient with diabetes with or without overt cardiovascular disease. Although the only trial of high-intensity statin therapy in primary prevention was performed in a population without diabetes, epidemiological evidence suggests that patients with diabetes are at substantially increased risk for atherosclerotic cardiovascular disease (ASCVD) during their lifetime, warranting an aggressive lipid-lowering strategy.[27] Indeed, the American Heart Association/American College of Cardiology guidelines identify diabetes, low-density lipoprotein (LDL) cholesterol 70–189 mg/dL, and age 40–75 years as indications for moderate-intensity statin therapy or high-intensity therapy if the estimated 10-year risk of ASCVD is ≥7.5%.[28] Although statins are efficacious in patients with T2DM, rates of cardiovascular events remain elevated in such patients even after statin treatment. Fibrate therapy in patients with T2DM reduced the rate of coronary heart disease events in the Veterans Affairs HDL Intervention Trial[29] but not in the Fenofibrate Intervention and

Event Lowering in Diabetes (FIELD) trial[30]; although when analyses in FIELD were adjusted for new interim statin use, fenofibrate did significantly reduce the risk of coronary heart disease and total cardiovascular disease (CVD) events by 19% and 15%, respectively. Furthermore, a post hoc analysis of data from the FIELD study suggested a benefit for patients with both elevated triglyceride levels and low HDL cholesterol levels.[31] In the ACCORD trial, 5,518 patients with type 2 diabetes were randomly assigned to open label simvastatin plus masked fenofibrate or placebo. After mean 4.7 years of follow-up, the combination of fenofibrate and simvastatin did not reduce the rate of death from cardiovascular causes, nonfatal myocardial infarction, or nonfatal stroke compared with simvastatin treatment alone.[32]

Biomarkers of Kidney Disease

Kidney disease is a common adverse health outcome associated with diabetes. Albuminuria (elevated albumin excretion in the urine) and impaired glomerular filtration rate (GFR; estimated from the serum creatinine level) are two measurable biomarkers that are independently and additively linked with adverse kidney and cardiovascular outcomes, including end-stage renal disease and cardiovascular events and death.[33] The American Diabetes Association recommends annual screening with urine albumin/creatinine ratio on a spot urine sample and estimated GFR assessment in all patients with T2DM, in patients with long-standing T1DM, and those with concomitant hypertension.[26] The prevalence of albuminuria (defined as a ratio of urine albumin to creatinine ≥30 mg/g) and impaired GFR (<60 mL/min · 1.73 m^{-2}) is 23.7% and 17.7%, respectively, among adults with diabetes in the US.[34] In a systematic review, patients with diabetes and micro-albuminuria had 2.4-fold increased risk of mortality.[35] Intensive glycemic control may delay the onset and progression of albuminuria.[11] The use of angiotensin-converting enzyme inhibitors or angiotensin receptor blockers also help to slow the progression of kidney disease in patients with diabetes and hypertension, and they are indicated in those patients with albuminuria and/or impaired GFR. For example, in the Heart Outcomes Prevention Evaluation study, 3,577 participants with diabetes and high cardiovascular risk were randomly assigned to ramipril or placebo.[36] Overt nephropathy, defined as a 24-hour urine albumin ≥300 mg, 24-hour urine total protein ≥500 mg, or a measured albumin/creatinine ratio >36 mg/mmol, was decreased by 24% in the ramipril-treated group, with a consistent effect between those with and without albuminuria at baseline.

Cystatin C is an important emerging biomarker linking kidney disease and cardiovascular risk. Cystatin C is a cysteine-protease inhibitor produced by nucleated cells that is freely filtered by the glomerulus and can be used to estimate GFR and detect early renal impairment.[37] In the Cardiovascular Health Study, a longitudinal study of adults over the age of 65 years of whom between 13% and 19% had diabetes, cystatin C was superior to creatinine as a predictor of risk of death and cardiovascular events.[38] In patients with diabetes, cystatin C has also been associated with increased arterial stiffness as well as greater epicardial adipose tissue burden.[39,40] Cystatin C may be an important biomarker of CVD risk in patients with diabetes in the future.

Myocardial Injury and Cardiac Troponin

The presence of detectable serum cardiac troponin (cTnT) has been an important marker of acute myocardial injury[41] and is increasingly being recognized as a marker of chronic myocardial injury and provides prognostic information for ASCVD.[42] Troponin molecules use calcium to modify downstream cardiac muscle contraction; loss of membrane integrity causes leakage of troponins into the blood.[43] In patients with irreversible, chronic myocardial injury, it is postulated that there may be a continuous release of troponin.[43] Prospective observational studies have detected circulating troponin in the general population, raising the possibility of chronic, subclinical myocardial injury in patients without overt cardiovascular disease. In the Dallas Heart Study, with a cohort of over 3,500 ambulatory adults aged 30–65 years, a detectable cTnT was found in 0.7% of patients and was independently associated with high-risk phenotypes, including DM (adjusted OR, 4.6; 95% CI, 1.8 to 11.6).[44]

The advent of a high-sensitivity cardiac troponin T assay (hs-cTnT) allows for troponin detection at a 10-fold lower level than the standard assays.[45] The 99th percentile of the hs-cTnT assay, considered the upper reference limit for clinical use, is reported at 14 ng/L with a lower limit of detection <3 ng/L,[46] compared with the lower limit of detection of <10 ng/L for standard assays. A significant proportion of individuals have a detectable hs-cTnT below the detection of the standard assay, which has allowed significant exploration of hs-cTnT as a biomarker of subclinical cardiovascular dysfunction in multiple populations. The association of hs-cTnT with prediabetes and DM in the general population was evaluated in an analysis from the Atherosclerosis Risk in Communities study which included 9,051 participants who underwent measurement of hs-cTnT at two time points, 6 years apart.[47] The probability of having subclinical myocardial injury was ~2.5-fold higher among those with diabetes than with individuals free of diabetes. Furthermore, patients with diabetes and elevated hs-cTnT were at substantially higher risk of all-cause death (HR, 4.36; 95% CI, 3.14 to 6.07), coronary heart disease (HR, 3.84; 95% CI, 2.52 to 5.84), and heart failure (HR, 6.37; 95% CI, 4.27 to 9.51) than persons without diabetes and no incident elevation in hs-cTnT (Fig. 4.3).

In patients with diabetes and increased cardiovascular risk, hs-cTnT has increased prognostic value. In a nested case-cohort study of the ADVANCE trial, 62% of the participants had detectable levels (≥3 ng/L) of hs-cTnT.[48] Even after adjustment, hs-cTnT was a strong predictor of cardiovascular events and death, and the addition of hs-cTnT to the baseline clinical model improved 5-year risk classification for cardiovascular events by 46%. In a substudy of the Examination of Cardiovascular Outcomes with Alogliptin versus Standard of Care (EXAMINE) trial that assessed the cardiovascular safety of alogliptin in patients with diabetes and a recent acute coronary syndrome, acute coronary syndrome, high-sensitivity cardiac troponin I (hs-cTnI) was detectable (≥1.9 ng/L) in 93% of participants, and the 7% of study participants with undetectable hs-cTnI had the lowest risk of future cardiovascular events.[49] Finally, in an analysis of the SGLT2i canagliflozin in older patients with diabetes, those who received canagliflozin had hs-cTnI levels that remained unchanged or even decreased

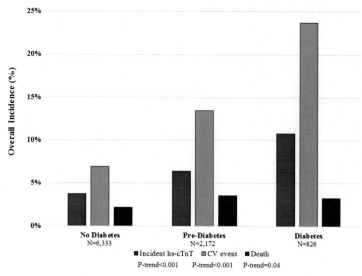

FIG. 4.3 Incidence of elevated high-sensitivity troponin, cardiovascular events, and death among study participants without diabetes, with prediabetes, and with diabetes in the atherosclerosis risk in communities study. (Data from Selvin E, et al. Diabetes, pre-diabetes, and incidence of subclinical myocardial damage. *Circulation.* October 2014;130(16):1374–82.)

compared with increasing hs-cTnI levels among those treated with placebo providing further evidence supporting the use of SGLT2i in DM.[50]

cTnT measured by a highly sensitive assay has also been investigated as a risk stratification tool among individuals with diabetes and stable ischemic heart disease (SIHD) to identify those at high risk for CVD events who might benefit from prompt coronary revascularization. In the Bypass Angioplasty Revascularization Investigation in Type 2 Diabetes trial, more than 2,000 patients with T2DM and SIHD were randomly assigned to medical therapy plus revascularization or medical therapy alone.[51] Over 99% of patients had detectable hs-cTnT and 39% had elevated hs-cTnT (≥14 ng/L) at baseline. The 5-year rate of the composite outcome cardiovascular death, myocardial infarction, or stroke was 27.1% in study participants who had baseline abnormal hs-cTnT concentrations versus 12.9% of those without baseline abnormal hs-cTnT (HR, 1.85; 95% CI, 1.48 to 2.32). Random assignment to revascularization, as compared with medical therapy alone, did not result in a significant reduction in the rate of the composite end point, suggesting that although hs-cTnT was an independent predictor of death from cardiovascular causes, myocardial infarction, or stroke in patients with both T2DM and SIHD, an abnormal value of ≥14 ng/L did not necessarily aid in the decision-making for revascularization with regard to outcomes.

Hemodynamic Stress and Natriuretic Peptides

Natriuretic peptides are a family of proteins that act in the maintenance of cardio-renal homeostasis through natriuretic, vasodilatory, and diuretic effects.[52] B-type natriuretic peptide (BNP) is manufactured in ventricular myocytes and released into the blood stream. Atrial natriuretic peptide is also found mainly in the heart. These markers have been shown to be prognostic in patients with acute decompensated heart failure (HF),[53] and attempts have been made to use BNP to guide therapy in HF patients with varying degrees of success.[54,55] Both BNP and NT-proBNP (biologically inert circulating prohormone of BNP) are used regularly in clinical settings for evaluation and treatment of patients with both systolic and diastolic heart failure. Plasma levels of the two molecules are closely correlated ($r = 0.90$, $P < .001$) and have similar efficacy in predicting clinical severity of heart failure and prediction of event-free survival.[56]

In a study of patients with diabetes at the San Diego Veterans Affairs Medical Center, the prognostic role of BNP was examined.[57] Participants were divided into those who were referred for echocardiography due to suspicion for cardiac dysfunction and those who were randomly recruited from a diabetes clinic. Regardless if participants were referred or not for echocardiography, individuals with BNP > 120 pg/mL had worsened survival.

The prognostic role of NT-proBNP in patients with diabetes and various amounts of albuminuria was evaluated at a tertiary referral center in Denmark.[58] After median follow-up of 15.5 years, NT-proBNP was a strong predictor of all-cause and cardiovascular death independent of urinary albumin excretion rate and traditional cardiovascular risk factors. In a substudy of the ADVANCE trial, the predictive ability of NT-proBNP for cardiovascular events and all-cause mortality was examined.[48] After a 5-year median follow-up period, the HR for cardiovascular events and death was 1.95 (95% CI, 1.72 to 2.20) and 1.97 (95% CI, 1.73 to 2.24) per 1-SD increase in NT-proBNP level, respectively. Five-year risk classification for cardiovascular events improved by 39% with the addition of NT-proBNP to the baseline clinical model. In the canagliflozin biomarker substudy of older patients with diabetes, similar results were seen with NT-proBNP as they were with hs-cTnI such that canagliflozin attenuated the increase in NT-proBNP.[50] A report from the ADVANCE study showed that NT-proBNP enhanced incident heart failure prediction in patients with T2DM independent of traditional cardiovascular risk factors and biomarkers.[59] The HR per 1-SD increase in NT-proBNP for incident or progressive HF was 3.06 (95% CI, 2.37 to 3.96).

Inflammation and C-Reactive Protein

Considerable evidence suggests that chronic, low-grade inflammation plays a role in diabetes and ASCVD. Visceral adipose tissue accumulation is a major risk factor for both incident T2DM[60] and ASCVD[61] and is associated with markers of inflammation and macrophage infiltration, suggesting a possible link with the proinflammatory state seen in diabetes. Obesity in general, visceral adiposity specifically, is associated with higher levels of high-sensitivity C-reactive protein (hs-CRP), an inflammatory biomarker that independently predicts future cardiovascular events regardless of the LDL cholesterol level. A study comparing levels of inflammatory biomarkers in patients with T1DM and those without diabetes suggest that higher levels of acute phase proteins, including hs-CRP, are found among those with diabetes (0.23 vs. 0.14 mg/dL).[62]

More recent data contribute new insights regarding whether targeting inflammation itself can alter the natural history of CVD in patients with diabetes. The Canakinumab Antiinflammatory Thrombosis Outcome Study tested the hypothesis whether targeting the inflammatory pathway in atherothrombosis directly using the novel interleukin-1β antagonist canakinumab would prevent recurrent vascular events in individuals with prior myocardial infarction and persistently elevated hs-CRP ≥ 2 mg/L, and 40% of study participants had diabetes at baseline.[63] In a secondary analysis, higher hs-CRP was associated with increased risk of developing diabetes,[64] but inhibition of interleukin-1β with canakinumab did not lower the rate of incident diabetes. In addition, patients with and without diabetes who were randomized to receive canakinumab had similar reductions in major cardiovascular events.

Subclinical Coronary Artery Disease and Coronary Artery Calcium

Coronary artery calcium (CAC) is a subclinical marker of intracoronary atherosclerosis and can be measured with computed tomography. Subclinical atherosclerotic imaging is an important marker of cardiovascular disease in patients with diabetes but beyond the scope of this book.[65–69]

NOVEL AND EMERGING CARDIOVASCULAR BIOMARKERS IN DIABETES

Several novel and emerging biomarkers have been recently investigated to improve risk stratification and individualize preventive strategies for patients with diabetes at risk for cardiovascular disease. Growth differentiation factor 15 (GDF-15) is a marker of stress and inflammation produced by cardiomyocytes that belongs to the transforming growth factor β super family.[70] The prognostic role of GDF-15 in patients with T2DM was evaluated in a substudy of the sulodexide macroalbuminuria (Sun-MACRO) trial, a study evaluating the ability of sulodexide to reduce progression of nephropathy.[71,72] In this post hoc analysis, 862 patients with T2DM were analyzed for associations of biomarker levels with renal and cardiovascular events.[72] GDF-15 was independently associated with renal events (HR, 1.83; 95% CI, 1.02 to 3.28) but not cardiovascular events (HR, 1.19; 95% CI, 0.77 to 1.86).

Another emerging cardiovascular biomarker with potential use among patients with diabetes is microRNA (miRNA). These are small, noncoding, single-stranded RNA molecules that modify gene expression.[73] Owing to the ability to modify gene expression at the posttranscriptional level, miRNAs are involved in many physiologic and pathologic processes, including complications of diabetes. Circulating levels of a specific miRNA, miR-126, have been shown to distinguish patients with T2DM with and without coronary artery disease from healthy individuals suggesting its role as a possible biomarker.[74]

Osteoprotegerin (OPG) is a member of the tumor necrosis factor receptor superfamily that is emerging as a novel biomarker for cardiovascular diseases.[75] OPG is a soluble decoy receptor that mediates the interaction of the receptor activator of nuclear factor kappa B and its ligand, thus regulating inflammation. Among patients with T2DM, OPG levels were found to be significantly higher in patients with increased CAC (adjusted OR, 2.84; 95% CI, 2.2 to 3.67).[76] The associations of OPG with all-cause and cardiovascular death were evaluated in a prospective observational follow-up study with a median follow-up of 16.8 years in 283 patients with T2DM.[77] High versus low levels of OPG were associated with higher all-cause death (adjusted HR, 1.81; 95% CI, 1.21 to 2.69) but not cardiovascular death in an adjusted model.

CONCLUSIONS

Providers caring for patients with diabetes should be familiar with biomarkers already available in clinical practice. Plasma glucose and Hb A1c levels are part of the diagnostic criteria for diabetes and can be used as treatment targets. Screening for T2DM should be performed in adults of any age who are overweight or obese with at least 1 risk factor for diabetes or, among those with normal weight, at age 45 years and repeated every 3 years if normal.[78] Targeting lower glucose and Hb A1c levels with intensive glycemic control lowers the risk for microvascular complications but does not improve mortality or major cardiovascular end points. Controlling comorbid conditions that contribute to overall atherosclerotic cardiovascular risk, such as dyslipidemia, is key to the management of patients of with diabetes. Lipid profiles seen in diabetes are often abnormal, and providers should be familiar with total and HDL cholesterol levels as these are included in 10-year ASCVD risk calculations.

The ADA has recommendations for checking specific biomarkers such as urine albumin and serum creatinine, but there is less guidance regarding the evaluation of other prognostic biomarkers. cTnT and natriuretic peptides are commonly used in the evaluation of comorbid conditions seen with diabetes, including acute coronary syndromes and heart failure, but their use in a stable outpatient setting is less clear. Future cardiovascular disease risk calculators may account for chronic myocardial injury with cTnT, hemodynamic stress with NT-proBNP, and inflammation with CRP. Novel biomarkers, such as GDF-15, miRNAs, and OPG, are being studied in diabetes and may augment risk assessment.

Evaluation and implementation of established and emerging cardiovascular risk biomarkers in patients with diabetes is a dynamic process. Guideline recommended biomarkers are being used globally, whereas others may remain as research tools to better understand the pathophysiology of cardiac disease in patients with diabetes. Ongoing cardiovascular outcomes trials of novel antihyperglycemic medications in patients with diabetes will also help to inform the use of biomarkers. Certainly, with the evolving understanding of diabetes pathogenesis and impact on the cardiovascular system, additional insights into existing biomarkers and discovery of new measures will continue to inform and improve the care of patients with diabetes.

REFERENCES

1. Wild S, et al. Global prevalence of diabetes: estimates for the year 2000 and projections for 2030. *Diabetes Care.* 2004;27(5):1047–1053.
2. Kochanek KD, et al. Deaths: final data for 2014. *Natl Vital Stat Rep.* 2016;65(4):1–122.
3. Hogan P, et al. Economic costs of diabetes in the US in 2002. *Diabetes Care.* 2003;26(3):917–932.
4. Classification and diagnosis of diabetes mellitus and other categories of glucose intolerance. *Natl Diabetes Data Group Diabetes.* 1979;28(12):1039–1057.
5. Report of the Expert Committee on the diagnosis and classification of diabetes mellitus. *Diabetes Care.* 1997;20(7):1183–1197.
6. McCance DR, et al. Comparison of tests for glycated haemoglobin and fasting and two hour plasma glucose concentrations as diagnostic methods for diabetes. *BMJ.* 1994;308(6940):1323–1328.
7. International Expert Committee. International Expert Committee report on the role of the A1C assay in the diagnosis of diabetes. *Diabetes Care.* 2009;32(7):1327–1334.
8. American Diabetes Association. Diagnosis and classification of diabetes mellitus. *Diabetes Care.* 2014;37(suppl 1):S81–S90.
9. Khalil H. Diabetes microvascular complications-A clinical update. *Diabetes Metab Syndr.* 2017;11(suppl 1):S133–S139.
10. Intensive blood-glucose control with sulphonylureas or insulin compared with conventional treatment and risk of complications in patients with type 2 diabetes (UKPDS 33). UK Prospective Diabetes Study (UKPDS) Group. *Lancet.* 1998;352(9131):837–853.
11. Diabetes C, et al. The effect of intensive treatment of diabetes on the development and progression of long-term complications in insulin-dependent diabetes mellitus. *N Engl J Med.* 1993;329(14):977–986.
12. Ismail-Beigi F, et al. Effect of intensive treatment of hyperglycaemia on microvascular outcomes in type 2 diabetes: an analysis of the ACCORD randomised trial. *Lancet.* 2010;376(9739):419–430.
13. Action to Control Cardiovascular Risk in Diabetes Study, G, et al. Effects of intensive glucose lowering in type 2 diabetes. *N Engl J Med.* 2008;358(24):2545–2559.

14. Group AS, et al. Effects of medical therapies on retinopathy progression in type 2 diabetes. *N Engl J Med.* 2010;363(3):233–244.

15. Group AC, et al. Intensive blood glucose control and vascular outcomes in patients with type 2 diabetes. *N Engl J Med.* 2008;358(24):2560–2572.

16. Hemmingsen B, et al. Intensive glycaemic control for patients with type 2 diabetes: systematic review with meta-analysis and trial sequential analysis of randomised clinical trials. *BMJ.* 2011;343:d6898.

17. Kelly TN, et al. Systematic review: glucose control and cardiovascular disease in type 2 diabetes. *Ann Intern Med.* 2009;151(6):394–403.

18. Zinman B, Wanner C, Lachin JM, et al. Empagliflozin, Cardiovascular Outcomes, and Mortality in Type 2 Diabetes. *N Engl J Med.* 2015;373(22):2117–2128.

19. Neal B, et al. Canagliflozin and cardiovascular and renal events in type 2 diabetes. *N Engl J Med.* 2017;377(7):644–657.

20. Marso SP, et al. Liraglutide and cardiovascular outcomes in type 2 diabetes. *N Engl J Med.* 2016;375(4):311–322.

21. Marso SP, et al. Semaglutide and cardiovascular outcomes in patients with type 2 diabetes. *N Engl J Med.* 2016;375(19):1834–1844.

22. Patel KV, de Albuquerque Rocha N, McGuire DK. Diabetes medications and cardiovascular outcome trials: lessons learned. *Cleve Clin J Med.* 2017;84(10):759–767.

23. Lachin JM, et al. Effect of glycemic exposure on the risk of microvascular complications in the diabetes control and complications trial–revisited. *Diabetes.* 2008;57(4):995–1001.

24. Cohen RA, et al. Determinants of retinopathy progression in type 1 diabetes mellitus. *Am J Med.* 1999;107(1):45–51.

25. Mooradian AD. Dyslipidemia in type 2 diabetes mellitus. *Nat Clin Pract Endocrinol Metab.* 2009;5(3):150–159.

26. Chamberlain JJ, et al. Diagnosis and management of diabetes: synopsis of the 2016 American diabetes association standards of medical care in diabetes. *Ann Intern Med.* 2016;164(8):542–552.

27. Ridker PM, et al. Rosuvastatin to prevent vascular events in men and women with elevated C-reactive protein. *N Engl J Med.* 2008;359(21):2195–2207.

28. Stone NJ, et al. 2013 ACC/AHA guideline on the treatment of blood cholesterol to reduce atherosclerotic cardiovascular risk in adults: a report of the American College of Cardiology/American Heart Association Task Force on Practice Guidelines. *J Am Coll Cardiol.* 2014;63(25 Pt B):2889–2934.

29. Rubins HB, et al. Diabetes, plasma insulin, and cardiovascular disease: subgroup analysis from the Department of Veterans Affairs high-density lipoprotein intervention trial (VA-HIT). *Arch Intern Med.* 2002;162(22):2597–2604.

30. Keech A, et al. Effects of long-term fenofibrate therapy on cardiovascular events in 9795 people with type 2 diabetes mellitus (the FIELD study): randomised controlled trial. *Lancet.* 2005;366(9500):1849–1861.

31. Sacks FM. After the fenofibrate intervention and event lowering in diabetes (FIELD) study: implications for fenofibrate. *Am J Cardiol.* 2008;102(12A):34L–40L.

32. Group AS, et al. Effects of combination lipid therapy in type 2 diabetes mellitus. *N Engl J Med.* 2010;362(17):1563–1574.

33. Fox CS, et al. Associations of kidney disease measures with mortality and end-stage renal disease in individuals with and without diabetes: a meta-analysis. *Lancet.* 2012;380(9854):1662–1673.

34. de Boer IH, et al. Temporal trends in the prevalence of diabetic kidney disease in the United States. *JAMA.* 2011;305(24):2532–2539.

35. Dinneen SF, Gerstein HC. The association of microalbuminuria and mortality in non-insulin-dependent diabetes mellitus. A systematic overview of the literature. *Arch Intern Med.* 1997;157(13):1413–1418.

36. Effects of ramipril on cardiovascular and microvascular outcomes in people with diabetes mellitus: results of the HOPE study and MICRO-HOPE substudy. Heart Outcomes Prevention Evaluation Study Investigators. *Lancet.* 2000;355(9200):253–259.

37. Coll E, et al. Serum cystatin C as a new marker for noninvasive estimation of glomerular filtration rate and as a marker for early renal impairment. *Am J Kidney Dis.* 2000;36(1):29–34.

38. Shlipak MG, et al. Cystatin C and the risk of death and cardiovascular events among elderly persons. *N Engl J Med.* 2005;352(20):2049–2060.

39. Chung YK, et al. Serum cystatin C is associated with subclinical atherosclerosis in patients with type 2 diabetes: a retrospective study. *Diab Vasc Dis Res.* 2017: 1479164117738156.

40. Murai T, et al. Association of epicardial adipose tissue with serum level of cystatin C in type 2 diabetes. *PLoS One.* 2017;12(9):e0184723.

41. Jneid H, et al. Redefining myocardial infarction: what is new in the ESC/ACCF/AHA/WHF Third Universal Definition of myocardial infarction? *Methodist Debakey Cardiovasc J.* 2013;9(3):169–172.

42. de Lemos JA, et al. Multimodality strategy for cardiovascular risk assessment: performance in 2 population-based cohorts. *Circulation.* 2017;135(22):2119–2132.

43. Sato Y, Fujiwara H, Takatsu Y. Cardiac troponin and heart failure in the era of high-sensitivity assays. *J Cardiol.* 2012;60(3):160–167.

44. Wallace TW, et al. Prevalence and determinants of troponin T elevation in the general population. *Circulation.* 2006;113(16):1958–1965.

45. Reichlin T, et al. Early diagnosis of myocardial infarction with sensitive cardiac troponin assays. *N Engl J Med.* 2009;361(9):858–867.

46. Giannitsis E, et al. Analytical validation of a high-sensitivity cardiac troponin T assay. *Clin Chem.* 2010;56(2):254–261.

47. Selvin E, et al. Diabetes mellitus, prediabetes, and incidence of subclinical myocardial damage. *Circulation.* 2014;130(16):1374–1382.

48. Hillis GS, et al. The relative and combined ability of high-sensitivity cardiac troponin T and N-terminal pro-B-type natriuretic peptide to predict cardiovascular events and death in patients with type 2 diabetes. *Diabetes Care.* 2014;37(1):295–303.

49. Cavender MA, et al. Serial measurement of high-sensitivity troponin I and cardiovascular outcomes in patients with type 2 diabetes mellitus in the EXAMINE trial (examination of cardiovascular outcomes with alogliptin versus standard of care). *Circulation.* 2017;135(20):1911–1921.

50. Januzzi Jr JL, et al. Effects of canagliflozin on cardiovascular biomarkers in older adults with type 2 diabetes. *J Am Coll Cardiol.* 2017;70(6):704–712.

51. Everett BM, et al. Troponin and cardiac events in stable ischemic heart disease and diabetes. *N Engl J Med.* 2015;373(7):610–620.

52. Volpe M, Rubattu S, Burnett Jr J. Natriuretic peptides in cardiovascular diseases: current use and perspectives. *Eur Heart J.* 2014;35(7):419–425.

53. Masson S, et al. Prognostic value of changes in N-Terminal pro-brain natriuretic peptide in Val-HeFT (valsartan heart failure trial). *J Am Coll Cardiol.* 2008;52(12):997–1003.

54. Sanders-van Wijk S, et al. Long-term results of intensified, N-Terminal-Pro-B-Type natriuretic peptide–guided versus symptom-guided treatment in elderly patients with heart failure. *Circ Heart Fail.* 2014;7(1):131.

55. Gaggin HK, et al. Heart failure outcomes and benefits of NT-proBNP-guided management in the elderly: results from the prospective, randomized ProBNP outpatient tailored chronic heart failure therapy (PROTECT) study. *J Cardiac Fail.* 2012;18(8):626–634.

56. Richards M, et al. Comparison of B-Type natriuretic peptides for assessment of cardiac function and prognosis in stable ischemic heart disease. *J Am Coll Cardiol.* 2006;47(1):52–60.

57. Bhalla MA, et al. Prognostic role of B-type natriuretic peptide levels in patients with type 2 diabetes mellitus. *J Am Coll Cardiol.* 2004;44(5):1047–1052.

58. Tarnow L, et al. Plasma N-terminal pro-B-type natriuretic peptide and mortality in type 2 diabetes. *Diabetologia.* 2006;49(10):2256–2262.

59. Ohkuma T, et al. Cardiac stress and inflammatory markers as predictors of heart failure in patients with type 2 diabetes: the ADVANCE trial. *Diabetes Care.* 2017;40(9):1203–1209.

60. Neeland IJ, et al. Dysfunctional adiposity and the risk of prediabetes and type 2 diabetes in obese adults. *JAMA.* 2012;308(11):1150–1159.

61. Neeland IJ, et al. Body fat distribution and incident cardiovascular disease in obese adults. *J Am Coll Cardiol.* 2015;65(19):2150–2151.

62. Gomes MB, et al. Acute-phase proteins among patients with type 1 diabetes. *Diabetes Metab.* 2003;29(4 Pt 1):405–411.

63. Ridker PM, et al. Antiinflammatory therapy with canakinumab for atherosclerotic disease. *N Engl J Med.* 2017;377(12):1119–1131.

64. Everett BM, Donath MY, Pradhan AD, et al. Anti-Inflammatory Therapy With Canakinumab for the Prevention and Management of Diabetes. *J Am Coll Cardiol.* 2018;71(21):2392–2401.

65. Wong ND, et al. Metabolic syndrome, diabetes, and incidence and progression of coronary calcium: the Multiethnic Study of Atherosclerosis study. *JACC Cardiovasc Imaging.* 2012;5(4):358–366.

66. Elkeles RS, et al. Coronary calcium measurement improves prediction of cardiovascular events in asymptomatic patients with type 2 diabetes: the PREDICT study. *Eur Heart J.* 2008;29(18):2244–2251.

67. Blaha MJ, et al. Role of coronary artery calcium score of zero and other negative risk markers for cardiovascular disease: the multi-ethnic study of atherosclerosis (MESA). *Circulation.* 2016;133(9):849–858.

68. Fox CS, et al. Update on prevention of cardiovascular disease in adults with type 2 diabetes mellitus in light of recent evidence: a scientific statement from the American heart association and the American diabetes association. *Circulation.* 2015;132(8):691–718.

69. Greenland P, et al. 2010 ACCF/AHA guideline for assessment of cardiovascular risk in asymptomatic adults: a report of the American College of Cardiology Foundation/American heart association Task Force on Practice guidelines. *Circulation.* 2010;122(25):e584–636.

70. Adela R, Banerjee SK. GDF-15 as a target and biomarker for diabetes and cardiovascular diseases: a Translational prospective. *J Diabetes Res.* 2015;2015:490842.

71. Packham DK, et al. Sulodexide fails to demonstrate renoprotection in overt type 2 diabetic nephropathy. *J Am Soc Nephrol.* 2012;23(1):123–130.

72. Bidadkosh A, et al. Predictive properties of biomarkers GDF-15, NTproBNP, and hs-TnT for Morbidity and mortality in patients with type 2 diabetes with nephropathy. *Diabetes Care.* 2017;40(6):784–792.

73. Ding Y, Sun X, Shan PF. MicroRNAs and cardiovascular disease in diabetes mellitus. *Biomed Res Int.* 2017;2017:4080364.

74. Al-Kafaji G, et al. Circulating endothelium-enriched microRNA-126 as a potential biomarker for coronary artery disease in type 2 diabetes mellitus patients. *Biomarkers.* 2017;22(3–4):268–278.

75. Perez de Ciriza C, Lawrie A, Varo N. Osteoprotegerin in cardiometabolic disorders. *Int J Endocrinol.* 2015;2015:564934.

76. Anand DV, et al. The relationship between plasma osteoprotegerin levels and coronary artery calcification in uncomplicated type 2 diabetic subjects. *J Am Coll Cardiol.* 2006;47(9):1850–1857.

77. Reinhard H, et al. Osteoprotegerin and mortality in type 2 diabetic patients. *Diabetes Care.* 2010;33(12):2561–2566.

78. American Diabetes Association. Erratum. Classification and diagnosis of diabetes. Sec. 2. In standards of medical care in Diabetes-2016. *Diabetes Care.* 2016;39(suppl 1):S13–S22. *Diabetes Care.* 2016;39(9):1653.

CHAPTER 5

Advanced Lipid Testing

ANUM SAEED, MD • VIJAY NAMBI, MD, PHD • PETER H. JONES, MD

INTRODUCTION

Cardiovascular disease (CVD) is a leading cause of morbidity and mortality in the United States and worldwide.[1] CVD risk assessment and management rely on quantification of risk factors such as hyperlipidemia, hypertension, and diabetes mellitus. A routine lipid profile is the most commonly used laboratory measure to evaluate a patient's atherogenic risk, and it measures the total cholesterol, low-density lipoprotein cholesterol (LDL-C), high-density lipoprotein cholesterol (HDL-C), and triglycerides (TGs). In most cases, this basic lipid panel can provide valuable information about possible genetic and/or environmental causes of dyslipidemia. Measurements of causal lipid parameters (LDL-C) and risk markers for CVD (i.e., HDL-C and TGs) inform clinicians of an individual's risk for atherosclerotic CVD events and, in some cases, the risk for acute pancreatitis by very high TGs. LDL-C, a major causal factor for CVD, is most frequently used as the guideline recommended benchmark for initiation and intensification of preventive therapy.[2,3] However, a routine lipid profile only measures the cholesterol/lipid content of lipoproteins and has lead to an interest in whether further risk information could be gleaned from additional "advanced" lipid measures.

The lipoprotein particles, which are diverse in size, density, charge, core lipid composition, specific apolipoproteins, and function, carry cholesterol and TGs in the bloodstream.[4] Many lipoprotein assays have been established that can fractionate lipoprotein particles according to their specific properties and conformations. Some of these particle measurements may provide additional information that can influence clinical decisions about CVD risk and potential therapeutic options. These measurements are usually referred to as advanced lipid testing.

In this chapter, we review the availability of advanced lipid testing for use in clinical lipidology, as well as their applications.

Non–High-Density Lipoprotein Cholesterol

Non–HDL-C depicts the cholesterol transported by all potentially atherogenic and apoprotein B–containing particles, including low-density lipoprotein (LDL), intermediate-density lipoprotein (IDL), very-low-density lipoprotein (VLDL) and VLDL remnants, chylomicron particles and chylomicron remnants, and lipoprotein(a) [Lp(a)]. There is robust evidence that non–HDL-C is a superior predictor of atherosclerotic CVD events than measured LDL-C and does not require fasting.[5–8] Furthermore, changes in the on-treatment levels of non–HDL-C are associated with CVD risk as strongly as LDL-C.[9] The plausible reason for the association of non–HDL-C with atherosclerotic CVD risk prediction stems from the inclusion of atherogenic remnant cholesterol (discussed elsewhere in the article) and triglyceride-rich lipoproteins (TGRLs), which are not captured with LDL-C measurements.

Non–HDL-C does not require additional assay methodology for measurements. It is calculated as the "*total cholesterol minus the HDL-C*" obtained in the routine lipid profile, making this test very cost-efficient. It is specifically useful when LDL-C cannot be calculated or is inaccurate (e.g., in cases with high chylomicronemia/hypertriglyceridemia and in patients with diabetes mellitus).

As a result, non–HDL-C has been identified as a secondary target of therapy by the European Atherosclerosis Society[10] and National Lipid Association (NLA)[11] guidelines, as well as the Expert Consensus Decision Pathway on the Role of Non-Statin Therapies (in diabetes).[12]

LDL Particle Size and Concentration (Number)

The measured cholesterol in plasma is held within lipoprotein particles. For a given total cholesterol value, if the lipoprotein particles are smaller, in order for them to hold that amount of cholesterol, there needs to be an increased number of particles. There have been

Biomarkers in Cardiovascular Disease. https://doi.org/10.1016/B978-0-323-54835-9.00005-3

studies to evaluate whether the low-density lipoprotein particle (LDL-P) number or its size can better predict risk than the cholesterol content of LDL because it is the lipoprotein particle that enters the subintimal space of the vessel wall to initiate atherosclerosis. The small-sized and dense (more concentrated with cholesterol) LDL-P are many times associated with elevated TG levels and may be more atherogenic[13,14] than large, less dense LDL-P which are usually associated with lower TG levels.[15,16]

In some patients who have achieved the guideline recommended level of LDL-C on optimal statin dosing, there may be residual lipid risk for CVD events. Calculated or directly measured LDL-C does not equate to uniform risk in each patient because each particle of LDL carries a variable amount of cholesterol.[17] Each person has a range of LDL-P sizes; hence, for any given measured cholesterol content within the LDL fraction, one person can have a greater number of small LDL-P, whereas another may have a lower number of larger LDL-P. In large cohort studies,[13,18] including the Atherosclerosis Risk in Communities (ARIC) and the Multi-Ethnic Study of Atherosclerosis, higher levels of small dense LDL-C levels (fourth vs. first quartile) conferred an added risk for incident coronary heart disease (CHD) among individuals with LDL-C of less than 100 mg/dL.

Although small dense LDL particles may indicate a more atherogenic risk than larger LDL particles, once the LDL particle concentration or number is taken into account, the LDL particle size does not appear to be independently associated with CVD risk.[19,20] Several epidemiologic studies have shown the independent role of LDL-P as a predictor of CVD risk, including the Women's Health Initiative and the Framingham cohort study.[21]

Generally, in discordant situations between LDL-C and LDL-P (above or below the median), CVD risk may be better predicted by LDL-P number. The European Atherosclerosis Society and National Lipid Association have endorsed the measurement of LDL-P to inform clinical treatment decisions in special clinical situations, such as patients with atherosclerotic cardiovascular disease (ASCVD) and diabetes or with elevated TGs, especially those with recurrent CVD events on optimal statin treatment.[11]

Apolipoprotein B-100

Because each chylomicron, VLDL, IDL, LDL, and Lp(a) particle has one molecule of apolipoprotein B-100 (apoB),[17] measuring this apoprotein can provide an estimate of the total burden of atherogenic particles in the bloodstream. ApoB is a better measure of these atherogenic particles in patients with diabetes than the LDL-C because the calculated LDL-C underestimates the real cholesterol content of LDL at low levels and when TG are >150 mg/dL.[15,22–26] Furthermore, because statin therapy reduces LDL-C more than it reduces LDL particle number, apoB measurement is a better assessment of on-treatment residual risk than LDL-C.[27] It should be noted that in the ARIC study, apoB was not superior to non–HDL-C as a marker of incident CHD risk in patients with diabetes or metabolic syndrome.[28]

The 2013 American College of Cardiology (ACC)/American Heart Association (AHA) cholesterol guidelines state that the apoB measurement for assessment of ASCVD risk is of uncertain value,[3] whereas in the 2016 European Guidelines on Cardiovascular Disease Prevention, apoB was not recommended as superior to LDL-C for routine ASCVD risk prediction.[29] On the other hand, for patients with diabetes mellitus or metabolic syndrome, apoB <100 mg/dL in high risk and <80 mg/dL in very high risk are recommended as secondary goals by the European Society of Cardiology, and the American Association of Clinical endocrinologists has recommended a goal of <70 mg/dL in extreme risk patients with diabetes.[30,31]

Although several recent guidelines have recommended apoB measurement for risk assessment, there remains lack of harmonization in apoB testing methods.[32] Immunoturbidimetry or immunonephelometry, relying on light-scattering measurements, are the primary methods for measuring apoB in clinical laboratories today. These assays, based on antibody-antigen complex identification, are less useful to determining apoB on lipoprotein particles of various configurations.[32] Antigenic sites of apoB may be less discrete for identification on VLDL, IDL, and LDL. Efforts such as addition of detergents to reduce nonspecific light scattering for evaluation of various shapes and sizes of lipoprotein particles and unmasking antigenic sites to improve the assay performance have also resulted in erroneous calculations.[33] The method-specific differences in apoB measurements were recently analyzed by Cao et al., and they highlighted an essential need for harmonization efforts for between-method comparability improvements.[34] At the present time, further efforts are required to standardize apoB measurements. In summary, apo B is equivalent to non–HDL-C and LDL-P in risk prediction and may be an option in selected clinical situations to assess on-treatment decisions.

Remnant-like Particle Cholesterol

TGRLs are the source of delivering fatty acids for energy to peripheral tissues or for storage in adipose tissue. TGRLs originate from the intestines (chylomicrons) and the liver (VLDL). Increased production rates and delayed catabolism of TGRLs lead to increased TG-enriched remnant lipoproteins, with increased levels of remnant-like particle cholesterol (RLP-C). In the hypertriglyceridemic state, increased transfer of TGs from chylomicrons and VLDL to LDL and HDL takes place and results in extensive lipoprotein remodeling with TG enrichment of remnant lipoproteins, including VLDL remnants, IDL, and LDL, as well as the formation of small dense LDL particles. Numerous studies have focused on the atherogenic potential of remnant lipoproteins and RLP-C.[35-39] RLP-C has been shown to be an independent risk factor for CVD in women,[40] and multi-directional Mendelian randomization and prospective cohort studies have found strong relationships between RLP-C elevations and incident CVD events.[35,36,41]

RLP-C increases the susceptibility of the coronary endothelium to oxidative stress by inhibiting the NO-mediated arterial dilation[36] and upregulates endothelial expression of intracellular adhesion molecule-1 and vascular cell adhesion molecule-1, which are responsible for monocyte recruitment into the arterial wall, as well as tissue factor, which is essential for thrombotic events. Thus, these proinflammatory and proatherothrombogenic effects of RLP-C may explain the association with an increased CVD event incidence.

RLP-C can be easily calculated because it represents all the cholesterol that is not in the LDL and HDL fraction, that is, total cholesterol minus LDL cholesterol minus HDL cholesterol.[36,42,43] Ultracentrifugation, nuclear magnetic resonance (NMR) spectroscopy, and, a recently approved, fully automated detergent-based homogeneous method[44] are the other available options for measurement of RLP-C. RLP-C levels can be reduced by lifestyle interventions, improvements in insulin resistance, and medications that lower TGs.[41]

Although numerous studies show the association of RLP-C with incident CVD events, a recent analysis in the ARIC study did not show an association of RLP-C with incident CHD or stroke in models fully adjusted for traditional CVD risk factors.[44] Currently, due to the lack of clinical trial data indicating any CVD benefit by a targeted reduction in RLP-C with either lifestyle interventions and/or pharmacotherapy, there are no recommended thresholds for RLP-C levels and hence no clear clinical reason to use this parameter for clinical decisions.

Lipoprotein (a)

Lp(a) is a complex lipoprotein, first identified in 1963, which has been associated with CHD and stroke.[45,46] There has been an increased interest in Lp(a) research since robust evidence from Mendelian randomization studies[47] and large cohort studies showed the causal association of the *LPA* gene and Lp(a) levels with CVD events.[48,49] Elevated Lp(a) levels are a significant contributor to premature CHD[50] and have also been shown to correlate strongly with aortic stenosis.[36-38]

Apolipoprotein a [apo(a)] is covalently bound to apo B and accounts for the distinction between LDL and Lp(a) particles. Apo(a), which is different than apo A-1 found in HDL and responsible for reverse cholesterol transport, has a highly heterogeneous nature. The apo(a) kringle IV–like sequences are grouped into 10 types depending on the amino acid sequence (KIV1 to KIV10). All KIV kringle types are present in a single molecule of apo(a) except KIV2, which is present in variable number of identically repeated copies usually ranging from 3 to more than 40. Indeed, variations in the kringle type IV–2 repeats has been the primary challenge in the development of immunoassays to measure Lp(a) in the plasma. Besides the variations in KIV-2, alterable glycosylation occurs in the core of the KIV motifs, as well as in the sequences linking the kringles. Apo(a) confers various synthetic and catabolic properties to Lp(a). It is structurally similar to plasminogen, and thus, Lp(a) hinders fibrinolysis by competing with plasminogen binding to molecules and cells. As a result, plasminogen activation, plasmin generation, and fibrinolysis are impaired in the presence of elevated Lp(a).[22,23] Lp(a) can also bind to macrophages via a high-affinity receptor that promotes foam cell formation within atherosclerotic plaques.[15] Because of its combined prothrombotic and proatherogenic properties, Lp(a) may influence CVD development, progression, and events through multiple mechanisms.

In a combined cohort of individuals (n = 77,860) from the Copenhagen City Heart and Copenhagen General Population studies, there was an incremental risk in aortic stenosis noted across percentile increases in Lp(a) levels. The hazards ratios of association between Lp(a) percentiles and aortic stenosis were 2.0 (95% confidence interval [CI], 1.2–3.4) for 90th–95th percentile of Lp(a) levels (65–90 mg/dL) and 2.9 (95% CI, 1.8–4.9) for Lp(a) levels > 95th percentile (>90 mg/dL) when compared with levels <22nd percentile (<5 mg/dL; p-trend <0.001).[51]

Currently, the standardization of Lp(a) measurements are challenging due to different analytical methods, which include assignment of a uniform target value to the assay calibrators, assessment of Lp(a) mass (typically in mg/dL) versus particle number (in nmol/L), and an absence of guidelines for validation of methodical approaches.[52] Lp(a) measured as mg/dL usually includes apoB-100, apo(a), cholesterol, cholesteryl esters, phospholipids, TGs, and carbohydrates attached to apo(a). Levels of Lp(a) measured as nmol/L reflect the number of apo(a) and, therefore, the number of Lp(a) particles.[53] Lp(a) measured by either technique is not thought to be affected by fasting and does not seem to fluctuate significantly throughout lifetime without a specific intervention.[54]

A conversion factor of 2.85 for small isoforms and 1.85 for large isoforms, with a mean of 2.4 nmol/L for every 1 mg/dL, has been recommended for the interchange of the two measurements.[55] Of note, this conversion factor, if not calibrated meticulously, may result in incorrect Lp(a) interpretation.[52] A recently developed assay[56] can deliver a precise analytical method for Lp(a) measurement, and it reports Lp(a) concentrations in nmol/L (referenced to the World Health Organization [WHO]/International Federation of Clinical Chemistry and Laboratory Medicine reference materials).[52] The *NHLBI Working Group Recommendations to Reduce Lipoprotein(a)-Mediated Risk of Cardiovascular Disease and Aortic Stenosis*" has endorsed standardized assays to report Lp(a) levels and recommends the apo(a) particle number, measured in nmol/L.

Lp(a) mean concentrations vary among different ethnicities, as well as geographic regions, and have different thresholds for predicting CVD risk.[57-59] Given this interracial variability of Lp(a), there have been calls to measure race-specific Lp(a) values. For example, in Caucasians, a value of Lp(a) greater than the 75th–80th population percentile is suggestive of increased risk of CVD,[52] whereas for individuals of black or Japanese inheritance, no specific cut points have been established. At the present time, Lp(a) levels of >30 mg/dL and >75 nmol/L are identified as a cutoff for "high" in most laboratories.

Owing to the lack of clinical trial evidence showing a direct association between targeted Lp(a) reduction and associated decrease in CVD endpoints, the ACC/AHA guidelines[3] do not recommend universal Lp(a) screening. Other organizations, including the National Lipid Association[11] and the European Society of Cardiology/European Atherosclerosis Society[31] do recommend Lp(a) measurement for patients with familial hypercholesterolemia, family history of premature CVD and/or elevated Lp(a) levels, personal history of premature CVD, recurrent CVD despite optimal statin treatment, inadequate percent LDL-C reduction response to statins, and ≥10% 10-year risk of fatal or nonfatal CHD (per NLA) or ≥3% 10-year risk of fatal CVD (per the European guidelines). Other important reasons for screening Lp(a) levels include the following: (1) cascade screening of offspring of individuals with elevated Lp(a) given there is an autosomal dominant pattern of inheritance of Lp(a)[60,61] and (2) the use of aspirin in those with elevated Lp(a) levels because this may lower the risk for CVD events.[62]

Ultimately, Lp(a) measurements may become standardized and more prevalent in clinical practice given recent efforts to increase collaborative research and physiological understanding of Lp(a)-associated CVD and aortic stenosis.[63] Furthermore, newer therapies like the proprotein convertase subtilisin/kexin kinase type 9 (PCSK9) inhibitors have shown beneficial lowering of Lp(a) levels. Approximately 30% lowering of Lp(a) levels has been reported with the use of PCSK9 inhibitors.[29] PCSK9 inhibitors–associated Lp(a) lowering is mechanistically unclear at this time; however, it has been hypothesized that at extremely low levels of LDL-C (which can be obtained with PCSK9 inhibition), LDL-R may be involved in the clearance of Lp(a). Currently, PCSK9 inhibitors are not approved for treatment of elevated Lp(a).

Although niacin and PCSK9 inhibitors lower Lp(a), emerging therapies aimed at lowering Lp(a) are in clinical development at this time as well. An antisense oligonucleotide agent (IONIS-APO(a)-LRx) is currently undergoing a phase 2 randomized clinical trial (clinicaltrials.gov Identifier:NCT03070782) to assess the mean reduction of Lp(a) and the safety and tolerability in patients with established CVD. This subcutaneously injected investigational agent is an N-acetyl-galactosamine conjugated molecule designed to be selectively taken up by hepatocytes to inhibit apo(a) synthesis.

METHODOLOGY OF ADVANCED LIPID TESTING

Currently, there are several methodologies used to quantify the specialized lipid parameters discussed here, and they include (but not limited to) vertical auto profile (also known as VAP),[60,64] NMR (discussed previously), liquid chromatography isotopic-dilution mass spectrometry,[61,65] and, most recently, electrospray differential mobility analysis.[66] Several other unique assays to isolate novel parameters of lipids biomarkers are currently in the translational phases[18,67] which may be available for clinical use in the near future. The various analytical methods are summarized in the table. NMR profile, which is a commonly used method for advanced lipid testing and clinical testing, is detailed in the following section (Table 5.1).

NMR Profile

Proton NMR was first described in 1991 as a novel spectroscopic method for measurement of lipoproteins.[68,69] This method was automated and commercialized as the NMR LipoProfile (LabCorp, Burlington, NC, USA).

NMR profile testing is a unique and, now, routinely used method for quantification of lipoprotein particle number and size. This procedure is completed by measuring the amplitude of the proton NMR signal produced by each discrete lipoprotein under predefined conditions.[69] NMR identifies different lipoprotein sizes (diameter) and concentrations based on the signals produced. Furthermore, the amplitude of the lipid resonance signal accounts for the amount of lipids in the particle.[68] Components of the NMR profile include LDL-C, LDL-P, small LDL-P, and LDL size which have been discussed previously and HDL-C and HDL-P. The role of HDL-C and HDL-P as well as their clinical use in atherosclerotic CVD is discussed elsewhere.

Density Gradient Ultracentrifugation

This method, also known as VAP II, provides the cholesterol content within different lipoprotein subtractions.[32] The measured cholesterol content within the VLDL, IDL, Lp(a), and HDL subclasses can be quantified, and in addition, apoB levels are also reported with the VAP II testing. The VAP II also determine the

TABLE 5.1
Commonly Used Lipoprotein Measurement Techniques and Methods

Technique	Methodology and Analysis	Reference	Clinical Use
Tube gel electrophoresis	Separation of particles based on size and surface charge; Use of cholesterol-specific dye; Lipoproteins are detected by densitometry for profiling; Automated data-processing software; Concentration: lipoprotein fractions with value assigned total cholesterol	Externally calibrated and very few data available on calibration methodology used	Lipoprotein profiles are obtained in less than 3 hours
Nuclear magnetic resonance (NMR)	Proton resonance for analysis; measures the proton resonance of lipids within lipoproteins; software-associated deconvolution of lipoproteins	WHO reference materials; proprietary library of fractionated lipoproteins	Widely used for ALT
Vertical auto profile (VAP-II)	2-step process: plasma density adjustment and ultracentrifugation; lipoproteins separated by density; cholesterol quantification by continuous enzymatic reaction assay; UV visible absorbance	WHO reference materials	
Ion mobility/electrospray differential mobility analysis (ES-DMA)	Selection and counting of lipoprotein particles in aerosol phase; based on lipoprotein electrical mobility diameter; measures full intact lipoprotein and externally calibrated	Certified reference materials of inorganic nanoparticles	Most recent advanced lipid testing method; harmonization of the process to derive aerosol phase particle concentration into liquid (original) sample phase is not uniform
Apolipoprotein profiling by liquid chromatography isotopic-dilution mass spectrometry (LC-ID/MS)	Enzymatic trypsin digestion of serum apolipoproteins; analysis by chromatographic separation and mass spectrometry	IN and IT assays (endorsed by the WHO)	High accuracy and good comparability for apo B and apo A-1 quantifications; expensive

ALT, advanced lipid testing; *apo A-1*, apolipoprotein A-1; *apo B*, apolipoprotein B-100; *IN*, Immunonephelometric; *IT*, Immunoturbidimetric; *UV*, ultraviolet; *WHO*, World Health Organization.

relative phenotype of the LDL size (e.g., A, AB, or B phenotype); however, it does not quantify the LDL particle concentration.

Limitations

Most of the methods of advanced lipid quantifications have not been uniformly correlated together, have only been tested against one-another,[70] and lack standardization. Most of the methods do use WHO-certified reference materials as standards to guarantee traceability of results but may use different calibrators, which results in numerous traceability chains and eventual nonstandardization of results. Therefore the lack of harmonious standardization of the advanced lipids discussed here, combined with a lack of evidence targeting these lipid parameters in randomized clinical trials, has resulted in guidelines and recommendations that limit the use of advanced lipid testing to a select minority of high-risk patients.

CONCLUSIONS

There are several available advanced lipid-testing assays that can be clinically relevant in assessing residual atherogenic risk as well as informing the options for pharmacotherapy initiation, titration, and/or add-on therapy. Advanced lipid testing is most useful in scenarios where there is discordance with LDL-C and non–HDL-C after statin therapy. Specifically, apoB, LDL-P, and Lp(a) levels can be conveniently quantified and may influence clinical decision-making for risk stratification as well as changes in therapies. There is no evidence to show that LDL-P size or charge or the RLP-C level add any further information once these other measures of atherogenic particle number are known.

It must be stated that routine testing of *"advanced"* lipids has not been uniformly endorsed in current guidelines. However, given the advance in the analytical techniques and emerging evidence on therapies that target these lipid parameters in high-risk patients, it is possible that advanced lipid testing may be harmoniously adopted as routine clinical testing in the near future.

REFERENCES

1. Benjamin EJ, Blaha MJ, Chiuve SE, et al. Heart disease and stroke statistics-2017 update: a report from the American heart association. *Circulation*. 2017;135:e146–e603.
2. Goff Jr DC, Lloyd-Jones DM, Bennett G, et al. 2013 ACC/AHA guideline on the assessment of cardiovascular risk: a report of the American College of Cardiology/American heart association task force on practice guidelines. *J Am Coll Cardiol*. 2013;63:2935–2959.
3. Stone NJ, Robinson JG, Lichtenstein AH, et al. 2013 ACC/AHA guideline on the treatment of blood cholesterol to reduce atherosclerotic cardiovascular risk in adults: a report of the American College of Cardiology/American Heart Association Task Force on Practice Guidelines. *J Am Coll Cardiol*. 2014;63:2889–2934.
4. Mudd JO, Borlaug BA, Johnston PV, et al. Beyond low-density lipoprotein cholesterol: defining the role of low-density lipoprotein heterogeneity in coronary artery disease. *J Am Coll Cardiol*. 2007;50:1735–1741.
5. Nordestgaard BG. A test in context: lipid profile, fasting versus nonfasting. *J Am Coll Cardiol*. 2017;70:1637–1646.
6. Pischon T, Girman CJ, Sacks FM, Rifai N, Stampfer MJ, Rimm EB. Non-high-density lipoprotein cholesterol and apolipoprotein B in the prediction of coronary heart disease in men. *Circulation*. 2005;112:3375–3383.
7. Blaha MJ, Blumenthal RS, Brinton EA, Jacobson TA. The importance of non-HDL cholesterol reporting in lipid management. *J Clin Lipidol*. 2008;2:267–273.
8. Rallidis LS, Pitsavos C, Panagiotakos DB, Sinos L, Stefanadis C, Kremastinos DT. Non-high density lipoprotein cholesterol is the best discriminator of myocardial infarction in young individuals. *Atherosclerosis*. 2005;179:305–309.
9. Boekholdt SM, Arsenault BJ, Mora S, et al. Association of LDL cholesterol, non-HDL cholesterol, and apolipoprotein B levels with risk of cardiovascular events among patients treated with statins: a meta-analysis. *Jama*. 2012;307:1302–1309.
10. Catapano AL, Reiner Z, De Backer G, et al. ESC/EAS guidelines for the management of dyslipidaemias the task force for the management of dyslipidaemias of the European Society of Cardiology (ESC) and the European atherosclerosis Society (EAS). *Atherosclerosis*. 2011;217:3–46.
11. Jacobson TA, Ito MK, Maki KC, et al. National lipid association recommendations for patient-centered management of dyslipidemia: part 1–full report. *J Clin Lipidol*. 2015;9:129–169.
12. Lloyd-Jones DM, Morris PB, Ballantyne CM, et al. 2016 ACC Expert Consensus decision Pathway on the role of non-statin therapies for LDL-cholesterol lowering in the management of atherosclerotic cardiovascular disease risk: a report of the American College of Cardiology task force on clinical Expert Consensus Documents. *J Am Coll Cardiol*. 2016;68:92–125.
13. Tsai MY, Steffen BT, Guan W, et al. New automated assay of small dense low-density lipoprotein cholesterol identifies risk of coronary heart disease: the Multi-ethnic Study of Atherosclerosis. *Arterioscler Thromb Vasc Biol*. 2014;34:196–201.
14. Kuller L, Arnold A, Tracy R, et al. Nuclear magnetic resonance spectroscopy of lipoproteins and risk of coronary heart disease in the cardiovascular health study. *Arterioscler Thromb Vasc Biol*. 2002;22:1175–1180.
15. Kathiresan S, Otvos JD, Sullivan LM, et al. Increased small low-density lipoprotein particle number: a prominent feature of the metabolic syndrome in the Framingham Heart Study. *Circulation*. 2006;113:20–29.

16. Mora S, Wenger NK, Demicco DA, et al. Determinants of residual risk in secondary prevention patients treated with high- versus low-dose statin therapy: the Treating to New Targets (TNT) study. *Circulation.* 2012;125:1979–1987.

17. Sniderman A, Williams K, Cobbaert C. ApoB versus non-HDL-C: what to do when they disagree. *Curr Atheroscler Rep.* 2009;11:358–363.

18. Ito Y, Fujimura M, Ohta M, Hirano T. Development of a homogeneous assay for measurement of small dense LDL cholesterol. *Clin Chem.* 2011;57:57–65.

19. Mora S, Szklo M, Otvos JD, et al. LDL particle subclasses, LDL particle size, and carotid atherosclerosis in the Multi-Ethnic Study of Atherosclerosis (MESA). *Atherosclerosis.* 2007;192:211–217.

20. Mora S, Otvos JD, Rifai N, Rosenson RS, Buring JE, Ridker PM. Lipoprotein particle profiles by nuclear magnetic resonance compared with standard lipids and apolipoproteins in predicting incident cardiovascular disease in women. *Circulation.* 2009;119:931–939.

21. Cromwell WC, Otvos JD, Keyes MJ, et al. LDL particle number and risk of future cardiovascular disease in the Framingham offspring study - implications for LDL management. *J Clin Lipidol.* 2007;1:583–592.

22. Sattar N, Williams K, Sniderman AD, D'Agostino Jr R, Haffner SM. Comparison of the associations of apolipoprotein B and non-high-density lipoprotein cholesterol with other cardiovascular risk factors in patients with the metabolic syndrome in the Insulin Resistance Atherosclerosis Study. *Circulation.* 2004;110:2687–2693.

23. Garvey WT, Kwon S, Zheng D, et al. Effects of insulin resistance and type 2 diabetes on lipoprotein subclass particle size and concentration determined by nuclear magnetic resonance. *Diabetes.* 2003;52:453–462.

24. Walldius G, Jungner I, Holme I, Aastveit AH, Kolar W, Steiner E. High apolipoprotein B, low apolipoprotein A-I, and improvement in the prediction of fatal myocardial infarction (AMORIS study): a prospective study. *Lancet.* 2001;358:2026–2033.

25. van Lennep JE, Westerveld HT, van Lennep HW, Zwinderman AH, Erkelens DW, van der Wall EE. Apolipoprotein concentrations during treatment and recurrent coronary artery disease events. *Arterioscler Thromb Vasc Biol.* 2000;20:2408–2413.

26. Sathiyakumar V, Park J, Golozar A, et al. Fasting versus nonfasting and low-density lipoprotein cholesterol accuracy. *Circulation.* 2018;137:10–19.

27. Sniderman AD. Differential response of cholesterol and particle measures of atherogenic lipoproteins to LDL-lowering therapy: implications for clinical practice. *J Clin Lipidol.* 2008;2:36–42.

28. Ndumele CE, Matsushita K, Astor B, et al. Apolipoproteins do not add prognostic information beyond lipoprotein cholesterol measures among individuals with obesity and insulin resistance syndromes: the ARIC study. *Eur J Prev Cardiol.* 2014;21:866–875.

29. Sixth Joint Task Force of the European Society of Cardiology and other societies on cardiovascular disease prevention in clinical practice. 2016 European guidelines on cardiovascular disease prevention in clinical practice. *Eur Heart J.* 2016;37:2315–2381.

30. Jellinger PS, Handelsman Y, Rosenblit PD, et al. American association of clinical endocrinologists and American College of endocrinology guidelines for management of dyslipidemia and prevention of cardiovascular disease. *Endocr Pract Off J Am Coll Endocrinol Am Assoc Clin Endocrinol.* 2017;23:1–87.

31. Task Force for the Management of Dyslipidaemias of the European Society of Cardiology (ESC) and European Atherosclerosis Society (EAS). *ESC/EAS Guidelines for the Management of Dyslipidaemias.* Eur Heart J 2016 prepub; 2016.

32. Contois JH, Delatour V. Apolipoprotein B measurement: need for standardization. *J Clin Lipidol.* 2018;12:264–265.

33. Albers JJ, Kennedy H, Marcovina SM. Evaluation of a new homogenous method for detection of small dense LDL cholesterol: comparison with the LDL cholesterol profile obtained by density gradient ultracentrifugation. *Clin Chim Acta.* 2011;412:556–561.

34. Cao J, Steffen BT, Guan W, et al. A comparison of three apolipoprotein B methods and their associations with incident coronary heart disease risk over a 12-year follow-up period: the Multi-Ethnic Study of Atherosclerosis. *J Clin Lipidol.* 2018;12:300–304.

35. Varbo A, Nordestgaard BG. Remnant cholesterol and triglyceride-rich lipoproteins in atherosclerosis progression and cardiovascular disease. *Arterioscler Thromb Vasc Biol.* 2016;36:2133–2135.

36. Varbo A, Benn M, Tybjaerg-Hansen A, Jorgensen AB, Frikke-Schmidt R, Nordestgaard BG. Remnant cholesterol as a causal risk factor for ischemic heart disease. *J Am Coll Cardiol.* 2013;61:427–436.

37. Joshi PH, Khokhar AA, Massaro JM, et al. Remnant lipoprotein cholesterol and incident coronary heart disease: the Jackson heart and Framingham offspring cohort studies. *J Am Heart Assoc.* 2016;5.

38. Jorgensen AB, Frikke-Schmidt R, West AS, Grande P, Nordestgaard BG, Tybjaerg-Hansen A. Genetically elevated non-fasting triglycerides and calculated remnant cholesterol as causal risk factors for myocardial infarction. *Eur Heart J.* 2013;34:1826–1833.

39. Imke C, Rodriguez BL, Grove JS, et al. Are remnant-like particles independent predictors of coronary heart disease incidence? The Honolulu Heart study. *Arterioscler Thromb Vasc Biol.* 2005;25:1718–1722.

40. McNamara JR, Shah PK, Nakajima K, et al. Remnant-like particle (RLP) cholesterol is an independent cardiovascular disease risk factor in women: results from the Framingham Heart Study. *Atherosclerosis.* 2001;154:229–236.

41. Varbo A, Benn M, Nordestgaard BG. Remnant cholesterol as a cause of ischemic heart disease: evidence, definition, measurement, atherogenicity, high risk patients, and present and future treatment. *Pharmacol Ther.* 2014;141:358–367.

42. Nordestgaard BG, Benn M, Schnohr P, Tybjaerg-Hansen A. Nonfasting triglycerides and risk of myocardial infarction, ischemic heart disease, and death in men and women. *Jama*. 2007;298:299–308.

43. Freiberg JJ, Tybjaerg-Hansen A, Jensen JS, Nordestgaard BG. Nonfasting triglycerides and risk of ischemic stroke in the general population. *Jama*. 2008;300:2142–2152.

44. Saeed A, Ballantyne C, Sun W, et al. Association of remnant-like particle cholesterol and low-density lipoprotein triglyceride with incidence of cardiovascular events: the ARIC study. *J Am Coll Cardiol*. 2017;69:1721.

45. Kamstrup PR, Benn M, Tybjaerg-Hansen A, Nordestgaard BG. Extreme lipoprotein(a) levels and risk of myocardial infarction in the general population: the Copenhagen City Heart Study. *Circulation*. 2008;117:176–184.

46. Tsimikas S, Brilakis ES, Miller ER, et al. Oxidized phospholipids, Lp(a) lipoprotein, and coronary artery disease. *N Engl J Med*. 2005;353:46–57.

47. Kamstrup PR, Tybjaerg-Hansen A, Steffensen R, Nordestgaard BG. Genetically elevated lipoprotein(a) and increased risk of myocardial infarction. *Jama*. 2009;301:2331–2339.

48. Erqou S, Kaptoge S, Perry PL, et al. Lipoprotein(a) concentration and the risk of coronary heart disease, stroke, and nonvascular mortality. *Jama*. 2009;302:412–423.

49. Clarke R, Peden JF, Hopewell JC, et al. Genetic variants associated with Lp(a) lipoprotein level and coronary disease. *N Engl J Med*. 2009;361:2518–2528.

50. Genest JJ, Martin-Munley SS, McNamara JR, et al. Familial lipoprotein disorders in patients with premature coronary artery disease. *Circulation*. 1992;85:2025–2033.

51. Kamstrup PR, Tybjaerg-Hansen A, Nordestgaard BG. Elevated lipoprotein(a) and risk of aortic valve stenosis in the general population. *J Am Coll Cardiol*. 2014;63:470–477.

52. Marcovina SM, Albers JJ. Lipoprotein (a) measurements for clinical application. *J Lipid Res*. 2016;57:526–537.

53. Tsimikas SA. Test in context: lipoprotein(a): diagnosis, prognosis, controversies, and emerging therapies. *J Am Coll Cardiol*. 2017;69:692–711.

54. Rifai N, Heiss G, Doetsch K. Lipoprotein(a) at birth, in blacks and whites. *Atherosclerosis*. 1992;92:123–129.

55. Brown WV, Ballantyne CM, Jones PH, Marcovina S. Management of Lp(a). *J Clin Lipidol*. 2010;4:240–247.

56. Marcovina SM, Albers JJ, Scanu AM, et al. Use of a reference material proposed by the International Federation of Clinical Chemistry and Laboratory Medicine to evaluate analytical methods for the determination of plasma lipoprotein(a). *Clin Chem*. 2000;46:1956–1967.

57. Saleheen D, Zaidi M, Rasheed A, et al. The Pakistan Risk of Myocardial Infarction Study: a resource for the study of genetic, lifestyle and other determinants of myocardial infarction in South Asia. *Eur J Epidemiol*. 2009;24:329–338.

58. Waldeyer C, Makarova N, Zeller T, et al. Lipoprotein(a) and the risk of cardiovascular disease in the European population: results from the BiomarCaRE consortium. *Eur Heart J*. 2017.

59. Virani SS, Brautbar A, Davis BC, et al. Associations between lipoprotein(a) levels and cardiovascular outcomes in black and white subjects: the Atherosclerosis Risk in Communities (ARIC) Study. *Circulation*. 2012;125:241–249.

60. Cone JT, Segrest JP, Chung BH, Ragland JB, Sabesin SM, Glasscock A. Computerized rapid high resolution quantitative analysis of plasma lipoproteins based upon single vertical spin centrifugation. *J Lipid Res*. 1982;23:923–935.

61. Cohen A, Hertz HS, Mandel J, et al. Total serum cholesterol by isotope dilution/mass spectrometry: a candidate definitive method. *Clin Chem*. 1980;26:854–860.

62. Suk Danik J, Rifai N, Buring JE, Ridker PM. Lipoprotein(a), measured with an assay independent of apolipoprotein(a) isoform size, and risk of future cardiovascular events among initially healthy women. *JAMA*. 2006;296(11):1363–1370.

63. Tsimikas S, Fazio S, Ferdinand KC, et al. NHLBI working Group recommendations to reduce lipoprotein(a)-mediated risk of cardiovascular disease and aortic stenosis. *J Am Coll Cardiol*. 2018;71:177–192.

64. Chung BH, Segrest JP, Cone JT, Pfau J, Geer JC, Duncan LA. High resolution plasma lipoprotein cholesterol profiles by a rapid, high volume semi-automated method. *J Lipid Res*. 1981;22:1003–1014.

65. Ellerbe P, Sniegoski LT, Welch MJ. Isotope dilution mass spectrometry as a candidate definitive method for determining total glycerides and triglycerides in serum. *Clin Chem*. 1995;41:397–404.

66. Musunuru K, Orho-Melander M, Caulfield MP, et al. Ion mobility analysis of lipoprotein subfractions identifies three independent axes of cardiovascular risk. *Arterioscler Thromb Vasc Biol*. 2009;29:1975–1980.

67. Ito Y, Ohta M. Development of a new homogeneous assay for LDL-Triglyceride (abstract A-95). *Clin Chem*. 2012;58:A29.

68. Otvos JD. Measurement of lipoprotein subclass profiles by nuclear magnetic resonance spectroscopy. *Clin Lab*. 2002;48:171–180.

69. Otvos JD, Jeyarajah EJ, Bennett DW. Quantification of plasma lipoproteins by proton nuclear magnetic resonance spectroscopy. *Clin Chemistry*. 1991;37:377–386.

70. Clouet-Foraison N, Gaie-Levrel F, Gillery P, Delatour V. Advanced lipoprotein testing for cardiovascular diseases risk assessment: a review of the novel approaches in lipoprotein profiling. *Clin Chem Lab Med*. 2017;55:1453–1464.

CHAPTER 6

High-Density Lipoprotein and High-Density Lipoprotein Cholesterol

KAYLA A. RIGGS, MD • ANAND ROHATGI, MD

INTRODUCTION

High-density lipoprotein (HDL) is one of the five major classes of lipoproteins, which vary in density, size, and protein composition. HDL is the most dense and smallest lipoprotein, containing the most protein and the least amount of lipid. Apolipoproteins are the proteins associated with lipoproteins. The two most common apolipoproteins associated with HDL are ApoA-I, found on essentially all HDL particles, and ApoA-II, found on two-thirds of HDL particles.

HDL-C Epidemiology

The first large-scale measurements of HDL assessed the cholesterol content, HDL-C, which allowed for epidemiological studies of the relationship of HDL-C with atherosclerotic cardiovascular disease (ASCVD). The Framingham Heart Study was the first study to show that the incidence of coronary heart disease (CHD) was highest in subjects with low HDL-C. Subjects with HDL-C less than 40 mg/dL had the highest CHD risk, whereas those with high HDL-C (greater than 50 mg/dL) had the lowest CHD risk. This established the concept that HDL cholesterol was "good cholesterol." The Lipid Research Clinics Coronary Primary Prevention Trial and Multiple Risk Factor Intervention Trial along with The Framingham Heart study estimated approximately 2%–3% decrease in CHD risk associated with 1 mg/dL increase in HDL-C level.[1] Recent observational studies suggest that the inverse relationship curve between HDL-C levels and CHD and mortality is present only below 40 mg/dL, becomes flat in the normal range up to 70 mg/dL, and then inflects upward with increased risk at extreme elevations in HDL-C.[2]

Multiple intrinsic and extrinsic factors affect the concentration of HDL-C. Age and alcohol consumption are positively associated with increasing HDL-C.[3,4] Black ethnicity is associated with higher HDL-C levels than white ethnicity.[5] On the other hand, male sex, central abdominal weight, increasing body mass index (BMI), smoking, and liver failure are negatively associated with HDL-C.[6–10]

Genes, HDL-C, and Cardiovascular Disease

Efforts to understand the causal role of HDL-C on ASCVD using genetic mutations in key enzymes related to HDL metabolism have been mixed. Individuals with ABCA1 mutations and subsequent lower HDL-C levels have larger atherosclerotic burden and risk for cardiovascular disease.[11] Individuals with ApoA-1 mutations have increased endothelial dysfunction, arterial wall thickness, and coronary artery disease risk.[12] In contrast, a Mendelian randomization study assessing the impact of mutations in endothelial lipase, which raises HDL-C levels, did not reveal an expected protective effect on coronary disease.[13] Paradoxically, mutations in the scavenger receptor B1 (SR-B1) which lead to marked increases in HDL-C levels have been linked to increased ASCVD risk.[14] Similarly, mutations in cholesteryl ester transfer protein (CETP) also lead to marked increases in HDL-C levels but have mixed associations with ASCVD, with benefits likely due to lowering of apolipoprotein B and not related to HDL-C.[15]

Interventions Affecting HDL-C Levels and Outcomes

Gemfibrozil

Gemfibrozil is in the fibric acid derivatives drug class, which inhibits the production of very-low-density lipoproteins (VLDLs) and enhances VLDL clearance by stimulating lipoprotein lipase activity. This primarily results in reducing triglycerides and raising HDL-C.[16] One of the earlier trials, the Helsinki Heart Study, assessed the impact of gemfibrozil in middle-aged men with dyslipidemia (non-HDL ≥ 200 mg/dL). In this placebo-controlled randomized control trial 600 mg of gemfibrozil two times daily for 5 years resulted in an increase of HDL-C by more than 10% and a reduction in total cholesterol, LDL cholesterol, non-HDL cholesterol, and triglycerides by 8%, 8%, 12%, and 35%, respectively. The primary end points of coronary heart disease—fatal and nonfatal myocardial infarction and cardiac death—incidence was reduced by 34%.[17] The Veterans Affairs High-Density

Biomarkers in Cardiovascular Disease. https://doi.org/10.1016/B978-0-323-54835-9.00006-5

Lipoprotein Cholesterol Intervention Trial (VA-HIT) trial studied gemfibrozil in men with known CHD and low HDL-C and LDL-C. Gemfibrozil's primary effect on lipids was improvements in plasma HDL-C and triglyceride levels with little effect on LDL-C. This study found that randomization to gemfibrozil was associated with a 22% decrease in the rate of death from CHD or nonfatal myocardial infarction.[18]

Niacin

Niacin increases HDL-C levels and decreases LDL-C, triglyceride, and lipoprotein (a) levels.[19] A metaanalysis of niacin studies with and without statin treatment revealed that niacin treatment reduced myocardial infarction and coronary revascularization but did not have a significant benefit in mortality.[20] The addition of niacin to statin therapy, currently the established treatment of choice for decreasing ASCVD risk, did not produce increased benefit in two trials, Atherothrombosis Intervention in Metabolic Syndrome with Low HDL/High Triglycerides: Impact on Global Health Outcomes (AIM-HIGH) and Heart Protection Study 2-Treatment of HDL to Reduce the Incidence of Vascular Events (HPS2-THRIVE). AIM-HIGH studied adults with established cardiovascular disease and low HDL-C. Treatment of niacin in addition to statin therapy produced 25% increase in baseline HDL-C after 2 years, but there was no significant difference in the primary end point of cardiovascular death or vascular-related hospitalization by trial conclusion at 3 years.[21] HPS2-THRIVE assessed the addition of niacin with laropiprant to statin therapy in adults with known vascular disease. Laropiprant reduces niacin's side effect of flushing to improve adherence of niacin therapy. There was no significant reduction in the incidence of major vascular events.[22]

Pioglitazone

Pioglitazone is a glucose-lowering medication that works as an agonist of peroxisome proliferator–activated receptor gamma. The Prospective Pioglitazone Clinical Trial in Macrovascular Events (PROActive) trial in 2005 reported that pioglitazone had a beneficial effect on cardiovascular disease through reduction in all-cause mortality, nonfatal myocardial infarction, and stroke in patients with type 2 diabetes with a history of macrovascular disease. This study randomized participants to 45 mg pioglitazone or placebo with a mean follow-up of 34.5 months.[23] A post hoc analysis suggested that the cardiovascular impact of pioglitazone was through an increase in HDL-C by a median of 19% from baseline.[24] Pioglitazone Randomised Italian Study on Metabolic Syndrome (PRISMA): Effect of pioglitazone with metformin on HDL-C levels in Type 2 diabetic patients reinforced the findings from PROActive.

In this trial HDL-C significantly increased at 6 months compared with baseline levels by 6.31 mg/dL with pioglitazone compared with 3.02 mg/dL with placebo. This difference was independent of statin use.[25] A metaanalysis on the impact of diabetes medications on lipids revealed that both acarbose (difference in means 0.04) and pioglitazone (difference in means 0.093) increase HDL-C levels, whereas sulfonylureas (difference in means –0.024) decrease HDL-C levels.[26]

CETP inhibitors

CETP inhibitors raise HDL-C by decreasing the transfer of cholesteryl esters to other lipoprotein particles such as LDL, thereby retaining more cholesterol in HDL. Because most cholesteryl esters originate in HDL, decreasing the transfer to other non-HDL particles and increasing the protective HDL concentration is a promising cardioprotective approach.[27]

Four recent phase 3 randomized control trials studied CETP inhibitors: torcetrapib, dalcetrapib, evacetrapib, and anacetrapib (Table 6.1). These trials included patients with known atherosclerotic cardiovascular disease or history of cardiovascular disease. The first CETP inhibitor, torcetrapib, increased HDL-C but also increased the risk of death and cardiovascular events. The trial ended early due to the increased harm to patients. The hazard ratio for major cardiovascular events was 1.25 and for death was 1.58 in torcetrapib group.[28,29] Dalcetrapib increased HDL-C but did not reduce the risk of cardiovascular events and was terminated due to futility.[30] In dal-OUTCOMES, dalcetrapib was not associated with a reduction in the primary outcome; however, a post hoc analysis revealed a pharmacogenomic interaction. The homozygous AA genotype had increased cholesterol efflux capacity (CEC), discussed in the following section, and a reduction in cardiovascular events compared with the heterozygous or homozygous GG allele genotype.[31] The phase 2 trial of evacetrapib monotherapy and combined therapy with statins increased total CEC.[32] Evacetrapib in the phase 3 trial decreased LDL-C and increased HDL-C but had no significant difference in cardiovascular event rate compared with placebo.[33] Anacetrapib is the only CETP inhibitor to have beneficial cardiovascular effects. This CETP inhibitor decreased the incidence of major coronary events compared with placebo. At the midpoint of the study, HDL was 43 mg/dL higher in the test group than in the placebo group. Anacetrapib also decreased the mean level of non-HDL cholesterol by 17 mg/dL. The primary outcome, first major coronary event, was significantly reduced in anacetrapib group, but there was no significant effect on the rates of death

TABLE 6.1
CETP Inhibitors

CETP Inhibitor	Population	Effect on HDL-C[a]	Primary End Point	Primary End Point Result
Torcetrapib	• Cardiovascular disease or diabetes • N = 7,533; atorvastatin + torcetrapib • N = 7,534; atorvastatin + placebo	72.1% increase	First major cardiovascular event (coronary death: MI, stroke, hospitalization for unstable angina) • Median length of follow-up: 18.3 months (550 days)	Primary end point elevated • 6.2% torcetrapib vs 5% atorvastatin only • Hazard ratio of 1.25 (95% CI, 1.09 to 1.44)
Dalcetrapib	• Recent coronary syndrome on evidence-based LDL-lowering treatment • N = 7,938; dalcetrapib • N = 7,933; placebo	31%–40% increase	Death from coronary heart disease, nonfatal myocardial infarction, ischemic stroke, unstable angina, cardiac arrest with resuscitation • Median length of follow-up: 31 months	No significant effect • 8.3% dalcetrapib group vs 8.0% placebo • Hazard ratio of 1.04 (95% CI, 0.93 to 1.16)
Evacetrapib	• Atherosclerotic vascular disease • N = 6,038; evacetrapib • N = 6,054; placebo	133.2% increase	First major cardiovascular end point (death from cardiovascular causes: MI, stroke, coronary revascularization, hospitalization from unstable angina) • Median length of follow-up: 28 months	No significant effect • 12.9% evacetrapib group vs 12.8% placebo group • Hazard ratio of 1.01 (95% CI, 0.91 to 1.11)
Anacetrapib	• Atherosclerotic vascular disease on intensive statin therapy • N = 15,225; anacetrapib • N = 15,224; placebo	104% relative difference	First major coronary event (coronary death: MI, coronary revascularization) • Median length of follow-up: 49.2 months (4.1 years)	Primary end point lowered • 10.8% in anacetrapib vs 11.8% in placebo • Rate ratio 0.91 (95% CI, 0.85 to 0.97)

[a]Percentages are placebo-corrected increases.

from cardiovascular causes. The mechanism by how anacetrapib reduced the primary outcomes was unable to be determined due to the combination of increased HDL-C and decreased non-HDL cholesterol.[34]

HDL Particle Number
Epidemiology of HDL particle number and cardiovascular disease
Apart from the cholesterol content of HDL, the number of particles can also be measured, typically by nuclear magnetic resonance (NMR), and may be a useful marker of HDL metabolism. Ancillary studies within the population-based cohort of the Multi-Ethnic Study of Atherosclerosis (MESA) and the Justification for the Use of Statin in Prevention: An Intervention Trial Evaluating Rosuvastatin (JUPITER) randomized trial revealed that HDL-P was inversely associated with incident ASCVD. However, when adjusting for HDL-P, HDL-C was not associated with cardiovascular disease, whereas HDL-P remained significantly associated with

cardiovascular disease, suggesting that HDL-P may be a more robust marker of ASCVD risk than HDL-C levels.[35,36] The Dallas Heart Study (DHS) reinforced the association of HDL-P with CHD. In this cohort, HDL-P, and not HDL-C, was inversely associated with coronary artery calcium and incident CHD (Fig. 6.1).[5]

The European Prospective Investigation into Cancer and Nutrition-Norfolk (EPIC-Norfolk) cohort and Incremental Decrease in End Points through Aggressive Lipid Lowering (IDEAL) randomized trial used different populations but had similar findings. The EPIC-Norfolk study had lower risk participants without prior myocardial infarction or stroke, and participants were not using lipid-lowering medications. The IDEAL trial participants had a prior history of myocardial infarction. Both studies found an inverse association between ApoA-I levels and incident cardiac events. When adjusting for ApoA-I and ApoB, two lipoproteins associated with HDL and LDL, respectively, the association for HDL-P with major coronary event—fatal or nonfatal CAD in EPIC-Norfolk—was significantly higher with larger HDL-P size.[37,38]

The metabolic syndrome is affiliated with increased cardiovascular risk, and studies have assessed the protection of HDL-P in developing metabolic syndrome and in developing CHD in participants with metabolic syndrome. In participants without the metabolic syndrome the DHS found that low HDL-P doubles the risk of developing metabolic syndrome.[39] In the MESA cohort, HDL-P was inversely associated with incident coronary disease among those with diabetes but not among those with metabolic syndrome.[40]

Interventions and effects on HDL particles

Niacin is known to increase HDL-C concentration, but niacin's effect on particles differs. Le et al. studied type IIa and IIb hyperlipidemic patients and noted that combination therapy of niacin with ezetimibe and simvastatin had the greatest and most significant increase in HDL-P. In individuals with a history of cardiovascular disease, niacin with statin therapy did not increase HDL-P or improve ABCA-1 specific efflux but did increase HDL-C and global macrophage efflux. These heterogeneous effects on different aspects of HDL composition and function may explain in part the lack of benefit on ASCVD.[41,42]

With regard to statins, on treatment, HDL-P but not HDL-C or ApoA-I is inversely associated with ASCVD. In JUPITER, HDL-P increased by 3.8% compared with baseline after 1 year of rosuvastatin therapy.[36,43]

HDL FUNCTION
Cholesterol Efflux
Cholesterol efflux epidemiology
Cholesterol efflux capacity (CEC) is one of HDL's key functions involved in reverse cholesterol transport. Reverse cholesterol transport is the movement of cholesterol from peripheral vessels to the liver, the opposite of the formation of atherosclerosis. Cholesterol efflux is the transport of cholesterol from macrophages to HDL, the first step in reverse cholesterol transport. CEC is measured through blood samples with radiolabeled or fluorescent-labeled cholesterol. Observational studies have revealed that efflux capacity is a strong inverse predictor of coronary disease status (Fig. 6.2).[44,45]

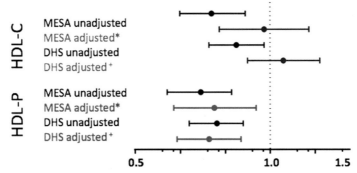

FIG. 6.1 Hazard ratios for high density lipoprotein cholesterol content (HDL-C) and high density lipoprotein particles (HDL-P) for incident coronary heart disease. Hazard ratios and 95% confidence intervals from Cox-proportional hazards models for 1 standard deviation increase in HDL-C or HDL-P. Adjusted = adjusted for base covariates and for each other, HDL-P or HDL-C, respectively. *MESA base covariates = adjusted for age, sex, ethnicity, hypertension, smoking, LDL-P, log triglyceride. +DHS base covariates = adjusted for age, sex, ethnicity, hypertension, diabetes, smoking, BMI, non-HDL-C, log triglyceride, any lipid-lowering therapy, hormone replacement therapy, menopause, alcohol intake, history of CHD at baseline.

Khera et al. found an inverse cross-sectional relationship between CEC and carotid intima-media thickness, even when adjusted for HDL-C and ApoA-I levels. The study found no association between HDL-C and carotid intima-media thickness. They also found a similar inverse cross-sectional association between CEC and severity of coronary atherosclerosis.[44]

In the DHS, among participants without cardiovascular disease, there was an inverse step-wise association between increasing CEC at baseline and reduced ASCVD risk, even with adjustment for HDL-C and HDL-P.[45] A subsequent analysis in the DHS demonstrated that CEC improved risk prediction beyond not only traditional risk factors but also coronary calcium, family history, and C-reactive protein (CRP).[46] A study in Europe assessed the utility of CEC in a higher risk population, patients scheduled for coronary angiography. Low CEC was found to be an independent risk factor for cardiovascular death.[47-49]

In patients without cardiovascular disease, CEC is similar in men and woman but significantly lower in blacks than in nonblacks. In individuals without CVD, CEC is positively correlated with alcohol, male sex, HDL-C, and total cholesterol and negatively with black ethnicity.[45] On the other hand, in patients with CVD, CEC is positively correlated with HDL-C, ApoA-I, LDL-C, and alcohol consumption[48,49] and negatively correlated with type II diabetes, blood glucose, and CRP.[49]

Interventions and effects on efflux
As many treatments that increase HDL-C did not show significant improvement in cardiovascular events,

research has targeted interventions affecting HDL function. The four recent CETP inhibitors have various effects on cholesterol efflux. Both dalcetrapib and torcetrapib increased cholesterol efflux capacity but predominately non–ABCA1-specific CEC.[28,50,51] Dalcetrapib increased non–ABCA1-specific CEC by 9.5%.[50] High-dose torcetrapib (120 mg) increased non–ABCA1-specific CEC, whereas low dose (60 mg) did not, but the ILLUMINATE trial to assess torcetrapib's efficacy used 60 mg daily dosing.[28,51,52]

Evacetrapib increased both non–ABCA1- and ABCA1-specific CEC by a currently unknown mechanism. Evacetrapib monotherapy increased total CEC and non–ABCA1-specific CEC in a dose-dependent manner, but not for ABCA1-specific efflux. Total efflux increased by 18% with 30 mg and 34% with 500 mg. Non–ABCA1-specific efflux increased by up to 47% with 500 mg. ABCA1-specific efflux increased up to 26%. The addition of statin therapy blunted the increase in CEC.[32,52]

Anacetrapib, the only current CETP inhibitor associated with decreased ASCVD risk, has been shown to increase cholesterol efflux in a small study with 18 patients. The increased CEC was related to increased lecithin-cholesterol acyltransferase (LCAT) and dependent on ABCA1 and ABCG1, ATP-binding cassette transporters.[53]

The Mediterranean diet, particularly enriched with virgin olive oil, improved several metrics of HDL function, including CEC.[54] The addition of niacin to statin therapy in patients with carotid atherosclerosis increased HDL-C but did not have an impact on CEC.[55]

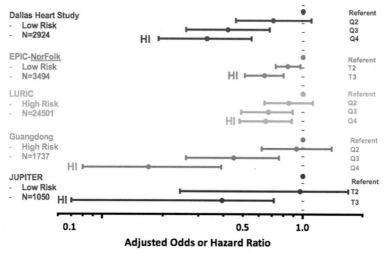

FIG. 6.2 Efflux and incident CV events.

Endothelial nitric oxide

Nitric oxide (NO) is a signaling molecule that causes endothelial vasodilation. Among healthy individuals, HDL increases NO production and phosphorylation of endothelial nitric oxide synthase (eNOS).[56] HDL activates eNOS through SR-B1. Impairment of NO leads to atherogenesis.[57]

Patients with CAD have increased inhibitory phosphorylation of eNOS and reduced paraoxonase 1 (PON1), an HDL-associated enzyme, activity leading to increased endothelial inflammation and decreased endothelial repair.[56] Patients with diabetes do not have HDL's endothelial protective features. Diabetic HDL does not have a dose-dependent increase in NO-mediated vasodilation of vessels or reduction in tumor necrosis factor alpha–stimulated superoxide production.[58]

Interventions and effect on NO

HDL in children with CKD did not produce the endothelial protective features found in HDL without CKD. HDL in CKD patients inhibited NO production and cholesterol efflux and promoted superoxide and vascular cell adhesion molecule-1 production. The endothelial dysfunction correlated with the stage of CKD; children on dialysis had the most significant changes in HDL function. After kidney transplantation, HDL function recovered.[59]

The Mediterranean diet has been shown to improve HDL function.[54] The Prevencion con Dieta Mediterranea (PREDIMED) trial studied the Mediterranean diet's effect on plasma NO and blood pressure. The Mediterranean diet had a significant increase in total polyphenol excretion that was positively correlated with plasma NO. With these increases in NO, there was an associated decrease in systolic and diastolic blood pressure promoting future cardiovascular protection.[60]

Oxidation

HDL plays an important role in protecting against macrophage-mediated LDL oxidation through PON1. This enzyme promotes cholesterol efflux and increases HDL binding to macrophages.[61] As myeloperoxidase is prooxidative and associated with systemic inflammation, a study revealed that independent of PON1, the increasing ratio of myeloperoxidase to HDL-P is associated with increased incidence and risk of cardiovascular disease.[62] Furthermore, in diabetic patients, abnormal PON1 is associated with increased atherosclerosis.[63]

Suppressing platelet production

In diabetic patients, reconstituted HDL reduced platelet membrane cholesterol content through cholesterol efflux subsequently reducing the reactivity of platelets.[64] Reconstituted HDL reduced megakaryocyte progenitor proliferation and platelet count through ABCG4 and the promotion of cholesterol efflux. ABCG4 is essential in the ability of the reconstituted HDL to suppress platelet production. Without ABCG4, there was prominent thrombocytosis.[65]

POSSIBLE NEW HDL HYPOTHESIS

The recent research surrounding HDL function has had many physician scientists question the current HDL hypothesis' utility in cardiovascular risk estimation. The ASCVD risk calculator, one of the most prominent cardiovascular risk estimation calculations, continues to have HDL cholesterol (HDL-C) as a component in the calculation. In 2016 Mody et al. assessed that cholesterol efflux improved the ASCVD risk prediction beyond coronary artery calcium, family history of myocardial infarction, and high-sensitivity CRP.[46] As many reviews and editorials have questioned the future measurement of HDL in risk calculations, the current evidence suggests that HDL function as opposed to HDL-C may prove to be a better measurement and target for cardiovascular risk reduction.[46,66,67]

SUMMARY

In summary, the relationship between HDL metabolism and ASCVD is complex. Although HDL-C continues to be considered the "good cholesterol," there are many facets of HDL to understand. HDL-C through observational studies is associated with decreased ASCVD; however, most therapies to raise HDL-C have not decreased ASCVD. HDL-P remains associated with ASCVD despite adjustment for HDL-C, suggesting that HDL-P may be a more meaningful measurement of HDL. HDL's functions, cholesterol efflux, endothelial nitric oxide, oxidation, and platelet suppression all contribute to HDL's prevention of atherosclerosis. Studies are continuing to elucidate the impact of HDL in cardiovascular disease.

REFERENCES

1. Gordon DJ, Probstfield JL, Garrison RJ, et al. High-density lipoprotein cholesterol and cardiovascular disease. Four prospective American studies. *Circulation*. 1989;79(1):8–15.
2. Madsen CM, Varbo A, Nordestgaard BG. Extreme high high-density lipoprotein cholesterol is paradoxically associated with high mortality in men and women: two prospective cohort studies. *Eur Heart J*. 2017;38(32):2478–2486.

3. de Backer G, de Bacquer D, Kornitzer M. Epidemiological aspects of high density lipoprotein cholesterol. *Atherosclerosis*. 1998;137 suppl:S1–6.

4. De Oliveira ESER, Foster D, McGee Harper M, et al. Alcohol consumption raises HDL cholesterol levels by increasing the transport rate of apolipoproteins A-I and A-II. *Circulation*. 2000;102(19):2347–2352.

5. Chandra A, Neeland IJ, Das SR, et al. Relation of black race between high density lipoprotein cholesterol content, high density lipoprotein particles and coronary events (from the Dallas Heart Study). *Am J Cardiol*. 2015;115(7):890–894.

6. Etogo-Asse FE, Vincent RP, Hughes SA, et al. High density lipoprotein in patients with liver failure; relation to sepsis, adrenal function and outcome of illness. *Liver Int*. 2012;32(1):128–136.

7. Gossett LK, Johnson HM, Piper ME, Fiore MC, Baker TB, Stein JH. Smoking intensity and lipoprotein abnormalities in active smokers. *J Clin Lipidol*. 2009;3(6):372–378.

8. Lamon-Fava S, Wilson PW, Schaefer EJ. Impact of body mass index on coronary heart disease risk factors in men and women. The Framingham Offspring Study. *Arterioscler Thromb Vasc Biol*. 1996;16(12):1509–1515.

9. Pietilainen KH, Soderlund S, Rissanen A, et al. HDL subspecies in young adult twins: heritability and impact of overweight. *Obesity*. 2009;17(6):1208–1214.

10. Solhpour A, Parkhideh S, Sarrafzadegan N, et al. Levels of lipids and apolipoproteins in three cultures. *Atherosclerosis*. 2009;207(1):200–207.

11. Bochem AE, van Wijk DF, Holleboom AG, et al. ABCA1 mutation carriers with low high-density lipoprotein cholesterol are characterized by a larger atherosclerotic burden. *Eur Heart J*. 2013;34(4):286–291.

12. Hovingh GK, Brownlie A, Bisoendial RJ, et al. A novel apoA-I mutation (L178P) leads to endothelial dysfunction, increased arterial wall thickness, and premature coronary artery disease. *J Am Coll Cardiol*. 2004;44(7):1429–1435.

13. Voight BF, Peloso GM, Orho-Melander M, et al. Plasma HDL cholesterol and risk of myocardial infarction: a mendelian randomisation study. *Lancet*. 2012;380(9841):572–580.

14. Zanoni P, Khetarpal SA, Larach DB, et al. Rare variant in scavenger receptor BI raises HDL cholesterol and increases risk of coronary heart disease. *Science*. 2016;351(6278):1166–1171.

15. Ference BA, Kastelein JJP, Ginsberg HN, et al. Association of genetic variants related to CETP inhibitors and statins with lipoprotein levels and cardiovascular risk. *JAMA*. 2017;318(10):947–956.

16. Zimetbaum P, Frishman WH, Kahn S. Effects of gemfibrozil and other fibric acid derivatives on blood lipids and lipoproteins. *J Clin Pharmacol*. 1991;31(1):25–37.

17. Frick MH, Elo O, Haapa K, et al. Helsinki Heart Study: primary-prevention trial with gemfibrozil in middle-aged men with dyslipidemia. Safety of treatment, changes in risk factors, and incidence of coronary heart disease. *N Engl J Med*. 1987;317(20):1237–1245.

18. Rubins HB, Robins SJ, Collins D, et al. Gemfibrozil for the secondary prevention of coronary heart disease in men with low levels of high-density lipoprotein cholesterol. Veterans Affairs High-Density Lipoprotein Cholesterol Intervention Trial Study Group. *N Engl J Med*. 1999;341(6):410–418.

19. Carlson LA. Nicotinic acid: the broad-spectrum lipid drug. A 50th anniversary review. *J Intern Med*. 2005;258(2):94–114.

20. Verdoia M, Schaffer A, Suryapranata H, De Luca G. Effects of HDL-modifiers on cardiovascular outcomes: a meta-analysis of randomized trials. *Nutr Metab Cardiovasc Dis*. 2015;25(1):9–23.

21. Investigators A-H, Boden WE, Probstfield JL, et al. Niacin in patients with low HDL cholesterol levels receiving intensive statin therapy. *N Engl J Med*. 2011;365(24):2255–2267.

22. Group HTC, Landray MJ, Haynes R, et al. Effects of extended-release niacin with laropiprant in high-risk patients. *N Engl J Med*. 2014;371(3):203–212.

23. Dormandy JA, Charbonnel B, Eckland DJ, et al. Secondary prevention of macrovascular events in patients with type 2 diabetes in the PROactive Study (PROspective pioglitAzone Clinical Trial in macroVascular Events): a randomised controlled trial. *Lancet*. 2005;366(9493):1279–1289.

24. Ferrannini E, Betteridge DJ, Dormandy JA, et al. High-density lipoprotein-cholesterol and not HbA1c was directly related to cardiovascular outcome in PROactive. *Diabetes Obes Metab*. 2011;13(8):759–764.

25. Genovese S, Passaro A, Brunetti P, et al. Pioglitazone Randomised Italian Study on Metabolic Syndrome (PRISMA): effect of pioglitazone with metformin on HDL-C levels in Type 2 diabetic patients. *J Endocrinol Invest*. 2013;36(8):606–616.

26. Monami M, Vitale V, Ambrosio ML, et al. Effects on lipid profile of dipeptidyl peptidase 4 inhibitors, pioglitazone, acarbose, and sulfonylureas: meta-analysis of placebo-controlled trials. *Adv Ther*. 2012;29(9):736–746.

27. Barter PJ, Rye KA. Cholesteryl ester transfer protein inhibition as a strategy to reduce cardiovascular risk. *J Lipid Res*. 2012;53(9):1755–1766.

28. Barter PJ, Caulfield M, Eriksson M, et al. Effects of torcetrapib in patients at high risk for coronary events. *N Engl J Med*. 2007;357(21):2109–2122.

29. Hovingh GK, Kastelein JJP, van Deventer SJH, et al. Cholesterol ester transfer protein inhibition by TA-8995 in patients with mild dyslipidaemia (TULIP): a randomised, double-blind, placebo-controlled phase 2 trial. *Lancet*. 2015;386(9992):452–460.

30. Schwartz GG, Olsson AG, Abt M, et al. Effects of dalcetrapib in patients with a recent acute coronary syndrome. *N Engl J Med*. 2012;367(22):2089–2099.

31. Tardif JC, Rhainds D, Brodeur M, et al. Genotype-dependent effects of dalcetrapib on cholesterol efflux and inflammation: concordance with clinical outcomes. *Circ Cardiovasc Genet*. 2016;9(4):340–348.

32. Nicholls SJ, Ruotolo G, Brewer HB, et al. Cholesterol efflux capacity and pre-beta-1 HDL concentrations are increased in dyslipidemic patients treated with evacetrapib. *J Am Coll Cardiol.* 2015;66(20):2201–2210.

33. Lincoff AM, Nicholls SJ, Riesmeyer JS, et al. Evacetrapib and cardiovascular outcomes in high-risk vascular disease. *N Engl J Med.* 2017;376(20):1933–1942.

34. Group HTRC, Bowman L, Hopewell JC, et al. Effects of anacetrapib in patients with atherosclerotic vascular disease. *N Engl J Med.* 2017;377(13):1217–1227.

35. Mackey RH, Greenland P, Goff Jr DC, Lloyd-Jones D, Sibley CT, Mora S. High-density lipoprotein cholesterol and particle concentrations, carotid atherosclerosis, and coronary events: MESA (multi-ethnic study of atherosclerosis). *J Am Coll Cardiol.* 2012;60(6):508–516.

36. Mora S, Glynn RJ, Ridker PM. High-density lipoprotein cholesterol, size, particle number, and residual vascular risk after potent statin therapy. *Circulation.* 2013;128(11):1189–1197.

37. Arsenault BJ, Lemieux I, Despres JP, et al. HDL particle size and the risk of coronary heart disease in apparently healthy men and women: the EPIC-Norfolk prospective population study. *Atherosclerosis.* 2009;206(1):276–281.

38. van der Steeg WA, Holme I, Boekholdt SM, et al. High-density lipoprotein cholesterol, high-density lipoprotein particle size, and apolipoprotein A-I: significance for cardiovascular risk: the IDEAL and EPIC-Norfolk studies. *J Am Coll Cardiol.* 2008;51(6):634–642.

39. Mani P, Ren HY, Neeland IJ, et al. The association between HDL particle concentration and incident metabolic syndrome in the multi-ethnic Dallas Heart Study. *Diabetes Metab Syndr.* 2017;11(suppl 1):S175–S179.

40. Tehrani DM, Zhao Y, Blaha MJ, et al. Discordance of low-density lipoprotein and high-density lipoprotein cholesterol particle versus cholesterol concentration for the prediction of cardiovascular disease in patients with metabolic syndrome and diabetes mellitus (from the multi-ethnic study of atherosclerosis [MESA]). *Am J Cardiol.* 2016;117(12):1921–1927.

41. Le NA, Jin R, Tomassini JE, Tershakovec AM, Neff DR, Wilson PW. Changes in lipoprotein particle number with ezetimibe/simvastatin coadministered with extended-release niacin in hyperlipidemic patients. *J Am Heart Assoc.* 2013;2(4):e000037.

42. Ronsein GE, Hutchins PM, Isquith D, Vaisar T, Zhao XQ, Heinecke JW. Niacin therapy increases high-density lipoprotein particles and total cholesterol efflux capacity but not ABCA1-specific cholesterol efflux in statin-treated subjects. *Arterioscler Thromb Vasc Biol.* 2016;36(2):404–411.

43. Khera AV, Demler OV, Adelman SJ, et al. Cholesterol efflux capacity, high-density lipoprotein particle number, and incident cardiovascular events: an analysis from the JUPITER trial (justification for the use of statins in prevention: an intervention trial evaluating rosuvastatin). *Circulation.* 2017;135(25):2494–2504.

44. Khera AV, Cuchel M, de la Llera-Moya M, et al. Cholesterol efflux capacity, high-density lipoprotein function, and atherosclerosis. *N Engl J Med.* 2011;364(2):127–135.

45. Rohatgi A, Khera A, Berry JD, et al. HDL cholesterol efflux capacity and incident cardiovascular events. *N Engl J Med.* 2014;371(25):2383–2393.

46. Mody P, Joshi PH, Khera A, Ayers CR, Rohatgi A. Beyond coronary calcification, family history, and C-Reactive protein: cholesterol efflux capacity and cardiovascular risk prediction. *J Am Coll Cardiol.* 2016;67(21):2480–2487.

47. Ritsch A, Scharnagl H, Marz W. HDL cholesterol efflux capacity and cardiovascular events. *N Engl J Med.* 2015;372(19):1870–1871.

48. Saleheen D, Scott R, Javad S, et al. Association of HDL cholesterol efflux capacity with incident coronary heart disease events: a prospective case-control study. *Lancet Diab Endocrinol.* 2015;3(7):507–513.

49. Liu C, Zhang Y, Ding D, et al. Cholesterol efflux capacity is an independent predictor of all-cause and cardiovascular mortality in patients with coronary artery disease: a prospective cohort study. *Atherosclerosis.* 2016;249:116–124.

50. Ray KK, Ditmarsch M, Kallend D, et al. The effect of cholesteryl ester transfer protein inhibition on lipids, lipoproteins, and markers of HDL function after an acute coronary syndrome: the dal-ACUTE randomized trial. *Eur Heart J.* 2014;35(27):1792–1800.

51. Yvan-Charvet L, Matsuura F, Wang N, et al. Inhibition of cholesteryl ester transfer protein by torcetrapib modestly increases macrophage cholesterol efflux to HDL. *Arterioscler Thromb Vasc Biol.* 2007;27(5):1132–1138.

52. Rohatgi A, Grundy SM. Cholesterol efflux capacity as a therapeutic target: rationale and clinical implications. *J Am Coll Cardiol.* 2015;66(20):2211–2213.

53. Yvan-Charvet L, Kling J, Pagler T, et al. Cholesterol efflux potential and antiinflammatory properties of high-density lipoprotein after treatment with niacin or anacetrapib. *Arterioscler Thromb Vasc Biol.* 2010;30(7):1430–1438.

54. Hernaez A, Castaner O, Elosua R, et al. Mediterranean diet improves high-density lipoprotein function in high-cardiovascular-risk individuals: a randomized controlled trial. *Circulation.* 2017;135(7):633–643.

55. Khera AV, Patel PJ, Reilly MP, Rader DJ. The addition of niacin to statin therapy improves high-density lipoprotein cholesterol levels but not metrics of functionality. *J Am Coll Cardiol.* 2013;62(20):1909–1910.

56. Besler C, Heinrich K, Rohrer L, et al. Mechanisms underlying adverse effects of HDL on eNOS-activating pathways in patients with coronary artery disease. *J Clin Invest.* 2011;121(7):2693–2708.

57. Yuhanna IS, Zhu Y, Cox BE, et al. High-density lipoprotein binding to scavenger receptor-BI activates endothelial nitric oxide synthase. *Nat Med.* 2001;7(7):853–857.

58. Sorrentino SA, Besler C, Rohrer L, et al. Endothelial-vasoprotective effects of high-density lipoprotein are impaired in patients with type 2 diabetes mellitus but are improved after extended-release niacin therapy. *Circulation.* 2010;121(1):110–122.

59. Shroff R, Speer T, Colin S, et al. HDL in children with CKD promotes endothelial dysfunction and an abnormal vascular phenotype. *J Am Soc Nephrol.* 2014;25(11): 2658–2668.
60. Medina-Remon A, Tresserra-Rimbau A, Pons A, et al. Effects of total dietary polyphenols on plasma nitric oxide and blood pressure in a high cardiovascular risk cohort. The PREDIMED randomized trial. *Nutr Metab Cardiovasc Dis.* 2015;25(1):60–67.
61. Efrat M, Aviram M. Paraoxonase 1 interactions with HDL, antioxidants and macrophages regulate atherogenesis - a protective role for HDL phospholipids. *Adv Exp Med Biol.* 2010;660:153–166.
62. Khine HW, Teiber JF, Haley RW, Khera A, Ayers CR, Rohatgi A. Association of the serum myeloperoxidase/high-density lipoprotein particle ratio and incident cardiovascular events in a multi-ethnic population: observations from the Dallas Heart Study. *Atherosclerosis.* 2017;263:156–162.
63. Rosenblat M, Karry R, Aviram M. Paraoxonase 1 (PON1) is a more potent antioxidant and stimulant of macrophage cholesterol efflux, when present in HDL than in lipoprotein-deficient serum: relevance to diabetes. *Atherosclerosis.* 2006;187(1):74–81.
64. Calkin AC, Drew BG, Ono A, et al. Reconstituted high-density lipoprotein attenuates platelet function in individuals with type 2 diabetes mellitus by promoting cholesterol efflux. *Circulation.* 2009;120(21):2095–2104.
65. Murphy AJ, Bijl N, Yvan-Charvet L, et al. Cholesterol efflux in megakaryocyte progenitors suppresses platelet production and thrombocytosis. *Nat Med.* 2013;19(5):586–594.
66. Mani P, Rohatgi A. Niacin therapy, HDL cholesterol, and cardiovascular disease: is the HDL hypothesis defunct? *Curr Atheroscler Rep.* 2015;17(8):43.
67. Vallejo-Vaz AJ, Ray KK. Cholesterol efflux capacity as a novel biomarker for incident cardiovascular events: has high-density lipoprotein been resuscitated? *Circ Res.* 2015;116(10):1646–1648.

CHAPTER 7

Blood Inflammatory Biomarkers of Cardiovascular Disease

ADITYA GOYAL, MD • AGASTYA D. BELUR, MD • AMIT K. DEY, MD •
NEHAL N. MEHTA, MD, MSCE

OVERVIEW

Inflammation is the change in vascular dynamics and recruitment of innate and adaptive immune cells after injury to tissue. Inflammation begins with an acute phase of increased vascular permeability, blood flow, and accumulation of various cytokines and leukocytes. If injury ensues, acute inflammation is followed by chronic inflammation, primarily comprised of specific humoral and cellular immune cells in contrast to acute inflammatory cells. Chronic systemic inflammation drives several human diseases. In the past 3 decades, chronic inflammation has been shown to drive initiation, progression, and sustainment of atherosclerotic cardiovascular diseases.

Atherosclerosis is the single most important contributor to cardiovascular (CV) disease burden, which remains the leading cause of death worldwide.[1] Extensive research studying atherosclerosis has unraveled that it involves a complex interplay of multiple factors, encompassing inflammation as the active driver in disease progression and surpassing our earlier belief of it being limited to lipid injury and infiltration.[2] Numerous lines of evidence exist in vitro and in vivo in mouse and human models which suggest inflammation potentially being causal in CV disease.[2-4]

Our understanding of atherosclerosis has evolved significantly over the past century, from cholesterol being the first culprit implicated in atherosclerosis to basic science research discovering the modulatory effects of proinflammatory cytokines including interferon-γ, tumor necrosis factor (TNF), and chemoattractant proteins such as monocyte chemoattractant protein-1 (MCP-1).[5,6] Several studies in mouse and human models have elucidated the role of active and innate immune systems, both stimulatory and inhibitory, acting at the center of atherosclerotic disease development and progression, thus determining its chronic inflammatory nature.[7,8] In conjunction with this, numerous epidemiological studies have demonstrated the association of inflammatory markers such as C-reactive protein (CRP), interleukin-6 (IL-6), interleukin-1 (IL-1), and TNF with atherosclerotic disease process.[9,10] Over the past 2 decades, multiple large-scale prospective trials not only highlighted the role of these biomarkers but also established their potential to independently predict CV events.[11-13] Finally a recent study, the Canakinumab Anti-Inflammatory Thrombosis Outcomes Study (CANTOS), provided compelling evidence for the inflammatory hypothesis of atherosclerosis by showing that inhibition of a proinflammatory cytokine IL-1β significantly lowered the rate of future CV events when compared with placebo.[14]

Systemic Inflammatory Diseases Associate with Early CV Disease in Humans

Inflammatory disease states have been shown to increase predisposition to adverse CV events.[15-17] For example, psoriasis, a chronic inflammatory disease, is associated with increased subclinical CV disease when compared with healthy controls by Fluorodeoxyglucose-Positron emission tomography/Computed tomography (FDG-PET/CT)[18,19] and coronary computed tomography angiography.[20,21] Indeed, consistent with the inflammatory hypothesis, psoriasis disease severity carries a dose-response relationship with subclinical vascular diseases [18] and early myocardial infarction (MI) (Fig. 7.1).[17] Similarly, in other inflammatory conditions such as rheumatoid arthritis (RA), systemic lupus erythematosus (SLE), chronic kidney disease, human immunodeficiency virus (HIV), and diabetes mellitus (DM), disease severity has been shown to be associated with an increase in inflammatory atherosclerotic burden.[16,22,23] Emerging literature in autoimmune diseases not only suggests that inflammation plays a significant role in development of CV disease but also demonstrates that treating inflammation in target tissues can potentially benefit vascular disease.[20,21]

Biomarkers in Cardiovascular Disease. https://doi.org/10.1016/B978-0-323-54835-9.00007-7

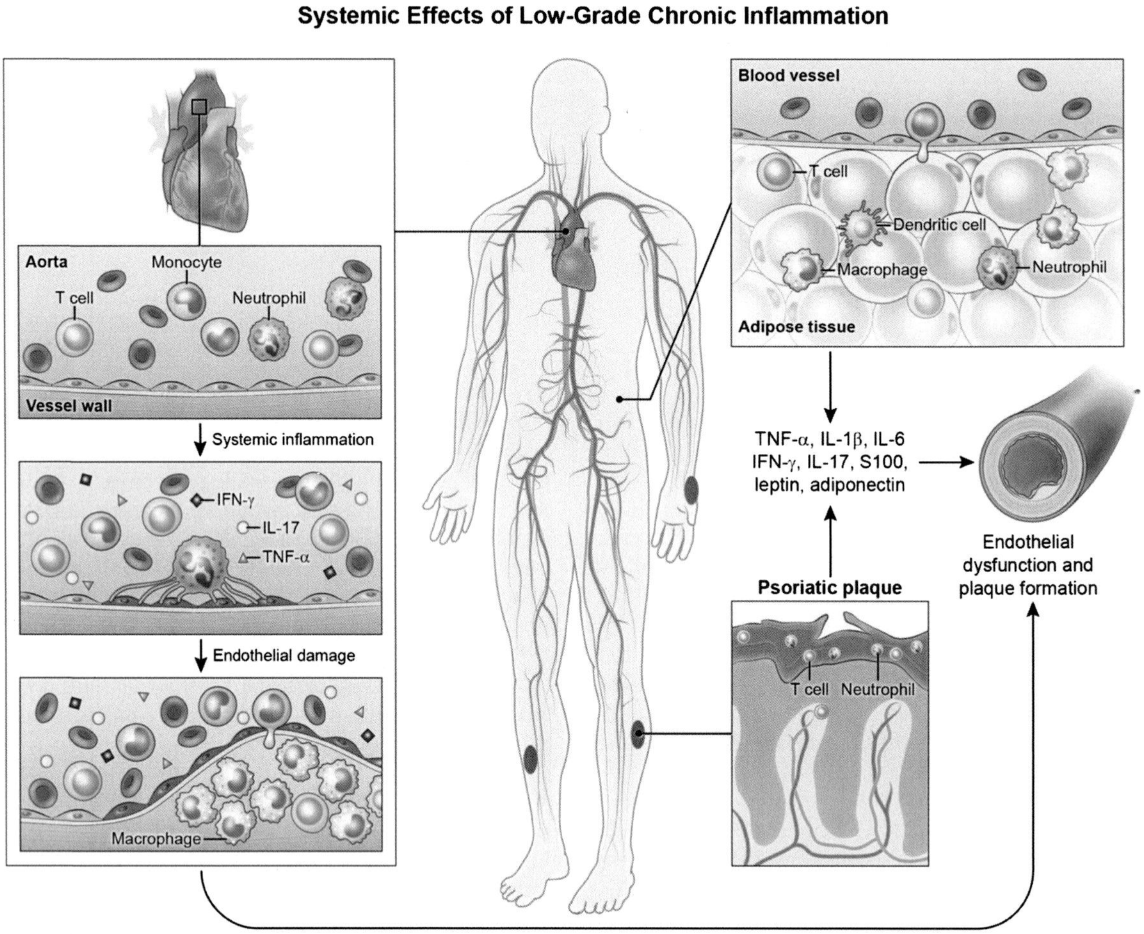

Systemic Effects of Low-Grade Chronic Inflammation

FIG. 7.1 Systemic effects of low-grade inflammation. Schematic representation of a psoriasis plaque, with various immune cells and activated keratinocytes, which secretes a vast array of proinflammatory cytokines, thus contributing to dysfunctional adipose tissue and release of proinflammatory adipokines. These pathways accelerate endothelial dysfunction, vascular inflammation, and atherosclerotic plaque buildup in the coronaries leading to incident myocardial infarction.

OVERVIEW OF EVOLUTION OF INFLAMMATORY BIOMARKERS

Traditional risk factors including age, sex, smoking, lipoprotein levels, hypertension, and diabetes have been widely used for predicting CV risk.[24] Given the high residual risk observed in CV disease despite standard CV risk calculators, blood biomarkers are increasingly being used in clinical care of patients. For example, CRP, an acute-phase reactant, has been shown to add an 8.5% risk on top of traditional risk factors for predicting residual CV risk.[25] In this section we describe the most common blood biomarkers being used in clinical practice or are on the horizon (Table 7.1).

Erythrocyte Sedimentation Rate

Erythrocyte sedimentation rate (ESR), a marker of erythrocyte aggregation influenced by blood proteins such as fibrinogen and immunoglobulins in a state of inflammation, was found to be potentially useful in CVD. Multiple validated methods exist for measuring ESR, and all of them allow for quick, cheap, and easy measurement using a small capillary blood sample.[26]

TABLE 7.1
Inflammatory Blood Biomarkers

Biomarkers	Description	Clinical Evidence in Cardiovascular Disease
Erythrocyte sedimentation rate	Sedimentation rate of RBCs over 1 h, governed by blood proteins such as fibrinogen and immunoglobulins. Raised in multiple conditions including inflammation, infections, and autoimmune diseases.	+
Fibrinogen	Acute-phase protein and coagulation factor responsible for formation of fibrin clot. Mainly used for evaluation of hemostasis.	None or little
White blood cell count	Total count of circulating white blood cells. Traditionally used as a measure of infection but also associated strongly with inflammation, however, nonspecific.	+
Neutrophils & monocytes	Major components of total white blood cell count. Neutrophils are now known to be first responders at atherosclerotic lesional sites. Both neutrophils and monocytes aid in atherosclerotic plaque development and progression.	++
Blood Proteins		
Uric acid	By-product of purine metabolism. Elevated in low-grade inflammatory conditions such as gout as well as metabolic syndrome.	+
Serum amyloid A	Acute-phase reactant found in tissues and blood in conditions of stress and inflammation. Laboratory measurement is difficult.	+
Cytokines	Cell signaling proteins released by immune cells in response to inflammation. Proinflammatory cytokines namely IL-6, TNF- α, IL-1β, and IL-18 have been implicated in atherosclerosis.	++
Chemokines	Cytokine subclass responsible for directing leukocytes to inflammatory sites. MCP-1, ICAM-1, and VCAM-1 among important chemokines with regard to cardiovascular disease.	+
C-reactive protein	Most widely studied acute-phase reactant. Synthesized in liver and extrahepatic tissues such as atherosclerotic plaques. A validated marker for predicting cardiovascular risk. High-sensitivity assay is a better marker than traditional measurement.	++
GlycA	Composite biomarker of a particular signal in NMR spectra. Neutrophils are major source. Raised in inflammatory conditions such as RA, SLE, and psoriasis. Emerging biomarker with promising evidence.	+

Elevated levels have been associated with heightened CV risk and mortality,[27] although some studies showed conflicting results.[28] Furthermore, ESR has not been used as a primary biomarker because its blood levels are known to be altered in several other disease states such as diabetes, end-stage renal disease, pregnancy, and obesity, thus reducing its specificity.[29] Therefore ESR measurement is usually performed in tandem with CRP levels when investigating inflammatory states.

Fibrinogen

Fibrinogen, a coagulation protein in plasma and an acute-phase reactant, serves as an important determinant of platelet aggregation[30] and has been found to associate with risk of coronary heart disease (CHD) in multiple prospective epidemiological studies.[31] By virtue of its role in the thrombotic cascade, fibrinogen carries an independent risk of propagating atherosclerosis and simultaneously influences the function of other markers of inflammation.[32] Even though fibrinogen has been shown to potentially capture CV risk efficiently,[33] studies have also reported that measuring fibrinogen levels provides no additional information over traditional risk and that plasma fibrinogen only reflects a general inflammatory state rather than directly influencing CV disease.[34,35] In present day clinical practice, routine measurement of fibrinogen is performed mostly for evaluating hemostasis.

White Blood Cell Count

White blood cell (WBC) count in blood, a commonly used measure of clinical disease states, was found to correlate with CHD in some small studies in the past.[36] Subsequent studies revealed that WBC count was strongly associated with inflammation as seen in atherosclerosis and could be a potential predictor of future CV events.[37,38] WBC count is an easy-to-measure marker in the blood, but the tight relation to CV risk factors and nonspecificity limits its use.[39]

Neutrophils and Monocytes

Among WBCs, two subsets of cells, namely monocytes and neutrophils, have been shown to be potentially related to CVD.[40] Monocytes are involved throughout the development of atherosclerosis; activated monocytes are released in the circulation which transform into macrophage foam cells after uptake of lipids in the vessel wall under the influence of MCP-1.[41,42] Neutrophils have been found to be the first responders in early atherosclerosis engaging monocyte recruitment and augmenting endothelial stress by releasing granule-based proteins.[43,44] Neutrophils also form neutrophil extracellular traps (NETosis), triggered by cholesterol crystals at lesional sites in atherosclerosis.[45] NETosis is associated with plaque development and progression.[46] Currently neither monocyte counts nor neutrophil frequencies are routinely checked in practice for CV disease but are increasingly the focus for ongoing research in inflammatory atherosclerosis to discover pathways to target with novel CVD therapeutics.

Proteins in Inflammatory Atherosclerosis

Proteins in the blood associated with acute inflammation have been evaluated in CVD. These include uric acid, cytokines, serum amyloid A (SAA), fibrinogen, high-sensitivity C-reactive protein (hsCRP), and GlycA; only hsCRP has been routinely used in clinical practice for CV risk prediction.[47]

Uric acid

Uric acid, an end product of purine metabolism, is associated with hypertension and metabolic syndrome.[48,49] Serum uric acid has been routinely used to evaluate gout, but cross-sectional studies have measured the impact of elevated serum uric acid on the cardiovascular disease. These have established an association with low-grade inflammation and potentially future CV events.[50] However, other studies failed to show an independent association of uric acid with CV disease along with questioning its role in pathogenesis of CV disease.[50] A recent study of colchicine showed

prospective reduction in CV risk in patients with gout. This risk reduction was in fact due to antiinflammatory effects of colchicine rather than its effect on serum uric acid, further suggesting the inflammatory hypothesis and lack of direct causality with uric acid.

Serum amyloid A

Another acute-phase reactant, SAA, has been used to characterize acute inflammation in recent translational studies. SAA is a highly inducible collection of small proteins[51] expressed in tissue macrophages in systemic diseases such as diabetes,[52] rheumatoid arthritis,[53] and atherosclerosis[54] as well as released in blood during phases of severe stress. It works by activating transcription factors, attracting phagocytes, and inhibiting neutrophilic apoptosis.[55] SAA has been found to be independently associated with future CV events.[56] Moreover, murine studies showed that SAA increased low-density lipoprotein (LDL) retention in macrophages early in the disease leading to atherosclerosis development.[57] SAA concentrations have associated with HDL functionality and have been a marker for CV mortality.[58] Use of SAA has been limited by its strenuous measurement in the clinical laboratory and lack of validation studies in diverse populations.

Cytokines

Cytokines are small, cell signaling proteins released by immune cells in response to various inflammatory and infectious stimuli and function as immunomodulators to maintain a balance between cellular and humoral immune systems.[59] In particular, proinflammatory cytokines have been critically implicated in the progression of atherosclerosis.[6] None are routinely used in practice owing to the nonstandardized measurement and high cost associated with testing.

Cytokines and innate immunity. TNF-α and IL-6, part of the innate immune system, are strongly implicated in inflammatory atherogenesis. TNF-α, a proinflammatory cytokine released early in inflammation from various cell types including macrophages, dendritic cells, and fibroblasts, directly leads to endothelial dysfunction, increases leukocyte recruitment, and aids in further synthesis and releases of acute-phase reactants, chemokines, and growth factors.[60] Increased plasma concentrations of TNF-α have been associated with premature CV disease in terms of CHD, MI, and peripheral artery disease (PAD).[61] Similarly, IL-6 is released from a variety of cells and also contributes to development and progression of atherosclerosis.[62] IL-6 is expressed in human atheromas and has been shown to be a strong predictor for future CV events.[63]

Cytokines and inflammasome activation. Part of the IL-1 family, IL-1α is present in healthy tissues unlike IL-1β.[64] In fact, IL-1β is a product of inflammatory cell types such as monocytes, macrophages, and dendritic cells and is induced by cytokines such as TNF-α, IL-18, IL-1α, and IL-1β itself.[65] Moreover, presence of caspase-1, a cysteine protease enzyme, is necessary for the intracellular cleavage and release of IL-1β.[66] Caspase-1 itself is activated after the assembly of a group of high-molecular-weight proteins called the inflammasome which is critical to production and subsequent release of IL-1β.[66] Studies in mouse and human models have demonstrated IL-1β as an active marker of ongoing inflammation in CV disease. In addition to this, IL-1β has also been shown to predict incident CV disease,[67] and concurrently blockade of IL-1β reduces CV events.[14]

Cytokines: chemokines related to vascular trafficking. Chemokines, a subclass of cytokines, are responsible for directing circulating leukocytes to inflammatory sites.[68] MCP-1, a principle chemokine mediator of monocyte and macrophage recruitment, is highly expressed in atherosclerotic plaques, is associated with inflammation, and is critical to all phases of atherosclerosis including formation, progression, and destabilization of plaques.[69] In fact, heightened expression of MCP-1 or its ligand-receptor CCR2 denotes a greater probability of developing atherosclerosis.[70] Moreover, studies have shown the presence of MCP-1 in atherosclerotic plaques[71] and have elucidated the mechanistic relationship of MCP-1 with future CV events independent of traditional risk factors.[72] Along with MCP-1, other chemokines that have been found useful in CVD are E-selectin, P-selectin, intercellular adhesion molecule-1 (ICAM-1), and vascular cell adhesion molecule (VCAM-1).[73] E-selectin and P-selectin are circulating adhesion molecules responsible for rolling of leukocytes along the endothelium and were shown to associate with the presence of CVD.[74] However, more recently, studies have provided contrasting evidence in which selectins were not found to predict CV risk independent of traditional risk factors, and some highlighted an absence of association with incident CHD.[75] Similarly, elevated levels of ICAM-1 and VCAM-1, responsible for firm attachment of leukocytes to vascular endothelium and subsequent transmigration, were found to be of risk in future vascular events.[76] However, owing to some contrasting evidence,[75] they are not used in routine clinical practice.

Therefore further research into novel cytokines and their ability to potentially predict residual inflammatory risk for atherosclerosis needs to be undertaken.

C-reactive protein

The most widely studied and reported marker of inflammation in CV risk prediction is CRP, an acute-phase reactant in blood released from the liver in states of both acute and chronic inflammation.[77] CRP belongs to the pentraxin protein group and is synthesized in hepatic and some extrahepatic tissues such as in atherosclerotic plaques and smooth muscle cells.[78] Mean CRP values in healthy blood samples are usually around 0.8 mg/L, and values lesser than that are hard to access using regular methods.[78] Thus a more accurate method and highly sensitive assay was designed to evaluate CRP levels less than 0.3 mg/L, an assay termed hsCRP.[77] High hsCRP has been associated with incident CV events in patients with and without history of prior CV disease.[47,79]

The Women's Health Study showed that hsCRP was a better marker for predicting CV events than LDL cholesterol or homocysteine in a group of healthy females.[80] Furthermore, hsCRP has been shown to provide additional prognostic value when combined with Framingham risk score, metabolic syndrome, and lipid concentration in predicting future CV events.[81] Based on these findings, recent CVD risk algorithms such as the Reynold's score now include hsCRP levels to better capture inflammation in CV risk but have not been tested in broad populations.[82] In addition to this, it has also been shown that CRP may lead to remodeling of atherosclerotic plaque through stimulation of release of various proinflammatory cytokines such as IL-1, IL-2, and TNF-α from macrophages and foam cells which further leads to plaque destabilization and rupture.[83] Despite these positive characteristics, acute-phase proteins including CRP have been shown to exhibit high intraindividual variability and may vary among genders as well as different ethnicities.[84] Furthermore, the clinical usefulness of CRP in cardiovascular disease has been challenged in utility for CV risk prediction in inflammatory disease conditions such as SLE,[85] psoriasis,[86] RA,[87] and HIV.[88] Despite these limitations, the recent American College of Cardiology/American Heart Association (ACC/AHA) guidelines recommend assessing hsCRP only if the decision remains uncertain after quantitative CV risk assessment in those who are at intermediate risk.[89]

GlycA

Given that hsCRP may not capture the heightened CV risk in inflammatory disease states,[90] novel biomarkers are emerging which may capture both systemic inflammation and risk for CVD. GlycA is a novel composite biomarker comprised of a particular signal in NMR spectra.[91] The GlycA Nuclear magnetic resonance (NMR) spectra arise largely from the N-acetyl glucosamine residues on the glycan portions of acute-phase proteins including alpha 1-acid glycoprotein (orosomucoid), haptoglobin, alpha1-antitrypsin, and alpha1-antichymotrypsin.[91,92] Neutrophils may be a potential source of GlycA beyond the liver.[92] GlycA is higher in patients with febrile illnesses, as well as chronic inflammatory disease states due to glycan formation augmented during inflammation along with acute-phase proteins.[92] Furthermore, GlycA is positively correlated with cardiometabolic risk factors such as body mass index, insulin resistance, and markers of metabolic syndrome in DM[93] and chronic inflammatory states.[94] In large cohort studies, GlycA has been associated with the presence of coronary artery disease defined as at least one coronary artery with significant stenosis[95] as well as prospective CV events independent of traditional CV risk factors.[96] Furthermore, GlycA has also been shown to be a robust biomarker for prediction of CV disease in type-2 DM, as well as risk of progression to incident type-2 DM.[97] GlycA may better highlight systemic inflammation and may not exhibit high intraindividual variability compared with hsCRP.[91] Indeed, GlycA is higher in patients with inflammatory conditions such as RA, SLE, and psoriasis.[94,98–100] For example, in psoriasis, a chronic inflammatory skin disease, GlycA predicted not only skin disease activity but also subclinical cardiovascular disease assessed by aortic vascular inflammation and noncalcified coronary plaque burden beyond hsCRP.[94] Although less than a decade old, GlycA may represent a reliable emerging inflammatory biomarker of CV risk in patients with inflammatory diseases, but more outcome studies are needed to understand risk discrimination.

In addition to this, the modulation of blood inflammatory markers in response to therapy has been shown in the past. Treatment with statins and lifestyle changes reduces hsCRP and incident CV events,[11] whereas GlycA levels decreased in response to biologic therapy for psoriasis.[94,100] Thus these may be markers of potential value in the future to monitor therapy.

FUTURE DIRECTIONS

Within the realm of CVD, several biomarkers will emerge in the future, and it is important that systematic characterization of biomarkers after rigorous interventional studies be performed. Recently the CANTOS trial demonstrated that in patients with a history of MI, antiinflammatory therapy with canakinumab (anti IL-1B) reduced the incidence of subsequent adverse CV events independent of lipid levels.[14] Only one in three patients responded. In those who responded, they had higher baseline hsCRP levels suggesting that inflammatory biomarkers more specific than hsCRP may better capture vascular risk.

CONCLUSION

Inflammation is a critical link between CVD, traditional risk factors, and atherosclerosis. How we use measurement of inflammation will certainly impact how we target antiinflammatory therapies for CVD. Established and emerging blood biomarkers identify patients at higher risk for CVD; however, their modulation after effective CV treatment is not well understood.

DISCLOSURES

Authors have no disclosures except Dr. Mehta who is a full-time US Government Employee and receives research grants to the NHLBI from AbbVie, Janssen, Celgene, and Novartis.

REFERENCES

1. Benjamin EJ, Blaha MJ, Chiuve SE, et al. Heart disease and stroke statistics-2017 update: a report from the American heart association. *Circulation.* 2017;135(10): e146–e603.
2. Libby P, Ridker PM, Hansson GK. Progress and challenges in translating the biology of atherosclerosis. *Nature.* 2011;473(7347):317–325.
3. Libby P, Lichtman AH, Hansson GK. Immune effector mechanisms implicated in atherosclerosis: from mice to humans. *Immunity.* 2013;38(6):1092–1104.
4. Hansson GK. Inflammatory mechanisms in atherosclerosis. *J Thromb Haemost.* 2009;7(Suppl. 1):328–331.
5. Buja LM, Nikolai N. Anitschkow and the lipid hypothesis of atherosclerosis. *Cardiovasc Pathol.* 2014;23(3): 183–184.
6. Ait-Oufella H, Taleb S, Mallat Z, Tedgui A. Recent advances on the role of cytokines in atherosclerosis. *Arterioscler Thromb Vasc Biol.* 2011;31(5):969–979.
7. Hansson GK, Hermansson A. The immune system in atherosclerosis. *Nat Immunol.* 2011;12(3):204–212.
8. Andersson J, Libby P, Hansson GK. Adaptive immunity and atherosclerosis. *Clin Immunol.* 2010;134(1): 33–46.
9. Ridker PM, Stampfer MJ, Rifai N. Novel risk factors for systemic atherosclerosis: a comparison of C-reactive protein, fibrinogen, homocysteine, lipoprotein(a), and standard cholesterol screening as predictors of peripheral arterial disease. *JAMA.* 2001;285(19):2481–2485.
10. Sattar N, Murray HM, Welsh P, et al. Are markers of inflammation more strongly associated with risk for fatal than for nonfatal vascular events? *PLoS Med.* 2009;6(6):e1000099.

11. Ridker PM, Danielson E, Fonseca FA, et al. Rosuvastatin to prevent vascular events in men and women with elevated C-reactive protein. *N Engl J Med.* 2008;359(21):2195–2207.

12. Boekholdt SM, Hack CE, Sandhu MS, et al. C-reactive protein levels and coronary artery disease incidence and mortality in apparently healthy men and women: the EPIC-Norfolk prospective population study 1993-2003. *Atherosclerosis.* 2006;187(2):415–422.

13. Downs JR, Clearfield M, Weis S, et al. Primary prevention of acute coronary events with lovastatin in men and women with average cholesterol levels: results of AFCAPS/TexCAPS. Air Force/Texas Coronary Atherosclerosis Prevention Study. *JAMA.* 1998;279(20):1615–1622.

14. Ridker PM, Everett BM, Thuren T, et al. Antiinflammatory therapy with canakinumab for atherosclerotic disease. *N Engl J Med.* 2017;377(12):1119–1131.

15. Mason JC, Libby P. Cardiovascular disease in patients with chronic inflammation: mechanisms underlying premature cardiovascular events in rheumatologic conditions. *Eur Heart J.* 2015;36(8):482–489.

16. Ogdie A, Yu Y, Haynes K, et al. Risk of major cardiovascular events in patients with psoriatic arthritis, psoriasis and rheumatoid arthritis: a population-based cohort study. *Ann Rheum Dis.* 2015;74(2):326–332.

17. Gelfand JM, Neimann AL, Shin DB, Wang X, Margolis DJ, Troxel AB. Risk of myocardial infarction in patients with psoriasis. *JAMA.* 2006;296(14):1735–1741.

18. Naik HB, Natarajan B, Stansky E, et al. Severity of psoriasis associates with aortic vascular inflammation detected by FDG PET/CT and neutrophil activation in a prospective observational study. *Arterioscler Thromb Vasc Biol.* 2015;35(12):2667–2676.

19. Mehta NN, Yu Y, Saboury B, et al. Systemic and vascular inflammation in patients with moderate to severe psoriasis as measured by [18F]-fluorodeoxyglucose positron emission tomography-computed tomography (FDG-PET/CT): a pilot study. *Arch Dermatol.* 2011;147(9):1031–1039.

20. Dey AK, Joshi AA, Chaturvedi A, et al. Association between skin and aortic vascular inflammation in patients with psoriasis: a case-cohort study using positron emission tomography/computed tomography. *JAMA Cardiol.* 2017;2(9):1013–1018.

21. Lerman JB, Joshi AA, Chaturvedi A, et al. Coronary plaque characterization in psoriasis reveals high-risk features that improve after treatment in a prospective observational study. *Circulation.* 2017;136(3):263–276.

22. Beckman JA, Creager MA, Libby P. Diabetes and atherosclerosis: epidemiology, pathophysiology, and management. *JAMA.* 2002;287(19):2570–2581.

23. Kaplan MJ. Premature vascular damage in systemic lupus erythematosus. *Autoimmunity.* 2009;42(7):580–586.

24. Wilson PW, D'Agostino RB, Levy D, Belanger AM, Silbershatz H, Kannel WB. Prediction of coronary heart disease using risk factor categories. *Circulation.* 1998;97(18):1837–1847.

25. Shah T, Casas JP, Cooper JA, et al. Critical appraisal of CRP measurement for the prediction of coronary heart disease events: new data and systematic review of 31 prospective cohorts. *Int J Epidemiol.* 2009;38(1):217–231.

26. Jou JM, Lewis SM, Briggs C, et al. ICSH review of the measurement of the erythrocyte sedimentation rate. *Int J Lab Hematol.* 2011;33(2):125–132.

27. Erikssen G, Liestol K, Bjornholt JV, Stormorken H, Thaulow E, Erikssen J. Erythrocyte sedimentation rate: a possible marker of atherosclerosis and a strong predictor of coronary heart disease mortality. *Eur Heart J.* 2000;21(19):1614–1620.

28. Reinhart WH. [Erythrocyte sedimentation rate–more than an old fashion?]. *Ther Umsch.* 2006;63(1):108–112.

29. Jurado RL. Why shouldn't we determine the erythrocyte sedimentation rate? *Clin Infect Dis.* 2001;33(4):548–549.

30. Ikeda Y, Handa M, Kawano K, et al. The role of von Willebrand factor and fibrinogen in platelet aggregation under varying shear stress. *J Clin Invest.* 1991;87(4):1234–1240.

31. Folsom AR, Wu KK, Rosamond WD, Sharrett AR, Chambless LE. Prospective study of hemostatic factors and incidence of coronary heart disease: the Atherosclerosis Risk in Communities (ARIC) Study. *Circulation.* 1997;96(4):1102–1108.

32. Levenson J, Giral P, Razavian M, Gariepy J, Simon A. Fibrinogen and silent atherosclerosis in subjects with cardiovascular risk factors. *Arterioscler Thromb Vasc Biol.* 1995;15(9):1263–1268.

33. Kannel WB, Wolf PA, Castelli WP, D'Agostino RB. Fibrinogen and risk of cardiovascular disease. The Framingham Study. *JAMA.* 1987;258(9):1183–1186.

34. Ndrepepa G, Braun S, King L, et al. Relation of fibrinogen level with cardiovascular events in patients with coronary artery disease. *Am J Cardiol.* 2013;111(6):804–810.

35. Appiah D, Schreiner PJ, MacLehose RF, Folsom AR. Association of plasma gamma' fibrinogen with incident cardiovascular disease: the atherosclerosis risk in Communities (ARIC) study. *Arterioscler Thromb Vasc Biol.* 2015;35(12):2700–2706.

36. Gillum RF, Ingram DD, Makuc DM. White blood cell count, coronary heart disease, and death: the NHANES I epidemiologic follow-up Study. *Am Heart J.* 1993;125(3):855–863.

37. Brown DW, Giles WH, Croft JB. White blood cell count: an independent predictor of coronary heart disease mortality among a national cohort. *J Clin Epidemiol.* 2001;54(3):316–322.

38. Cannon CP, McCabe CH, Wilcox RG, Bentley JH, Braunwald E. Association of white blood cell count with increased mortality in acute myocardial infarction and unstable angina pectoris. OPUS-TIMI 16 investigators. *Am J Cardiol.* 2001;87(5):636–639. A610.

39. Gillum RF, Mussolino ME, Madans JH. Counts of neutrophils, lymphocytes, and monocytes, cause-specific mortality and coronary heart disease: the NHANES-I epidemiologic follow-up study. *Ann Epidemiol.* 2005;15(4):266–271.

40. Horne BD, Anderson JL, John JM, et al. Which white blood cell subtypes predict increased cardiovascular risk? *J Am Coll Cardiol*. 2005;45(10):1638–1643.

41. Ghattas A, Griffiths HR, Devitt A, Lip GY, Shantsila E. Monocytes in coronary artery disease and atherosclerosis: where are we now? *J Am Coll Cardiol*. 2013;62(17): 1541–1551.

42. Moore KJ, Tabas I. Macrophages in the pathogenesis of atherosclerosis. *Cell*. 2011;145(3):341–355.

43. Drechsler M, Megens RT, van Zandvoort M, Weber C, Soehnlein O. Hyperlipidemia-triggered neutrophilia promotes early atherosclerosis. *Circulation*. 2010;122(18): 1837–1845.

44. Soehnlein O. Multiple roles for neutrophils in atherosclerosis. *Circ Res*. 2012;110(6):875–888.

45. Kaplan MJ, Radic M. Neutrophil extracellular traps: double-edged swords of innate immunity. *J Immunol*. 2012;189(6):2689–2695.

46. Sanda GE, Belur AD, Teague HL, Mehta NN. Emerging associations between neutrophils, atherosclerosis, and psoriasis. *Curr Atheroscler Rep*. 2017;19(12):53.

47. Ridker PM. High-sensitivity C-reactive protein, inflammation, and cardiovascular risk: from concept to clinical practice to clinical benefit. *Am Heart J*. 2004;148 (Suppl. 1):S19–S26.

48. Cannon PJ, Stason WB, Demartini FE, Sommers SC, Laragh JH. Hyperuricemia in primary and renal hypertension. *N Engl J Med*. 1966;275(9):457–464.

49. Lee JJ, Ahn J, Hwang J, et al. Relationship between uric acid and blood pressure in different age groups. *Clin Hypertens*. 2015;21:14.

50. Zalawadiya SK, Veeranna V, Mallikethi-Reddy S, et al. Uric acid and cardiovascular disease risk reclassification: findings from NHANES III. *Eur J Prev Cardiol*. 2015;22(4):513–518.

51. Uhlar CM, Whitehead AS. Serum amyloid A, the major vertebrate acute-phase reactant. *Eur J Biochem*. 1999;265(2):501–523.

52. Marzi C, Huth C, Herder C, et al. Acute-phase serum amyloid A protein and its implication in the development of type 2 diabetes in the KORA S4/F4 study. *Diabetes Care*. 2013;36(5):1321–1326.

53. Vallon R, Freuler F, Desta-Tsedu N, et al. Serum amyloid A (apoSAA) expression is up-regulated in rheumatoid arthritis and induces transcription of matrix metalloproteinases. *J Immunol*. 2001;166(4):2801–2807.

54. Wilson PG, Thompson JC, Webb NR, de Beer FC, King VL, Tannock LR. Serum amyloid A, but not C-reactive protein, stimulates vascular proteoglycan synthesis in a pro-atherogenic manner. *Am J Pathol*. 2008;173(6):1902–1910.

55. Ye RD, Sun L. Emerging functions of serum amyloid A in inflammation. *J Leukoc Biol*. 2015;98(6):923–929.

56. King VL, Thompson J, Tannock LR. Serum amyloid A in atherosclerosis. *Curr Opin Lipidol*. 2011;22(4):302–307.

57. O'Brien KD, McDonald TO, Kunjathoor V, et al. Serum amyloid A and lipoprotein retention in murine models of atherosclerosis. *Arterioscler Thromb Vasc Biol*. 2005;25(4):785–790.

58. Zewinger S, Drechsler C, Kleber ME, et al. Serum amyloid A: high-density lipoproteins interaction and cardiovascular risk. *Eur Heart J*. 2015;36(43):3007–3016.

59. Lackie J, Cytokines. In.

60. Zhang H, Park Y, Wu J, et al. Role of TNF-alpha in vascular dysfunction. *Clin Sci (Lond)*. 2009;116(3):219–230.

61. Schreyer SA, Peschon JJ, LeBoeuf RC. Accelerated atherosclerosis in mice lacking tumor necrosis factor receptor p55. *J Biol Chem*. 1996;271(42):26174–26178.

62. Rieckmann P, Tuscano JM, Kehrl JH. Tumor necrosis factor-alpha (TNF-alpha) and interleukin-6 (IL-6) in B-lymphocyte function. *Methods*. 1997;11(1):128–132.

63. Blake GJ, Ridker PM. Inflammatory bio-markers and cardiovascular risk prediction. *J Intern Med*. 2002;252(4): 283–294.

64. Berda-Haddad Y, Robert S, Salers P, et al. Sterile inflammation of endothelial cell-derived apoptotic bodies is mediated by interleukin-1alpha. *Proc Natl Acad Sci USA*. 2011;108(51):20684–20689.

65. Dinarello CA, Ikejima T, Warner SJ, et al. Interleukin 1 induces interleukin 1. I. Induction of circulating interleukin 1 in rabbits in vivo and in human mononuclear cells in vitro. *J Immunol*. 1987;139(6):1902–1910.

66. Martinon F, Mayor A, Tschopp J. The inflammasomes: guardians of the body. *Annu Rev Immunol*. 2009;27: 229–265.

67. Rader DJ. IL-1 and atherosclerosis: a murine twist to an evolving human story. *J Clin Invest*. 2012;122(1):27–30.

68. Gerard C, Rollins BJ. Chemokines and disease. *Nat Immunol*. 2001;2(2):108–115.

69. Gonzalez-Quesada C, Frangogiannis NG. Monocyte chemoattractant protein-1/CCL2 as a biomarker in acute coronary syndromes. *Curr Atheroscler Rep*. 2009;11(2):131–138.

70. Coll B, Alonso-Villaverde C, Joven J. Monocyte chemoattractant protein-1 and atherosclerosis: is there room for an additional biomarker? *Clin Chim Acta*. 2007; 383(1–2):21–29.

71. Yu X, Dluz S, Graves DT, et al. Elevated expression of monocyte chemoattractant protein 1 by vascular smooth muscle cells in hypercholesterolemic primates. *Proc Natl Acad Sci USA*. 1992;89(15):6953–6957.

72. Zungsontiporn N, Tello RR, Zhang G, et al. Non-classical monocytes and monocyte chemoattractant Protein-1 (MCP-1) correlate with coronary artery calcium progression in chronically HIV-1 infected adults on stable antiretroviral therapy. *PLoS One*. 2016;11(2):e0149143.

73. Jude EB, Douglas JT, Anderson SG, Young MJ, Boulton AJ. Circulating cellular adhesion molecules ICAM-1, VCAM-1, P- and E-selectin in the prediction of cardiovascular disease in diabetes mellitus. *Eur J Intern Med*. 2002;13(3):185–189.

74. Ridker PM, Buring JE, Rifai N. Soluble P-selectin and the risk of future cardiovascular events. *Circulation*. 2001;103(4):491–495.

75. Malik I, Danesh J, Whincup P, et al. Soluble adhesion molecules and prediction of coronary heart disease: a prospective study and meta-analysis. *Lancet*. 2001;358(9286):971–976.

76. Blankenberg S, Rupprecht HJ, Bickel C, et al. Circulating cell adhesion molecules and death in patients with coronary artery disease. *Circulation.* 2001;104(12): 1336–1342.

77. Yousuf O, Mohanty BD, Martin SS, et al. High-sensitivity C-reactive protein and cardiovascular disease: a resolute belief or an elusive link? *J Am Coll Cardiol.* 2013;62(5):397–408.

78. Casas JP, Shah T, Hingorani AD, Danesh J, Pepys MB. C-reactive protein and coronary heart disease: a critical review. *J Intern Med.* 2008;264(4):295–314.

79. Greenland P, Alpert JS, Beller GA, et al. 2010 ACCF/AHA guideline for assessment of cardiovascular risk in asymptomatic adults: executive summary: a report of the American College of Cardiology Foundation/American heart association task force on practice guidelines. *Circulation.* 2010;122(25):2748–2764.

80. Ridker PM, Hennekens CH, Buring JE, Rifai N. C-reactive protein and other markers of inflammation in the prediction of cardiovascular disease in women. *N Engl J Med.* 2000;342(12):836–843.

81. Corrado E, Novo S. Evaluation of C-reactive protein in primary and secondary prevention. *J Investig Med.* 2007;55(8):430–438.

82. Cook NR, Paynter NP, Eaton CB, et al. Comparison of the Framingham and Reynolds Risk scores for global cardiovascular risk prediction in the multiethnic Women's Health Initiative. *Circulation.* 2012;125(14):1748–1756. S1741-1711.

83. Calabro P, Golia E, Yeh ET. Role of C-reactive protein in acute myocardial infarction and stroke: possible therapeutic approaches. *Curr Pharm Biotechnol.* 2012; 13(1):4–16.

84. Clark GH, Fraser CG. Biological variation of acute phase proteins. *Ann Clin Biochem.* 1993;30(Pt 4):373–376.

85. Kay SD, Poulsen MK, Diederichsen AC, Voss A. Coronary, carotid, and lower-extremity atherosclerosis and their interrelationship in Danish patients with systemic lupus erythematosus. *J Rheumatol.* 2016;43(2): 315–322.

86. Staniak HL, Bittencourt MS, de Souza Santos I, et al. Association between psoriasis and coronary calcium score. *Atherosclerosis.* 2014;237(2):847–852.

87. Emami H, Vijayakumar J, Subramanian S, et al. Arterial 18F-FDG uptake in rheumatoid arthritis correlates with synovial activity. *JACC Cardiovasc Imaging.* 2014;7(9):959–960.

88. Subramanian S, Tawakol A, Burdo TH, et al. Arterial inflammation in patients with HIV. *JAMA.* 2012;308(4):379–386.

89. Goff Jr DC, Lloyd-Jones DM, Bennett G, et al. 2013 ACC/AHA guideline on the assessment of cardiovascular risk: a report of the American College of Cardiology/American heart association task force on practice guidelines. *J Am Coll Cardiol.* 2014;63(25 Pt B):2935–2959.

90. Alemao E, Cawston H, Bourhis F, et al. Comparison of cardiovascular risk algorithms in patients with vs without rheumatoid arthritis and the role of C-reactive protein in predicting cardiovascular outcomes in rheumatoid arthritis. *Rheumatol Oxf.* 2017;56(5):777–786.

91. Otvos JD, Shalaurova I, Wolak-Dinsmore J, et al. GlycA: a composite nuclear magnetic resonance biomarker of systemic inflammation. *Clin Chem.* 2015;61(5):714–723.

92. Ritchie SC, Wurtz P, Nath AP, et al. The biomarker GlycA is associated with chronic inflammation and predicts long-term risk of severe infection. *Cell Syst.* 2015;1(4):293–301.

93. Lorenzo C, Festa A, Hanley AJ, Rewers MJ, Escalante A, Haffner SM. Novel protein glycan-derived markers of systemic inflammation and C-Reactive protein in relation to glycemia, insulin resistance, and insulin secretion. *Diabetes Care.* 2017;40(3):375–382.

94. Joshi AA, Lerman JB, Aberra TM, et al. GlycA is a novel biomarker of inflammation and subclinical cardiovascular disease in psoriasis. *Circ Res.* 2016;119(11):1242–1253.

95. McGarrah RW, Kelly JP, Craig DM, et al. A novel protein glycan-derived inflammation biomarker independently predicts cardiovascular disease and modifies the association of HDL subclasses with mortality. *Clin Chem.* 2017;63(1):288–296.

96. Akinkuolie AO, Buring JE, Ridker PM, Mora S. A novel protein glycan biomarker and future cardiovascular disease events. *J Am Heart Assoc.* 2014;3(5):e001221.

97. Connelly MA, Gruppen EG, Wolak-Dinsmore J, et al. GlycA, a marker of acute phase glycoproteins, and the risk of incident type 2 diabetes mellitus: PREVEND study. *Clin Chim Acta.* 2016;452:10–17.

98. Ormseth MJ, Chung CP, Oeser AM, et al. Utility of a novel inflammatory marker, GlycA, for assessment of rheumatoid arthritis disease activity and coronary atherosclerosis. *Arthritis Res Ther.* 2015;17:117.

99. Durcan L, Winegar DA, Connelly MA, Otvos JD, Magder LS, Petri M. Longitudinal evaluation of lipoprotein variables in systemic lupus erythematosus reveals adverse changes with disease activity and prednisone and more favorable profiles with hydroxychloroquine therapy. *J Rheumatol.* 2016;43(4):745–750.

100. Connelly MA, Otvos JD, Shalaurova I, Playford MP, Mehta NN. GlycA, a novel biomarker of systemic inflammation and cardiovascular disease risk. *J Transl Med.* 2017;15(1):219.

CHAPTER 8

Cardiac Injury, Maladaptation, and Heart Failure Incidence

M. WESLEY MILKS, MD • VIJAY NAMBI, MD, PHD

INTRODUCTION

Heart failure (HF) is a complex clinical syndrome that results from impairment in ventricular filling or ejection. Dyspnea, fatigue, exercise intolerance, fluid retention, and congestion of the splanchnic and/or pulmonary vasculature, each manifests to a variable degree in a given individual.[1] HF affects approximately 5.8 million people in the United States, with an annual incidence of at least 550,000 and lifetime risk of approximately 20%.[2,3] Although certain HF syndromes may result from pericardial, endocardial, valvular, or great vessel disease, the majority of HF is attributed to impairment in left ventricular (LV) myocardial function.[1]

Historically, HF has been diagnosed and managed after the development of symptoms, but in doing so, identification of pivotal opportunities for disease prevention and modification of the natural pathophysiologic history may have been missed. Medicine continues to undergo a paradigm shift away from diagnosis to one of prediction, prevention, and early disease interruption.[1] To emphasize the preclinical spectrum of HF, the American College of Cardiology and American Heart Association proposed that "stage A" HF be defined as the presence of certain risk factors, such as diabetes mellitus and hypertension, without manifesting myocardial dysfunction.[2]

Various modalities continue to be explored to further stratify the risk of incident HF among individuals with risk factors, so that efforts such as targeted lifestyle or medical intervention can be evaluated in those who would derive the greatest benefit. Imaging assessments of subclinical myocardial dysfunction are developing rapidly. Myocardial strain imaging using speckle tracking echocardiography[4,5] has demonstrated tremendous promise in identifying the onset of myocardial disease among entities such as cancer therapeutics–related cardiac dysfunction,[6–12] aortic stenosis,[13] and hypertrophic cardiomyopathy,[14] examples of disease states which in early stages may involve myocardial dysfunction in the absence of clinical HF. Cardiovascular magnetic resonance imaging techniques such as T1 mapping[15,16] and myocardial feature–tracking strain imaging[17] hold similarly high potential. However, these approaches are not universally applied,[18] and any imaging-based screening modality carries a certain intrinsic cost and labor-intensiveness that may not be appropriate for widespread application to unselected populations.

The use of circulating biomarkers for the prediction of HF is amassing a perpetually expanding body of evidence. Whereas a myriad of substances are associated with incident HF, several leading entities have most closely approached the criteria of an ideal clinically useful biomarker, including the ability to provide predictive information not otherwise available and to undergo accurate, expeditious, and repeatable measurement at a reasonable cost.[19] Although short of an exhaustive list, this chapter will summarize the pathophysiologic basis and application of certain leading key biomarkers for the prediction of incident HF, several of which are depicted (Fig. 8.1).

THE ROLE OF STAGE A HF RISK FACTORS IN PATHOPHYSIOLOGY

While historically diagnosed only when LV dysfunction is present, HF was further defined in 2005 to encompass stage A disease, which represents risk factors for HF in the absence of known myocardial dysfunction or HF symptoms.[20] The principal risk factors identified to qualify as stage A HF include the presence of hypertension, atherosclerotic disease, diabetes mellitus, obesity, metabolic syndrome, potentially cardiotoxic chemical (e.g., chemotherapeutic) exposures, or a family history of cardiomyopathy.[20] In addition, incident HF exhibits a powerful age dependency, with incidence of 1.4/1000 person-years in individuals aged 55–59 years versus 47.4/1000 person-years in those aged ≥90 years.[21] Considering the implications for disease prevention or attenuation, this section will review the relationship between HF and several important modifiable risk factors.

Biomarkers in Cardiovascular Disease. https://doi.org/10.1016/B978-0-323-54835-9.00008-9

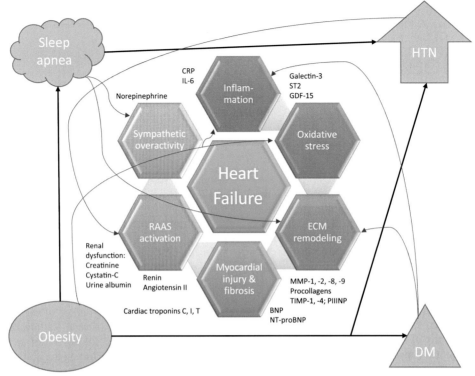

FIG. 8.1 Relationship between several modifiable risk factors, heart failure pathophysiology, and established or potential biomarkers [Original–Milks]. *BNP*, B-type natriuretic peptide; *CRP*, C-reactive protein; *DM*, diabetes mellitus; *GDF-15*, growth differentiation factor 15; *HTN*, hypertension; *IL*, interleukin; *MMP*, matrix metalloproteinase; *NT-proBNP*, amino-terminal proBNP; *RAAS*, renin-angiotensin-aldosterone system; *ST2*, suppressor of tumorgenicity 2; *TIMP*, tissue inhibitor of matrix metalloproteinase.

Diabetes Mellitus

Being a well-recognized, potent risk factor for atherosclerotic cardiovascular disease, diabetes mellitus (DM) is also associated with risk of HF far beyond that mediated by macrovascular events.[22] Most epidemiologic data support an age-adjusted hazard ratio (HR) between 1.2 and 1.7 for HF in those with prediabetes or diabetes,[23,24] with manifestation of DM conferring greater risk compared to prediabetes. In the Heart and Soul study of patients with stable coronary artery disease (CAD) and no baseline HF, the presence of DM was associated with a doubling of HF risk.[25]

The mechanism of HF risk not mediated by epicardial CAD events in DM has been the subject of intensive study. First of all it is well recognized that the myocardium exhibits hypertrophy and extracellular volume (ECV) expansion resulting from fibrosis, with collagen deposition, and possibly from triglyceride accumulation.[26] In fact, the degree of ECV expansion has exhibited an association with incident HF admissions and mortality.[27] Second, insulin resistance itself has been shown in experimental models to exacerbate myocyte hypertrophy and systolic dysfunction in DM[28]; cardiomyocytes are poorly adapted to store large amounts of lipid compounds.[22] The imbalance in bioenergetics with nutrient excess is depicted in Fig. 8.2. Third, signaling by the family of pattern recognition receptors that recognize advanced glycation end products leads to inflammatory signaling pathways and immune cell infiltration, such as via protein kinase C and nuclear factor-light-chain-enhancer of activated B cells (NF-κB).[29]

The debated term "diabetic cardiomyopathy" was introduced by Rubler et al. in the 1972 description of 27 patients with diabetic glomerulosclerosis and concurrent LV hypertrophy, fibrosis, and microangiopathy.[30] Regardless of whether diabetic cardiomyopathy should be recognized as its own entity, it is clear that myocyte hypertrophy, fibrosis, microcirculatory damage, inflammation, and extracellular matrix (ECM) remodeling are common final pathways in the diabetic heart which promote HF pathogenesis.

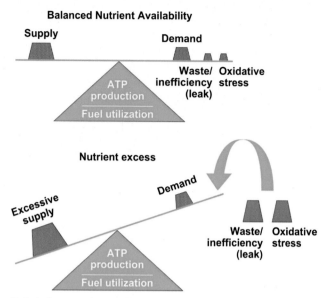

FIG. 8.2 Bioenergetic imbalance under conditions of nutrient excess. (From the study by Lehrke M and Marx N. Diabetes mellitus and heart failure. *Am J Cardiol*. 2017;120(1S):S37–S47.)[22] ATP, adenosine triphosphate.

Hypertension

Hypertension is a well-established HF risk factor, conferring a twofold to threefold increase in risk compared to normotensive individuals, as supported by data from the Framingham Heart Study (FHS).[31] Although conceptualized in a basic sense as a pure state of excessive afterload,[32] the details of the pathophysiologic relationship between hypertension and HF continues to be elucidated.[33] Arterial hypertension leads to coronary arteriolar constriction, myocardial ischemia, and endothelial dysfunction,[33] and changes in myocardial capillary density and arteriolar wall thickness may worsen ischemia. As a result of stress on the ECM, vascular smooth muscle hypertrophy and fibroblast hyperplasia ensue, leading to interstitial expansion and collagen deposition.[33–35] These compensatory mechanisms reduce ventricular wall stress in the short term,[36] which has been considered as a basis for their existence; however, progressive hypertrophy is clearly detrimental.[37]

On a multiorgan level, first of all, it is clear that sympathetic overactivity characterizes both hypertension and HF. The work by Hasking et al. highlighted the commonality of norepinephrine overproduction in both the heart and the kidneys[38] and the degree of sympathetic activity have been linked to worse HF outcomes in multiple studies.[39,40] Second, increased activity of the renin-angiotensin-aldosterone system (RAAS) serves as another central example of the unified nature of hypertension and HF pathophysiology. ATII exhibits

vasoconstrictor effects on multiple sites, including on subendocardial myocytes, contributing to ischemia, remodeling, and fibrosis.[33,41]

The high degree of population penetrance and potential for effective treatment make hypertension a prime target for amelioration of HF and other cardiovascular risk. Considering that (between 115/75 mmHg and 180/105 mmHg) each 20 mmHg increase in systolic or 10 mmHg increase in diastolic blood pressure (BP) results in a doubling of the risk of fatal CVD, current guidelines now recommend antihypertensive treatment when BP is at least 130/80 mmHg in individuals at 10-year atherosclerotic cardiovascular disease risk exceeding 10%.[42]

Obesity and Sleep-Disordered Breathing

Obesity is defined as a body mass index (BMI) of 30.0 kg/m² or greater, and class III obesity (BMI ≥ 40 kg/m²) in particular has been identified as an HF risk factor independent of comorbidities such as hypertension or CAD.[43,44] Data from the FHS support a 5% (men) to 7% (women) increase in HF risk for every 1 kg/m² increase in BMI, after adjustment for traditional risk factors.[43] Interestingly, individuals with HF who are overweight or have class I obesity (BMI 30.0–34.9 kg/m²) have a decreased risk of all-cause mortality in comparison with normal or underweight (BMI < 18.5 kg/m²) people.[45–47] This "obesity paradox" has been posited to exist due to a variety of factors including the

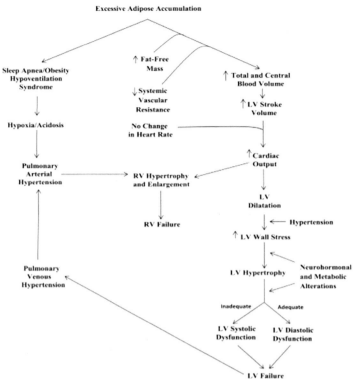

FIG. 8.3 Pathophysiology of obesity cardiomyopathy. (From the study by Alpert M.A., Lavie CJ, Agrawal H, Aggarwal KB, Kumar SA. Obesity and heart failure: epidemiology, pathophysiology, clinical manifestations, and management. *Transl Res.* 2014;164(4):345–356; Alpert MA. Obesity cardiomyopathy: pathophysiology and evolution of the clinical syndrome. *Am J Med Sci.* 2001;321(4):225–236). *LV,* left ventricular. *RV,* right ventricular.

unintended weight loss of catabolic diseases as well as covariate processes such as younger age at presentation underlying more severe disease (given a relationship between age and BMI), presence of smoking (inversely associated with obesity), and potential for successful medical treatment (given a relationship between BP and BMI).[48,49]

The pathophysiologic relationship between obesity and HF has been studied extensively and is depicted in Fig. 8.3. In a fundamental sense, obesity represents an excess cardiac workload as cardiac output increases in proportion to excess body weight.[50] LV mass is increased in obesity, particularly with concurrent hypertension,[51] although impairment in diastolic function may occur in obese patients in the absence of LV hypertrophy.[52] In the initial postmortem description in 1933, it was recognized that epicardial fat is increased in obesity, whereas the myocardial fat visible histologically did not significantly differ between obese and normal

weight individuals.[53] However, recently the concept of lipotoxicity has been introduced, whereby excess free fatty acids and triglycerides accumulate within cardiomyocytes in obesity.[54] Lipotoxic cardiomyopathy appears to be mediated in part by overexpression of acyl Co-A synthetase, a process that is attenuated by leptin and peroxisome proliferator-activated receptor gamma (PPAR-γ) agonists such as troglitazone.[55,56] Oxidation and inflammatory pathways driven by lipotoxicity eventually lead to increased ventricular wall stress and myocardial dysfunction.

The relationship between obesity and sleep-disordered breathing reveals important pathophysiologic pathways.[57] Obesity is a potent risk factor for obstructive sleep apnea (OSA), and OSA appears to exacerbate the degree of metabolic dysfunction in obesity.[58] Up to 35% of patients with HF have OSA, compared to 20% of the general population; however, OSA often remains undiagnosed in HF patients.[59,60]

The periodic hypoxemia and sudden swings of excessive intrathoracic negative pressure increase transmural pressure, afterload, and myocardial oxygen demand.[61] Over time, these events drive ventricular hypertrophy and adverse cardiac remodeling.[62] Clearly, obesity is associated with OSA, while each factor exhibits an independent contribution to HF pathogenesis.

COMPONENTS OF ADAPTATION AND MALADAPTATION IN HF AND THEIR POTENTIAL FOR USE AS BIOMARKERS

The risk factors examined previously contribute to multiple interrelated downstream pathophysiologic pathways resulting in cardiac dysfunction (Fig. 8.1). Several key axes of HF pathogenesis will be examined.

THE AUTONOMIC NERVOUS SYSTEM AND NEUROHORMONES

Neurohormonal signaling patterns are thought to possess a teleological basis as responses to intraarterial volume depletion, as can occur with hypotension or blood loss. However, these mechanisms may also be triggered by the state of hypoperfusion associated with HF and when chronically activated can lead to substantial maladaptation.

The Adrenergic and Cholinergic Nervous System

The cardiovascular effects of the adrenergic nervous system (ANS) include augmentation of heart rate (chronotropy), contractility (inotropy), and relaxation (lusitropy) while reducing the capacitance of the central venous system and constricting cutaneous vasculature. Such actions, mediated via the beta adrenergic receptor, make ready the body to utilize reserves of blood volume for the anticipated physiologic responses to stress.[63,64] In a counter-regulatory fashion, the cholinergic (parasympathetic) nervous system, via vagal cholinergic inputs to the atria and peripheral vasculature, can produce bradycardia and hypotension but has relatively little effect on ventricular contractility.[64,65] It has long been recognized that HF is associated with a state of increased catecholamine release[66]; generally, chronic beta adrenoceptor overstimulation is felt to underlie the pathophysiology of HF, whereas alpha adrenoceptor activity appears to have protective effects.[67] Direct measurement of plasma norepinephrine (NE) is a crude measure of ANS activity and is confounded by not only the rate of immediate NE release and reuptake but also by the rate of clearance from the circulation.[68] Cardiac-specific

adrenergic neuronal activity can be assessed using the radiolabeled NE analog ^{123}I-metaiodobenzylguanine,[69] which has been applied to patients with HF.[70]

Arguably one of the earliest classes of biomarkers in HF to be described,[66] adrenergic hyperactivity is recognized to be both a marker as well as a maladaptation to cardiac dysfunction. Excess circulating catecholamines may participate in the pathogenesis of HF, as suggested by the increased incidence of HF among patients with Parkinson's disease taking the non–ergot-derived dopamine agonist pramipexole.[71] In a cohort of individuals with end-stage renal disease free of HF at baseline, plasma NE was more strongly associated with incident adverse cardiovascular events than atrial natriuretic peptide.[72] As plasma NE chronically exceeds the upper limit of normal in >40% of patients receiving hemodialysis,[73] adrenergic overstimulation may play an especially important role in the development of cardiac dysfunction among those with advanced kidney disease.

Renin-Angiotensin-Aldosterone System

The RAAS also exists as an adaptive mechanism to counteract hypovolemia, renin release being triggered by hypoperfusion, as detected by baroreceptors of the renal afferent arteriole and by the macula densa of the distal tubule.[74] The majority of the end-organ effects of this process are mediated by angiotensin II (ATII), the production of which classically has been described via angiotensin-converting enzyme–related conversion of angiotensin I, although tissue-level (including cardiac) production of ATII has also been demonstrated.[74–76] ATII effects systemic and renal arteriolar vasoconstriction, aldosterone release from the adrenal glands, and renal tubular resorption of water and sodium.[74] Early descriptions of plasma renin and overall RAAS augmentation in HF revealed a clear inverse association between perfusion status and RAAS activity.[77]

MARKERS OF MYOCYTE INJURY AND CHAMBER WALL STRESS

Cardiac Troponins

Myocardial contraction occurs at the myofibrillar level by regulated interactions between actin and myosin. Cardiac troponins (cTns) serve various roles in such regulation, including troponin C (cTnC) in calcium binding, troponin I (cTnI) in inhibition, and troponin T (cTnT) in tropomyosin binding.[78] Proteins cTnT and cTnI can be released in patients with HF in the absence of an acute coronary ischemic event or underlying epicardial coronary artery stenosis. Subendocardial

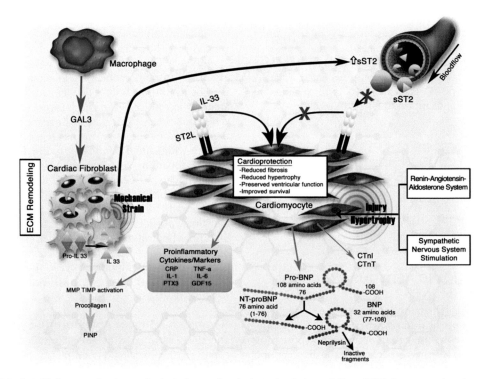

FIG. 8.4 Various mechanisms of adaptation and maladaptation in heart failure. *BNP*, B-type natriuretic peptide; *CRP*, C-reactive protein; *cTn*, cardiac troponin; *ECM*, extracellular matrix; *GAL3*, gelatinase-associated lipocain-3; *GDF-15*, growth differentiation factor 15; *IL*, interleukin; *MMP*, matrix metalloproteinase; *NT-proBNP*, amino-terminal pro -B-type natriuretic peptide; *PINP*, procollagen I intact N-terminal; *PTX3*, pentraxin 3; *sST2*, soluble suppressor of tumorgenicity 2; *ST2L*, ST2 membrane-bound receptor; *TIMP*, tissue inhibitor of matrix metalloproteinase; and *TNF-a*, tumor necrosis factor-alpha. (From the study by Chow SL, Maisel A, Anand I, et al. Role of biomarkers for the prevention, assessment, and management of heart failure: a scientific statement from the American Heart Association. *Circulation.* May 30, 2017;135(122):e1054–e1091.)

ischemia is thought to play a central role in this process.[79] Troponin assays have typically been used as part of the diagnosis of myocardial infarction in the emergency department or hospital. Recently, higher sensitivity cTn assays that have a 10-fold or greater sensitivity have been developed and quantitate the cTn level when it exceeds the 99th percentile of a reference population.[80] High-sensitivity (hs) assays can now quantitate cTn in 50% to greater than 95% of healthy individuals.[81]

cTns are now supported by a robust evidence basis in the prediction of HF.[82] In individuals at risk for HF (stage A HF) or asymptomatic individuals with ventricular dysfunction (stage B HF), cTn is detectable by standard modern assays in 1%–5%[83] and in 50%–80% with hs assays.[84,85] Importantly, elevated (≥0.003 ng/mL) hs-cTnT concentrations have a stronger

association with risk of incident HF (HR 5.95) rather than ischemic events (HR 2.29), as was demonstrated by Saunders et al. in an analysis of the Atherosclerosis Risk in Communities (ARIC) Study (Table 8.1).[85] Similarly, in the Prevention of Events with Angiotensin Converting Enzyme Inhibition (PEACE) trial, elevation of hs-cTnT in a general population with stable CAD was associated with HF and CV death but not with MI.[86] In the Cardiovascular Health Study (CHS), which included adults aged ≥65 years, hs-cTnT was measured at baseline and 2–3 years later; patients with the highest baseline hs-cTnT had the highest risk of incident HF, and there is a stepwise increase in adverse CV events when hs-cTnT exceeds 0.003 ng/mL[84,85,87]. Trends among repeated cTn values may carry particularly strong prognostic weight. In the CHS, among individuals with initially detectable hs-cTnT, a subsequent increase of more

TABLE 8.1
Summary of Key Established or Emerging Biomarkers for the Prediction of Heart Failure. Citations present in text

Key Pathway(s)	Biomarker	Example(s) of Predictive Capacity	Additional Comments
Inflammation & oxidative stress	Soluble ST2 (sST2)	sST2 > 26.5 ng/mL: OR 3.0 for acute HF in the emergency department setting	Exhibits less long-term interindividual variability (11%) than the NPs (33%–50%)
	GDF-15	GDF-15: HR 1.5 for each 1-SD increase in log10 units	Extracardiac production is well defined, especially in nonischemic cardiomyopathy
Extracellular matrix remodeling	Galectin-3	Gal-3: for incident HF, HR 1.28 for each 1-SD increase in log10 units	May exhibit less load dependency than NPs and track response to mineralocorticoid receptor antagonism
	Matrix metalloproteinases (MMP) and their tissue inhibitors (TIMP)	MMP-9: HR 3.73 for HF events	"Signature" of MMP and TIMP elevation pattern differs by HF etiology
Myocardial injury & fibrosis	Cardiac troponins: (cTn) C, I, T	hs-cTnT ≥0.003 ng/mL: HR 5.95 for incident HF	Isoforms have variable renal clearance
	Natriuretic peptides (NPs): BNP, NT-proBNP	Increase in NT-proBNP >25% and cTnT>50%: HR 3.56 for HF events	Obesity may affect NP clearance receptors and degradation
Renal dysfunction	Glomerular filtration rate (GFR) and serum creatinine	Each 1-SD decline in GFR: RR 1.24 for HF	In the CHS, serum creatinine >1.4 mg/dL: RR 1.5 for HF prediction
	Urinary albumin-to-creatinine ratio	HR 1.35 per log10 units for incident HF	Offers predictive information complementary to cTn and NPs

than 50% was associated with an increased risk for HF (adjusted HR [aHR] 1.61) and cardiovascular death (aHR 1.65), whereas a decrease of more than 50% was associated with a reduced risk of these outcomes (HF aHR 0.73, cardiovascular death aHR 0.71).[84]

It is noteworthy that cardiac troponin is also associated with other HF risk factors, such as increasing age, hypertension, diabetes, chronic renal failure, and LV hypertrophy.[83,88] Troponin elevation in kidney disease is particularly complex given that different cTn isoforms may demonstrate variable renal clearance, with cTnT felt to exhibit more dependence on renal clearance than cTnI, and that there is heterogeneity in renal clearance among different breakdown fragments of each isoform.[82,89,90] Despite some limitations, cardiac troponins remain a cornerstone of the prediction of HF using circulating biomarkers. In addition to de novo HF risk prediction, there is some evidence that trends in cTn values may be reliable for revised predictive estimates in the face of therapeutic lifestyle changes. An analysis of the CHS showed that higher physical activity was associated with reduced odds (odds ratio 0.50 [95% CI 0.33–0.77]) of cTnT increases as well as lower long-term incidence of HF.[91]

Natriuretic Peptides: B-type Natriuretic Peptide and NT-proBNP

B-type natriuretic peptide (BNP) and the amino-terminal cleavage equivalent NT-proBNP are released directly into the circulation from (predominantly ventricular) myocardium as a result of end-diastolic wall stress, in response to increased diastolic pressure.[92] BNP is synthesized in bursts, with the prohormone pre-proBNP being cleaved by proteolytic enzymes furin and corin to result in the formation of NT-proBNP and BNP, both of which can be measured accurately in clinical practice. The downstream adaptive effects of BNP include vasodilatation, natriuresis, and diuresis.[93] BNP and NT-proBNP have half-lives of 20 min and 1–2 h, respectively; BNP is cleared primarily by neutral endopeptidases and natriuretic peptide (NP) receptors, whereas NT-proBNP exhibits predominantly renal clearance.[94] Indeed the renal clearance of NPs has important diagnostic implications in chronic kidney disease. Importantly, marked decreases in measured NPs can be observed with obesity,[95] which has been suggested to relate to alterations in clearance receptors and NP degradation processes.[96,97] Additionally, the HF syndromes not associated with increased ventricular wall stress, such as pericardial constriction or cardiac tamponade, may not produce elevation of NP levels.[93]

The FHS first established NPs as biomarkers in the prediction of incident HF,[98] and multiple subsequent studies have confirmed or expanded on these findings. In an observational analysis of the CHS, adults with initially low biomarker concentrations and baseline risk of HF who exhibited rises in NT-proBNP >25% and cTnT >50% were found to have increased risk for systolic dysfunction, HF events (HR 3.56), and CV death (HR 2.98)[99]. Furthermore, in the 1024 participants of the Heart and Soul study, who had stable coronary heart disease, both BNP (c=0.72) and NT-proBNP (c=0.76) were significant predictors of the composite endpoint of HF hospitalization, nonfatal myocardial infarction, stroke or transient ischemic attack, or CV death.[100] Interestingly the test performance characteristics of NT-proBNP vary with age, and age-related cutoffs of 450 pg/mL for <50 years, 900 pg/mL for 50 -75 years, and 1800 pg/mL > 75 years have been proposed.[101]

Several large metaanalyses have summarized the use of the NPs in the diagnosis of incident HF.[102,103] In individuals presenting with undifferentiated dyspnea, elevated BNP or NT-proBNP demonstrated a sensitivity of 93% for the diagnosis of HF; one group advocates for NP assessment before echocardiography, deferring it if NP levels are normal, in patients without suggestive physical signs such as pulmonary rates or lower extremity edema.[102] BNP and NT-proBNP have shown superiority in their predictive capacity compared with other NPs such as atrial natriuretic peptide (ANP) and NT-proANP.[104]

In summary, the use of cardiac troponins and natriuretic peptides in the prediction of HF are supported by perhaps the most mature body of literature at this point in time. In the ARIC study an elegantly simple "lab report" HF prediction model based only on sex, age, race, hs-cTnT, and NT-proBNP provided most of the predictive capacity (in men, AUC=0.789; in women, AUC=0.767) of an extended model that included both the biomarkers in combination with the clinical variables of heart rate, BP, antihypertensive use, tobacco use, diabetes mellitus, and BMI which are part of the ARIC HF model (in men, c=0.836; in women, c=0.817).[105] Indeed a highly accurate prediction of HF

risk may be generated using easily accessible demographic and laboratory information available at the clinical level.

THE ROLE OF THE ECM
Matrix Metalloproteinases and Their Regulatory Factors

Extensive progress has been achieved in recent years to elucidate the critical role of the ECM not as a passive collagenous ultrastructure that houses cardiomyocytes but rather as an active tissue that demonstrates dynamic participation in both the mechanical and hormonal milieux.[106–108] Indeed, extracellular collagen is a major determinant of physical properties of the myocardium including elasticity and viscosity. Matrix metalloproteinases (MMPs) are a family of proteolytic enzymes that degrade collagen fibrils, and collagen degradation via plasmin-mediated endogenous MMP activation directly affects the elastic properties of the heart.[109]

Mechanistically the nature of the myocardial insult presented dictates the properties of the response by the ECM. With a chronic pressure overload, such as in aortic stenosis or arterial hypertension, collagen accumulation leads to myocardial stiffness, with severity of the disease process proportionate to levels of MMP-2, MMP-9, serum carboxy-terminal telopeptide of procollagen type I, and amino-terminal propeptide of procollagen type III.[110,111] The pattern of fibrosis and collagen volume fraction changes that occurs in HF appears to differ between HFrEF versus HFpEF, with reduction in ejection fraction (EF) being associated with a higher ratio of MMP-1 to TIMP-1, which is hypothesized to underlie a mechanism for systolic failure in hypertensive heart disease.[110]

The unique signature of the disruption in ECM homeostasis appears to have important implications regarding the particular etiology of HF.[106] MMPs, tissue inhibitors of matrix metalloproteinases (TIMPs), and procollagen III amino-terminal propeptide (PIIINP), as well as glycation and collagen breakdown products, among others, have been supported as having a key role in HF pathogenesis. The prodigious work of Zile et al.[112] has greatly elucidated the role of the ECM especially in HFpEF: In a group of 446 participants (241 control, 144 with LVH without HF, 61 with LVH and HFpEF), elevations in MMP-7, MMP-9, TIMP-1, PIIINP, and NT-proBNP predicted LVH (c=0.80), and elevations in MMP-2, TIMP-4, and PIIINP and decrease in MMP-8 predicted clinical HFpEF (c=0.79). In another study of patients with established HF, MMP-9 values independently predicted HF events (HR 3.73).[113] Clearly, maladaptive alterations in collagen turnover are continually becoming better defined as likely pathogenic as well as potential targets of therapeutic intervention in HF.[114,115]

Galectin-3

Galectin-3 (Gal-3) is a member of the galectin family, being a β-galactoside–binding lectin with an "atypical" N-terminal domain and C-terminal carbohydrate recognition domain.[116,117] Gal-3 exhibits release during the differentiation of monocytes into macrophages[118] and is thus involved in various inflammatory processes, including neutrophil adhesion and opsonization, monocyte chemoattraction, and mast cell activation.[119] Increased expression of Gal-3 in activated macrophages is thought to promote pathological remodeling by inducing fibroblast proliferation and collagen deposition.[120] Importantly, Gal-3 increases may demonstrate a lesser degree of load dependency than the NPs.[121]

A growing body of evidence supports the role of Gal-3 in HF pathophysiology as a pivotal link between inflammation and fibrosis.[122] In the Framingham Offspring Cohort, when added to a model fully adjusted for demographic variables and BNP, Gal-3 improved the ability to predict new-onset HF (HR 1.28, 95% CI 1.14–1.43, for each 1–standard deviation (SD) increase in log_{10}[Gal-3]) and was associated with increased mortality (adjusted HR 1.15, 95% CI 1.04–1.28).[123] In the population-based FINRISK cohort of 8444 patients, Gal-3 added modest but statistically significant predictive capacity as compared to NT-proBNP.[124] In Prevention of Vascular and Renal End Stage Disease (PREVEND), persistent Gal-3 elevations were more strongly predictive of incident HF than non-persistent elevations.[125] Peacock et al. showed that in patients presenting to the emergency department with dyspnea, Gal-3 had slightly better prognostic significance versus NT-proBNP.[126] Looking forward, Gal-3 is associated with certain profibrotic mediators such as aldosterone,[116] and there may be potential avenues for prevention or treatment of HF by specifically inhibiting Gal-3–induced cardiac remodeling.[127]

MARKERS OF INFLAMMATION AND OXIDATIVE STRESS

Since the seminal investigation by Levine et al. implicating cytokines in the cachectic state of advanced HF,[128] experimental and clinical evidence supporting heart failure as an inflammatory disease continues to grow.[129] Several important inflammatory markers in HF pathogenesis which have been well characterized to date are discussed here.

Suppressor of Tumorgenicity 2 and Interleukin 33

A member of the IL-1 receptor-like family of proteins, ST2, has been recognized as serving a role in inflammatory (including cardiovascular) disease states, especially those that involve type 2 CD4+ T-helper lymphocytes.[130-132] ST2 exists in both membrane-bound (ST2 ligand, i.e., ST2L) and soluble (sST2) forms,[133] and cardiomyocytes and fibroblasts express both ST2L and sST2 in response to increased tissue forces from wall stress.[134] Also induced by cellular stretch, IL-33 is thought to be protective against hypertrophy and fibrosis via downstream activation of MyD33, interleukin-1 receptor-associated kinase (IRAK), extracellular signal-regulated kinases (ERKs), and NF-κB.[135] IL-33/ST2L signaling underlies the adaptive processes to combat myocyte hypertrophy and enhanced ECM deposition in fibrosis. However, this protective process is counteracted by the activity of soluble ST2 (sST2), which appears to serve as a decoy protein to deleteriously prevent binding of IL-33 to (membrane-bound) ST2L.[136] Consequently, higher levels of sST2 are associated with myocardial fibrosis, adverse remodeling, and poorer clinical outcomes.[137]

Growth Differentiation Factor 15

Growth differentiation factor 15 (GDF-15) is a member of the TGF-β superfamily associated with inflammation and cellular injury.[133,138] Cardiomyocytes secrete GDF-15 in response to a variety of stimuli,[138] including oxidative stress,[139] proinflammatory cytokines, ATII, ischemia,[140] or mechanical stretch,[141] the association with stretch as support that GDF-15 shares certain upstream regulatory factors with the natriuretic peptides.[138] Various extracardiac cells also contribute to GDF-15 production, including macrophages,[142] vascular smooth muscle cells,[143] pulmonary endothelial cells,[144] and adipocytes[145] in response to oxidative stress or proinflammatory signaling molecules. Interestingly, while cardiomyocytes produce abundant GDF-15 in response to myocardial infarction, there is little to no cardiac production in nonischemic cardiomyopathy; however, serum GDF-15 levels are nevertheless markedly elevated in nonischemic cardiomyopathy, supporting extracardiac sources of GDF-15 production in this subgroup.[146]

APPLICATION OF INFLAMMATORY AND OXIDATIVE MARKERS

Inflammatory markers play a key role in igniting the process of remodeling in HF pathobiology. First of all, the role of CRP in the prediction of HF is well established, particularly in HFpEF[147] and in men.[148] In the

Health ABC (Health, Aging, and Body Composition) study, among candidate biomarkers IL-6, TNF-α, and CRP, previously shown to associate with incident adverse cardiovascular events,[149] only addition of IL-6 to a clinical model improved discrimination and fit for prediction specifically of HF.[150] Again, elevations in several inflammatory markers were more strongly associated with poorer outcomes in HFpEF than in HFrEF.[150]

GDF-15 adds incremental prognostic power beyond traditional risk factors, NT-proBNP, and CRP (c=0.815 vs. c=0.806, $P<.001$) for incident all-cause and cardiovascular mortality in older individuals in the community.[151] In fact, in this cohort, GDF-15 predicted all-cause mortality more strongly than NT-proBNP (HR 1.5 vs. 1.3 per SD log_{10} of GDF-15 level). Interestingly, GDF-15 also predicted noncardiovascular mortality in this cohort, with some evidence that GDF-15 is associated with cancer mortality.[151] One prospective population-based cohort study supported the improvement in model discrimination for the prediction of a composite adverse CV outcome while separately adding NT-proBNP (c=0.714; $P=.03$) or GDF-15 (c=0.721; $P=.02$) to traditional risk factors, medications, and echocardiographic measurements (c=0.703).[152] Cutoffs of normal GDF-15 of 1200 ng/L and 1800 ng/L have been proposed for presumed healthy and post-NSTE-ACS individuals, respectively.[153]

The clinical significance of sST2 level is supported by multiple other studies. In patients at risk for HF, increased sST2 levels are associated with greater LV dimension, poorer LV and RV function, and hemodynamic decompensation.[154,155] In post-MI patients at risk for developing HF, sST2 are significantly associated with infarct size, infarct transmurality, norepinephrine, and aldosterone, but not with NT-proBNP.[137] A threshold for abnormal sST2 has been proposed at 35 ng/mL, which represents the 90th to 95th percentile for normal individuals.[156] Interestingly, sST2 appears to demonstrate less long-term interindividual variability (11%) than the NPs (33%–50%),[157] which contributes to its candidacy as a promising clinical assay.

Using multibiomarker approaches that include inflammatory markers in addition to structural proteins or NPs, the goal is to capture unique predictive information in various aspects of HF pathogenesis. In the FHS, sST2, hs-cTnI, GDF-15, and BNP were independently associated with incident HF after 11 years of follow-up.[158] In patients presenting to the emergency department with dyspnea, Gal-3, sST2, and BNP were equally useful to predict all-cause mortality at 1 year.[159] In summary, the success of expanding the complement of predictive biomarkers to include inflammatory components defines inflammation as a key aspect of HF pathogenesis.

MARKERS OF RENAL DYSFUNCTION

In a general sense, renal dysfunction can be quantified in the laboratory by circulating either (1) substances such as serum creatinine or cystatin-C, which inappropriately accumulate with threatened kidney function or (2) urinary substances such as urinary albumin, which are not appropriately conserved or removed from the urinary space. CKD is defined as a glomerular filtration rate (GFR) of <60 mL/min/1.73 m² or urinary albumin-to-creatinine ratio of >30 mg/g.[160] However, even small declinations in renal function, termed worsening renal function and (variably) defined as serum creatinine increase by >0.3 mg/dL, estimated GFR decline of >5 mL/min/year, or cystatin-C increase by >0.3 mg/L, exhibit important prognostic implications for incident HF and poorer cardiovascular outcomes.[161] Certain other electrolyte disturbances such as hypomagnesemia, hyperphosphatemia, and hypercalcemia have also been associated with incident HF.[162]

As explored previously, renal dysfunction (encompassing CKD as well as worsening renal function that does not cross the threshold of CKD diagnosis) exhibits an important relationship with HF prediction and also covaries with certain other risk factors such as cardiac troponin.[83,88] In the FHS, urinary albumin-to-creatinine ratio was shown to be an independent predictor of incident HF, exhibiting an HR of 1.35 per log_{10} units.[98] In a substudy of FHS among older individuals (aged 76 ± 5 years), after adjustment for preceding systolic or diastolic dysfunction and excluding individuals with significant CKD (serum creatinine >2 mg/dL), subclinical renal dysfunction as quantified by each 1-SD decrease in GFR was associated with a 24% increase in HF risk.[163]

The excess risk of incident HF among patients with renal dysfunction was confirmed subsequently in large studies. In the CHS a serum creatinine that exceeded 1.4 mg/dL demonstrated a relative risk of 1.5 (95% CI 1.17–1.92, $P=.001$) in the prediction of HF, although this accounted for a smaller amount of the population-attributable risk (6.3%) than factors such as coronary heart disease (13.1%), hypertension (SBP > 140 mmHg; 12.8%), or elevated inflammatory markers (CRP > 7.0 mg/L, 9.7%).[164] The PREVEND study used a multibiomarker approach; among 13 candidate biomarkers using multivariate adjustments, the best model included NT-proBNP, high-sensitivity cTnT, cystatin-C, and urinary albumin excretion for the prediction of incident HF.[165] This suggests that renal dysfunction, NPs, and cTn offer complementary predictive information. The optimal metric that captures the risk of HF conferred by impairment in kidney function has yet to be definitively determined.[133]

CONCLUSIONS

The approach to HF management among populations is undergoing a transition away from identification in advanced stages to one of prediction, prevention, and early intervention. Identification of the pathophysiologic components in HF in various milieux, ranging from the autonomic drivers and neurohormonal and inflammatory mediators to ECM regulators, all may invite opportunities for biomarker application to targeted clinical HF prevention. Using biomarker data to augment the predictive capacity of demographic and clinical information alone is essential in identifying and implementing targeted risk factor modification strategies in individuals who are likely to develop HF in their lifetime.

REFERENCES

1. Writing Committee M, Yancy CW, Jessup M, et al. 2013 ACCF/AHA guideline for the management of heart failure: a report of the American College of Cardiology Foundation/American Heart Association Task Force on practice guidelines. *Circulation.* 2013;128(16):e240–e327.
2. Liu L, Eisen HJ. Epidemiology of heart failure and scope of the problem. *Cardiol Clin.* 2014;32(1):1–8, vii.
3. Roger VL, Go AS, Lloyd-Jones DM, et al. Executive summary: heart disease and stroke statistics–2012 update: a report from the American Heart Association. *Circulation.* 2012;125(1):188–197.
4. Gorcsan 3rd J, Tanaka H. Echocardiographic assessment of myocardial strain. *J Am Coll Cardiol.* 2011;58(14):1401–1413.
5. Collier P, Phelan D, Klein A. A test in context: myocardial strain measured by speckle-tracking echocardiography. *J Am Coll Cardiol.* 2017;69(8):1043–1056.
6. Cardinale DCA, Bacchiani G, et al. Early detection of anthracycline cardiotoxicity and improvement with heart failure therapy. *Circulation.* 2015;131(22):1981–1988.
7. Drafts BCTK, D'Agostino Jr R, et al. Low to moderate dose anthracycline-based chemotherapy is associated with early noninvasive imaging evidence of subclinical cardiovascular disease. *JACC Cardiovasc Imaging.* 2013;6(8):877–885.
8. Fallah-Rad N, Walker JR, Wassef A, et al. The utility of cardiac biomarkers, tissue velocity and strain imaging, and cardiac magnetic resonance imaging in predicting early left ventricular dysfunction in patients with human epidermal growth factor receptor II-positive breast cancer treated with adjuvant trastuzumab therapy. *J Am Coll Cardiol.* 2011;57(22):2263–2270.
9. Herrmann JLA, Sandhu NP, et al. Evaluation and management of patients with heart disease and cancer: cardio-oncology. *Mayo Clin Proc.* 2014;89(9):1287–1306.
10. Negishi KNT, Hare JL, et al. Independent and incremental value of deformation indices for prediction of trastuzumab-induced cardiotoxicity. *J Am Soc Echocardiogr.* May 2013;26(5):493–498.
11. Nolan MT, Plana JC, Thavendiranathan P, Shaw L, Si L, Marwick TH. Cost-effectiveness of strain-targeted cardioprotection for prevention of chemotherapy-induced cardiotoxicity. *Int J Cardiol.* 2016;212:336–345.
12. Plana JC, Galderisi M, Barac A, et al. Expert consensus for multimodality imaging evaluation of adult patients during and after cancer therapy: a report from the American Society of Echocardiography and the European Association of Cardiovascular Imaging. *J Am Soc Echocardiogr.* 2014;27(9):911–939.
13. Kearney LG, Lu K, Ord M, et al. Global longitudinal strain is a strong independent predictor of all-cause mortality in patients with aortic stenosis. *Eur Heart J Cardiovasc Imaging.* 2012;13(10):827–833.
14. Stokke TM, Hasselberg NE, Smedsrud MK, et al. Geometry as a confounder when assessing ventricular systolic function: comparison between ejection fraction and strain. *J Am Coll Cardiol.* 2017;70(8):942–954.
15. Jordan J, Vasu S, Morgan T, et al. Anthracycline-associated T1 mapping characteristics are elevated independent of the presence of cardiovascular comorbidities in cancer survivors. *Circ Cardiovasc Imaging.* 2016;9(8):e004325.
16. Lustberg M, Zareba K. Anthracycline cardiotoxicity: how do we move from diagnosis to prediction?. *Circ Cardiovasc Imaging.* 2016;9(8): e005324.
17. Taylor RJ, Moody WE, Umar F, et al. Myocardial strain measurement with feature-tracking cardiovascular magnetic resonance: normal values. *Eur Heart J Cardiovasc Imaging.* 2015;16(8):871–881.
18. Jovenaux LCJ, Resseguier N, et al. Practices in management of cancer treatment-related cardiovascular toxicity: a cardio-oncology survey. *Int J Cardiol.* 15, 2017;241:387–392.
19. Morrow DA, de Lemos JA. Benchmarks for the assessment of novel cardiovascular biomarkers. *Circulation.* 2007;115(8):949–952.
20. Hunt SA. American College of C, American Heart Association Task Force on practice G. ACC/AHA 2005 guideline update for the diagnosis and management of chronic heart failure in the adult: a report of the American College of Cardiology/American Heart Association Task Force on practice guidelines (Writing Committee to update the 2001 guidelines for the evaluation and management of heart failure). *J Am Coll Cardiol.* 2005;46(6):e1–e82.
21. Bleumink GS, Knetsch AM, Sturkenboom MC, et al. Quantifying the heart failure epidemic: prevalence, incidence rate, lifetime risk and prognosis of heart failure the Rotterdam Study. *Eur Heart J.* 2004;25(18):1614–1619.
22. Lehrke M, Marx N. Diabetes mellitus and heart failure. *Am J Cardiol.* 2017;120(1S):S37–S47.

23. Thrainsdottir IS, Aspelund T, Hardarson T, et al. Glucose abnormalities and heart failure predict poor prognosis in the population-based Reykjavik Study. *Eur J Cardiovasc Prev Rehabil.* 2005;12(5):465–471.

24. Thrainsdottir IS, Aspelund T, Thorgeirsson G, et al. The association between glucose abnormalities and heart failure in the population-based Reykjavik study. *Diabetes Care.* 2005;28(3):612–616.

25. van Melle JP, Bot M, de Jonge P, de Boer RA, van Veldhuisen DJ, Whooley MA. Diabetes, glycemic control, and new-onset heart failure in patients with stable coronary artery disease: data from the heart and soul study. *Diabetes Care.* 2010;33(9):2084–2089.

26. Levelt E, Mahmod M, Piechnik SK, et al. Relationship between left ventricular structural and metabolic remodeling in type 2 diabetes. *Diabetes.* 2016;65(1):44–52.

27. Wong TC, Piehler KM, Kang IA, et al. Myocardial extracellular volume fraction quantified by cardiovascular magnetic resonance is increased in diabetes and associated with mortality and incident heart failure admission. *Eur Heart Journal.* 2014;35(10):657–664.

28. Shimizu I, Minamino T, Toko H, et al. Excessive cardiac insulin signaling exacerbates systolic dysfunction induced by pressure overload in rodents. *J Clin Invest.* 2010;120(5):1506–1514.

29. Ramasamy R, Schmidt AM. Receptor for advanced glycation end products (RAGE) and implications for the pathophysiology of heart failure. *Curr Heart Fail Rep.* 2012;9(2):107–116.

30. Rubler S, Dlugash J, Yuceoglu YZ, Kumral T, Branwood AW, Grishman A. New type of cardiomyopathy associated with diabetic glomerulosclerosis. *Am J Cardiol.* 1972;30(6):595–602.

31. Levy D, Larson MG, Vasan RS, Kannel WB, Ho KK. The progression from hypertension to congestive heart failure. *JAMA.* 1996;275(20):1557–1562.

32. Johnson FL. Pathophysiology and etiology of heart failure. *Cardiol Clin.* 2014;32(1):9–19, vii.

33. Kannan A, Janardhanan R. Hypertension as a risk factor for heart failure. *Curr Hypertens Rep.* 2014;16(7):447.

34. Raman SV. The hypertensive heart. An integrated understanding informed by imaging. *J Am Coll Cardiol.* 2010;55(2):91–96.

35. Berenji K, Drazner MH, Rothermel BA, Hill JA. Does load-induced ventricular hypertrophy progress to systolic heart failure? *Am J Physiol Heart Circ Physiol.* 2005;289(1):H8–H16.

36. Grossman W, Jones D, McLaurin LP. Wall stress and patterns of hypertrophy in the human left ventricle. *J Clin Invest.* 1975;56(1):56–64.

37. Schillaci G, Verdecchia P, Porcellati C, Cuccurullo O, Cosco C, Perticone F. Continuous relation between left ventricular mass and cardiovascular risk in essential hypertension. *Hypertension.* 2000;35(2):580–586.

38. Hasking GJ, Esler MD, Jennings GL, Burton D, Johns JA, Korner PI. Norepinephrine spillover to plasma in patients with congestive heart failure: evidence of increased overall and cardiorenal sympathetic nervous activity. *Circulation.* 1986;73(4):615–621.

39. Cohn JN, Levine TB, Olivari MT, et al. Plasma norepinephrine as a guide to prognosis in patients with chronic congestive heart failure. *N Engl J Med.* 1984;311(13):819–823.

40. Kaye DM, Lefkovits J, Jennings GL, Bergin P, Broughton A, Esler MD. Adverse consequences of high sympathetic nervous activity in the failing human heart. *J Am Coll Cardiol.* 1995;26(5):1257–1263.

41. Hirsch AT, Pinto YM, Schunkert H, Dzau VJ. Potential role of the tissue renin-angiotensin system in the pathophysiology of congestive heart failure. *Am J Cardiol.* 1990;66(11):22D–30D; discussion 30D-32D.

42. Whelton PK, Carey RM, Aronow WS, et al. 2017 ACC/AHA/AAPA/ABC/ACPM/AGS/APhA/ASH/ASPC/NMA/PCNA guideline for the prevention, detection, evaluation, and management of high blood pressure in adults: a report of the American College of Cardiology/American Heart Association Task force on clinical practice guidelines. *Hypertension.* 2017.

43. Kenchaiah S, Evans JC, Levy D, et al. Obesity and the risk of heart failure. *N Engl J Med.* 2002;347(5):305–313.

44. Baena-Diez JM, Byram AO, Grau M, et al. Obesity is an independent risk factor for heart failure: Zona Franca Cohort study. *Clin Cardiol.* 2010;33(12):760–764.

45. Padwal R, McAlister FA, McMurray JJ, et al. The obesity paradox in heart failure patients with preserved versus reduced ejection fraction: a meta-analysis of individual patient data. *Int J Obes (Lond).* 2014;38(8):1110–1114.

46. Clark AL, Chyu J, Horwich TB. The obesity paradox in men versus women with systolic heart failure. *Am J Cardiol.* 2012;110(1):77–82.

47. Fonarow GC, Srikanthan P, Costanzo MR, et al. An obesity paradox in acute heart failure: analysis of body mass index and inhospital mortality for 108,927 patients in the Acute Decompensated Heart Failure National Registry. *Am Heart J.* 2007;153(1):74–81.

48. Lavie CJ, Alpert MA, Arena R, Mehra MR, Milani RV, Ventura HO. Impact of obesity and the obesity paradox on prevalence and prognosis in heart failure. *JACC Heart Fail.* 2013;1(2):93–102.

49. Lavie CJ, Milani RV, Ventura HO. Obesity and cardiovascular disease: risk factor, paradox, and impact of weight loss. *J Am Coll Cardiol.* 2009;53(21):1925–1932.

50. Alexander JK. Obesity and cardiac performance. *Am J Cardiol.* 1964;14:860–865.

51. Thakur V, Richards R, Reisin E. Obesity, hypertension, and the heart. *Am J Med Sci.* 2001;321(4):242–248.

52. Abel ED, Litwin SE, Sweeney G. Cardiac remodeling in obesity. *Physiol Rev.* 2008;88(2):389–419.

53. Smith HLW. F.A. Adiposity of the heart. *Arch Inter Med.* 1933;52:911–931.

54. McGavock JM, Victor RG, Unger RH, Szczepaniak LS. American College of P, the American physiological S. Adiposity of the heart, revisited. *Ann Internal Med.* 2006;144(7):517–524.

55. Alpert MA, Lavie CJ, Agrawal H, Aggarwal KB, Kumar SA. Obesity and heart failure: epidemiology, pathophysiology, clinical manifestations, and management. *Transl Res*. 2014;164(4):345–356.

56. Alpert MA. Obesity cardiomyopathy: pathophysiology and evolution of the clinical syndrome. *Am J Med Sci*. 2001;321(4):225–236.

57. Khayat R, Small R, Rathman L, et al. Sleep-disordered breathing in heart failure: identifying and treating an important but often unrecognized comorbidity in heart failure patients. *J Card Fail*. 2013;19(6):431–444.

58. Drager LF, Togeiro SM, Polotsky VY, Lorenzi-Filho G. Obstructive sleep apnea: a cardiometabolic risk in obesity and the metabolic syndrome. *J Am Coll Cardiol*. 2013;62(7):569–576.

59. Oldenburg O, Lamp B, Faber L, Teschler H, Horstkotte D, Topfer V. Sleep-disordered breathing in patients with symptomatic heart failure: a contemporary study of prevalence in and characteristics of 700 patients. *Eur J Heart Fail*. 2007;9(3):251–257.

60. Javaheri S, Caref EB, Chen E, Tong KB, Abraham WT. Sleep apnea testing and outcomes in a large cohort of Medicare beneficiaries with newly diagnosed heart failure. *Am J Respir Crit Care Med*. 2011;183(4):539–546.

61. Parker JD, Brooks D, Kozar LF, et al. Acute and chronic effects of airway obstruction on canine left ventricular performance. *Am J Respir Crit Care Med*. 1999;160(6):1888–1896.

62. Kasai T, Bradley TD. Obstructive sleep apnea and heart failure: pathophysiologic and therapeutic implications. *J Am Coll Cardiol*. 2011;57(2):119–127.

63. Lymperopoulos A, Rengo G, Koch WJ. Adrenergic nervous system in heart failure: pathophysiology and therapy. *Circ Res*. 2013;113(6):739–753.

64. Triposkiadis F, Karayannis G, Giamouzis G, Skoularigis J, Louridas G, Butler J. The sympathetic nervous system in heart failure physiology, pathophysiology, and clinical implications. *J Am Coll Cardiol*. 2009;54(19):1747–1762.

65. Zipes DP. Heart-brain interactions in cardiac arrhythmias: role of the autonomic nervous system. *Cleve Clin J Med*. 2008;75(suppl 2):S94–S96.

66. Chidsey CABE, Morrow AG, et al. Catecholamine excretion and cardiac stores of norepinephrine in congestive heart failure. *Am J Med*. 1965;39:442–451.

67. Jensen BC, O'Connell TD, Simpson PC. Alpha-1-adrenergic receptors in heart failure: the adaptive arm of the cardiac response to chronic catecholamine stimulation. *J Cardiovasc Pharmacol*. 2014;63(4):291–301.

68. Esler M, Jennings G, Lambert G, Meredith I, Horne M, Eisenhofer G. Overflow of catecholamine neurotransmitters to the circulation: source, fate, and functions. *Physiol Rev*. 1990;70(4):963–985.

69. Sisson JC, Shapiro B, Meyers L, et al. Metaiodobenzylguanidine to map scintigraphically the adrenergic nervous system in man. *J Nucl Med*. 1987;28(10):1625–1636.

70. Jacobson AF, Lombard J, Banerjee G, Camici PG. 123I-mIBG scintigraphy to predict risk for adverse cardiac outcomes in heart failure patients: design of two prospective multicenter international trials. *J Nucl Cardiol*. 2009;16(1):113–121.

71. Mokhles MM, Trifiro G, Dieleman JP, et al. The risk of new onset heart failure associated with dopamine agonist use in Parkinson's disease. *Pharmacol Res*. 2012;65(3):358–364.

72. Abd ElHafeez S, Tripepi G, Stancanelli B, et al. Norepinephrine, left ventricular disorders and volume excess in ESRD. *J Nephrol*. 2015;28(6):729–737.

73. Zoccali C, Mallamaci F, Parlongo S, et al. Plasma norepinephrine predicts survival and incident cardiovascular events in patients with end-stage renal disease. *Circulation*. 2002;105(11):1354–1359.

74. Sayer G, Bhat G. The renin-angiotensin-aldosterone system and heart failure. *Cardiol Clin*. 2014;32(1):21–32, vii.

75. Seikaly MG, Arant BS, Seney FD. Endogenous angiotensin concentrations in specific intrarenal fluid compartments of the rat. *J Clin Invest*. 1990;86(4):1352–1357.

76. van Kats JP, Danser AH, van Meegen JR, Sassen LM, Verdouw PD, Schalekamp MA. Angiotensin production by the heart: a quantitative study in pigs with the use of radiolabeled angiotensin infusions. *Circulation*. 1998;98(1):73–81.

77. Dzau VJ, Colucci WS, Hollenberg NK, Williams GH. Relation of the renin-angiotensin-aldosterone system to clinical state in congestive heart failure. *Circulation*. 1981;63(3):645–651.

78. Torre M, Jarolim P. Cardiac troponin assays in the management of heart failure. *Clin Chim Acta*. 2015;441:92–98.

79. De Boer RAPY, Van Veldhuisen DJ. The imbalance between oxygen demand and supply as a potential mechanism in the pathophysiology of heart failure: the role of microvascular growth and abnormalities. *Microcirculation*. 2003;10:113–126.

80. Wu AH, Christenson RH. Analytical and assay issues for use of cardiac troponin testing for risk stratification in primary care. *Clin Biochem*. 2013;46(12):969–978.

81. Apple FS, Collinson PO. Biomarkers ITFoCAoC. Analytical characteristics of high-sensitivity cardiac troponin assays. *Clin Chem*. 2012;58(1):54–61.

82. Sato Y, Fujiwara H, Takatsu Y. Cardiac troponin and heart failure in the era of high-sensitivity assays. *J Cardiol*. 2012;60(3):160–167.

83. Wallace TWAS, Drazner MH, et al. Prevalence and determinants of troponin T elevation in the general population. *Circulation*. April 25, 2006;113(16):1958–1965.

84. deFilippi CR, dLJ, Christenson RH, et al. Association of serial measures of cardiac troponin T using a sensitive assay with incident heart failure and cardiovascular mortality in older adults. *JAMA*. 2010;304(22):2494–2502.

85. Saunders JTNV, de Lemos JA, et al. Cardiac troponin T measured by a highly sensitive assay predicts coronary heart disease, heart failure, and mortality in the Atherosclerosis Risk in Communities Study. *Circulation*. 2011;123(13):1367–1376.

86. Omland T, de Lemos JA, Sabatine MS, et al. A sensitive cardiac troponin T assay in stable coronary artery disease. *N Engl J Med.* 2009;361(26):2538–2547.

87. de Lemos JA, Drazner MH, Omland T, et al. Association of troponin T detected with a highly sensitive assay and cardiac structure and mortality risk in the general population. *JAMA.* 2010;304(22):2503–2512.

88. Rubin J, Matsushita K, Lazo M, et al. Determinants of minimal elevation in high-sensitivity cardiac troponin T in the general population. *Clin Biochem.* 2016;49(9):657–662.

89. Diris JH, Hackeng CM, Kooman JP, Pinto YM, Hermens WT, van Dieijen-Visser MP. Impaired renal clearance explains elevated troponin T fragments in hemodialysis patients. *Circulation.* 2004;109(1):23–25.

90. Tsutamoto T, Kawahara C, Yamaji M, et al. Relationship between renal function and serum cardiac troponin T in patients with chronic heart failure. *Eur J Heart Fail.* 2009;11(7):653–658.

91. deFilippi CR, de Lemos J, Tkaczuk AT, et al. Physical activity, change in biomarkers of myocardial stress and injury, and subsequent heart failure risk in older adults. *J Am Coll Cardiol.* 2012;60(24):2539–2547.

92. Nakagawa OOY, Itoh H, et al. Rapid transcriptional activation and early mRNA turnover of brain natriuretic peptide in cardiocyte hypertrophy. Evidence for brain natriuretic peptide as an "emergency" cardiac hormone against ventricular overload. *J Clin Invest.* 1995;96(3):1280–1287.

93. Wettersten N, Maisel AS. Biomarkers for heart failure: an update for practitioners of internal medicine. *Am Journal Medicine.* 2016;129(6):560–567.

94. Daniels LB, Maisel AS. Natriuretic peptides. *J Am Coll Cardiol.* 2007;50(25):2357–2368.

95. Mehra MR, Uber PA, Park MH, et al. Obesity and suppressed B-type natriuretic peptide levels in heart failure. *J Am Coll Cardiol.* 2004;43(9):1590–1595.

96. Sarzani R, Dessi-Fulgheri P, Paci VM, Espinosa E, Rappelli A. Expression of natriuretic peptide receptors in human adipose and other tissues. *J Endocrinol Invest.* 1996;19(9):581–585.

97. Sengenes C, Berlan M, De Glisezinski I, Lafontan M, Galitzky J. Natriuretic peptides: a new lipolytic pathway in human adipocytes. *FASEB J.* 2000;14(10):1345–1351.

98. Velagaleti RSGP, Larson MG, et al. Multimarker approach for the prediction of heart failure incidence in the community. *Circulation.* 2010;122(17):1700–1706.

99. Glick DDC, Christenson R, et al. Long-term trajectory of two unique cardiac biomarkers and subsequent left ventricular structural pathology and risk of incident heart failure in community-dwelling older adults at low baseline risk. *JACC Heart Fail.* 2013;1(4):353–360.

100. Mishra RK, Beatty AL, Jaganath R, Regan M, Wu AH, Whooley MA. B-type natriuretic peptides for the prediction of cardiovascular events in patients with stable coronary heart disease: the Heart and Soul Study. *J Am Heart Assoc.* 2014;3(4).

101. Maisel A, Mueller C, Adams Jr K, et al. State of the art: using natriuretic peptide levels in clinical practice. *Eur J Heart Fail.* 2008;10(9):824–839.

102. Mant J, Doust J, Roalfe A, et al. Systematic review and individual patient data meta-analysis of diagnosis of heart failure, with modelling of implications of different diagnostic strategies in primary care. *Health Technol Assess.* 2009;13(32):1–207, iii.

103. Ewald B, Ewald D, Thakkinstian A, Attia J. Meta-analysis of B type natriuretic peptide and N-terminal pro B natriuretic peptide in the diagnosis of clinical heart failure and population screening for left ventricular systolic dysfunction. *Intern Med J.* 2008;38(2):101–113.

104. McKie PM, Cataliotti A, Sangaralingham SJ, et al. Predictive utility of atrial, N-terminal pro-atrial, and N-terminal pro-B-type natriuretic peptides for mortality and cardiovascular events in the general community: a 9-year follow-up study. *Mayo Clin Proc.* 2011;86(12):1154–1160.

105. Nambi V, Liu X, Chambless LE, et al. Troponin T and N-terminal pro-B-type natriuretic peptide: a biomarker approach to predict heart failure risk–the atherosclerosis risk in communities study. *Clin Chem.* 2013;59(12):1802–1810.

106. Spinale FG, Janicki JS, Zile MR. Membrane-associated matrix proteolysis and heart failure. *Circ Res.* 2013; 112(1):195–208.

107. Fomovsky GM, Thomopoulos S, Holmes JW. Contribution of extracellular matrix to the mechanical properties of the heart. *J Mol Cell Cardiol.* 2010;48(3):490–496.

108. Gillies AR, Lieber RL. Structure and function of the skeletal muscle extracellular matrix. *Muscle nerve.* 2011;44(3):318–331.

109. Stroud JD, Baicu CF, Barnes MA, Spinale FG, Zile MR. Viscoelastic properties of pressure overload hypertrophied myocardium: effect of serine protease treatment. *Am J Physiol Heart Circ Physiol.* 2002;282(6):H2324–H2335.

110. López B, González A, Querejeta R, Larman M, Díez J. Alterations in the pattern of collagen deposition may contribute to the deterioration of systolic function in hypertensive patients with heart failure. *J Am Coll Cardiol.* 2006;48(1):89–96.

111. Martos R, Baugh J, Ledwidge M, et al. Diastolic heart failure: evidence of increased myocardial collagen turnover linked to diastolic dysfunction. *Circulation.* 2007;115(7):888–895.

112. Zile MR, Desantis SM, Baicu CF, et al. Plasma biomarkers that reflect determinants of matrix composition identify the presence of left ventricular hypertrophy and diastolic heart failure. *Circ Heart Fail.* 2011;4(3):246–256.

113. Morishita T, Uzui H, Mitsuke Y, et al. Association between matrix metalloproteinase-9 and worsening heart failure events in patients with chronic heart failure. *ESC Heart Fail.* 2017;4(3):321–330.

114. Mak GJ, Ledwidge MT, Watson CJ, et al. Natural history of markers of collagen turnover in patients with early diastolic dysfunction and impact of eplerenone. *J Am Coll Cardiol.* 2009;54(18):1674–1682.

115. Lewis EF, Kim HY, Claggett B, et al. Impact of spirono-lactone on longitudinal changes in health-related quality of life in the treatment of preserved cardiac function heart failure with an aldosterone antagonist trial. *Circ Heart Fail.* 2016;9(3): e001937.

116. Filipe MD, Meijers WC, Rogier van der Velde A, de Boer RA. Galectin-3 and heart failure: prognosis, prediction & clinical utility. *Clin Chim Acta.* 2015;443:48–56.

117. Dumic J, Dabelic S, Flogel M. Galectin-3: an open-ended story. *Biochimica Biophys Acta.* 2006;1760(4):616–635.

118. Liu FT, Hsu DK, Zuberi RI, Kuwabara I, Chi EY, Henderson Jr WR. Expression and function of galectin-3, a beta-galactoside-binding lectin, in human monocytes and macrophages. *Am J Pathol.* 1995;147(4):1016–1028.

119. Henderson NC, Sethi T. The regulation of inflammation by galectin-3. *Immunol Rev.* 2009;230(1):160–171.

120. Sharma UCPS, van Brakel TJ, et al. Galectin-3 marks activated macrophages in failure-prone hypertrophied hearts and contributes to cardiac dysfunction. *Circulation.* 2004;110(19):3121–3128.

121. Carrasco-Sanchez FJ, Aramburu-Bodas O, Salamanca-Bautista P, et al. Predictive value of serum galectin-3 levels in patients with acute heart failure with preserved ejection fraction. *Int J Cardiol.* 2013;169(3):177–182.

122. Lala RI, Puschita M, Darabantiu D, Pilat L. Galectin-3 in heart failure pathology–"another brick in the wall"? *Acta Cardiol.* 2015;70(3):323–331.

123. Ho JE, Liu C, Lyass A, et al. Galectin-3, a marker of cardiac fibrosis, predicts incident heart failure in the community. *J Am Coll Cardiol.* 2012;60(14):1249–1256.

124. Jagodzinski A, Havulinna AS, Appelbaum S, et al. Predictive value of galectin-3 for incident cardiovascular disease and heart failure in the population-based FINRISK 1997 cohort. *Int J Cardiol.* 2015;192:33–39.

125. van der Velde AR, Meijers WC, Ho JE, et al. Serial galectin-3 and future cardiovascular disease in the general population. *Heart.* 2016;102(14):1134–1141.

126. Peacock WF, DiSomma S. Emergency department use of galectin-3. *Crit Pathw Cardiol.* 2014;13(2):73–77.

127. Liu YH, D'Ambrosio M, Liao TD, et al. N-acetyl-seryl-aspartyl-lysyl-proline prevents cardiac remodeling and dysfunction induced by galectin-3, a mammalian adhesion/growth-regulatory lectin. *Am J Physiol Heart Circ Physiol.* 2009;296(2):H404–H412.

128. Levine B, Kalman J, Mayer L, Fillit HM, Packer M. Elevated circulating levels of tumor necrosis factor in severe chronic heart failure. *N Engl J Med.* 1990;323(4):236–241.

129. Askevold ET, Gullestad L, Dahl CP, Yndestad A, Ueland T, Aukrust P. Interleukin-6 signaling, soluble glycoprotein 130, and inflammation in heart failure. *Curr Heart Fail Rep.* 2014;11(2):146–155.

130. Daniels LB, Bayes-Genis A. Using ST2 in cardiovascular patients: a review. *Future Cardiol.* 2014;10(4):525–539.

131. Yanagisawa K, Tsukamoto T, Takagi T, Tominaga S. Murine ST2 gene is a member of the primary response gene family induced by growth factors. *FEBS Lett.* 1992;302(1):51–53.

132. Coyle AJ, Lloyd C, Tian J, et al. Crucial role of the interleukin 1 receptor family member T1/ST2 in T helper cell type 2-mediated lung mucosal immune responses. *J Exp Med.* 1999;190(7):895–902.

133. Chow SLMA, Anand I, et al. Role of biomarkers for the prevention, assessment, and management of heart failure: a scientific statement from the American Heart Association. *Circulation.* 2017;135(122):e1054–e1091.

134. Weinberg EO, Shimpo M, De Keulenaer GW, et al. Expression and regulation of ST2, an interleukin-1 receptor family member, in cardiomyocytes and myocardial infarction. *Circulation.* 2002;106(23):2961–2966.

135. Schmitz J, Owyang A, Oldham E, et al. IL-33, an interleukin-1-like cytokine that signals via the IL-1 receptor-related protein ST2 and induces T helper type 2-associated cytokines. *Immunity.* 2005;23(5):479–490.

136. KRaL RT. The IL-33/ST2 pathway: therapeutic target and novel biomarker. *Nat Rev Drug Discov.* 2008;7(10):827–840.

137. Weir RA, Miller AM, Murphy GE, et al. Serum soluble ST2: a potential novel mediator in left ventricular and infarct remodeling after acute myocardial infarction. *J Am Coll Cardiol.* 2010;55(3):243–250.

138. Wollert KC, Kempf T. Growth differentiation factor 15 in heart failure: an update. *Curr Heart Fail Rep.* 2012;9(4):337–345.

139. Clerk A, Kemp TJ, Zoumpoulidou G, Sugden PH. Cardiac myocyte gene expression profiling during H2O2-induced apoptosis. *Physiol Genomics.* 2007;29(2):118–127.

140. Widera C, Giannitsis E, Kempf T, et al. Identification of follistatin-like 1 by expression cloning as an activator of the growth differentiation factor 15 gene and a prognostic biomarker in acute coronary syndrome. *Clin Chem.* 2012;58(8):1233–1241.

141. Frank D, Kuhn C, Brors B, et al. Gene expression pattern in biomechanically stretched cardiomyocytes: evidence for a stretch-specific gene program. *Hypertension.* 2008;51(2):309–318.

142. Schlittenhardt D, Schober A, Strelau J, et al. Involvement of growth differentiation factor-15/macrophage inhibitory cytokine-1 (GDF-15/MIC-1) in oxLDL-induced apoptosis of human macrophages in vitro and in arteriosclerotic lesions. *Cell Tissue Res.* 2004;318(2):325–333.

143. Bermudez B, Lopez S, Pacheco YM, et al. Influence of postprandial triglyceride-rich lipoproteins on lipid-mediated gene expression in smooth muscle cells of the human coronary artery. *Cardiovasc Res.* 2008;79(2):294–303.

144. Nickel N, Jonigk D, Kempf T, et al. GDF-15 is abundantly expressed in plexiform lesions in patients with pulmonary arterial hypertension and affects proliferation and apoptosis of pulmonary endothelial cells. *Respir Res.* 2011;12(62).

145. Ding Q, Mracek T, Gonzalez-Muniesa P, et al. Identification of macrophage inhibitory cytokine-1 in adipose tissue and its secretion as an adipokine by human adipocytes. *Endocrinology.* 2009;150(4):1688–1696.

146. Lok SI, Winkens B, Goldschmeding R, et al. Circulating growth differentiation factor-15 correlates with myocardial fibrosis in patients with non-ischaemic dilated cardiomyopathy and decreases rapidly after left ventricular assist device support. *Eur J Heart Fail.* 2012;14(11):1249–1256.

147. Williams ES, Shah SJ, Ali S, Na BY, Schiller NB, Whooley MA. C-reactive protein, diastolic dysfunction, and risk of heart failure in patients with coronary disease: heart and soul Study. *Eur J Heart Fail.* 2008;10(1):63–69.

148. Kardys I, Knetsch AM, Bleumink GS, et al. C-reactive protein and risk of heart failure. The Rotterdam Study. *Am Heart J.* 2006;152(3):514–520.

149. Cesari M, Penninx BW, Newman AB, et al. Inflammatory markers and onset of cardiovascular events: results from the Health ABC study. *Circulation.* 2003;108(19):2317–2322.

150. Kalogeropoulos AGV, Psaty BM, et al. Inflammatory markers and incident heart failure risk in older adults: the Health ABC (Health, Aging, and Body Composition) study. *J Am Coll Cardiol.* 2010;55(19):2129–2137.

151. Daniels LB, Clopton P, Laughlin GA, Maisel AS, Barrett-Connor E. Growth-differentiation factor-15 is a robust, independent predictor of 11-year mortality risk in community-dwelling older adults: the Rancho Bernardo Study. *Circulation.* 2011;123(19):2101–2110.

152. Pareek M, Bhatt DL, Vaduganathan M, et al. Single and multiple cardiovascular biomarkers in subjects without a previous cardiovascular event. *Eur J Prev Cardiol.* 2017;24(15):1648–1659.

153. Wollert KC, Kempf T, Peter T, et al. Prognostic value of growth-differentiation factor-15 in patients with non-ST-elevation acute coronary syndrome. *Circulation.* 2007;115(8):962–971.

154. Daniels LB, Clopton P, Iqbal N, Tran K, Maisel AS. Association of ST2 levels with cardiac structure and function and mortality in outpatients. *Am Heart J.* 2010;160(4):721–728.

155. Shah RV, Chen-Tournoux AA, Picard MH, van Kimmenade RR, Januzzi JL. Serum levels of the interleukin-1 receptor family member ST2, cardiac structure and function, and long-term mortality in patients with acute dyspnea. *Circ Heart Fail.* 2009;2(4):311–319.

156. Mueller T, Dieplinger B. The Presage((R)) ST2 Assay: analytical considerations and clinical applications for a high-sensitivity assay for measurement of soluble ST2. *Expert Rev Mol diagn.* 2013;13(1):13–30.

157. Wu AH, Wians F, Jaffe A. Biological variation of galectin-3 and soluble ST2 for chronic heart failure: implication on interpretation of test results. *Am Heart J.* 2013;165(6):995–999.

158. Wang TJWK, Larson MG, et al. Prognostic utility of novel biomarkers of cardiovascular stress: the Framingham Heart Study. *Circulation.* 2012;126(13):1596–1604.

159. Mueller TGA, Poelz W, et al. Diagnostic and prognostic accuracy of galectin-3 and soluble ST2 for acute heart failure. *Clin Chim Acta.* 2016;463:158–164.

160. Levey AS, de Jong PE, Coresh J, et al. The definition, classification, and prognosis of chronic kidney disease: a KDIGO Controversies Conference report. *Kidney Int.* 2011;80(1):17–28.

161. Filippatos G, Farmakis D, Parissis J. Renal dysfunction and heart failure: things are seldom what they seem. *Eur Heart J.* 2014;35(7):416–418.

162. Lutsey PL, Alonso A, Michos ED, et al. Serum magnesium, phosphorus, and calcium are associated with risk of incident heart failure: the Atherosclerosis Risk in Communities (ARIC) Study. *Am J Clin Nutr.* 2014;100(3):756–764.

163. Lam CS, Lyass A, Kraigher-Krainer E, et al. Cardiac dysfunction and noncardiac dysfunction as precursors of heart failure with reduced and preserved ejection fraction in the community. *Circulation.* 2011;124(1):24–30.

164. Gottdiener JS, Arnold AM, Aurigemma GP, et al. Predictors of congestive heart failure in the elderly: the Cardiovascular Health Study. *J Am Coll Cardiol.* 2000;35(6):1628–1637.

165. Brouwers FP, van Gilst GW, Damman K, et al. Clinical risk stratification optimizes value of biomarkers to predict new-onset heart failure in a community-based cohort. *Circ Heart Fail.* 2014;7(5):723–731.

CHAPTER 9

Biomarkers to Assess and Guide the Management of Heart Failure

PAVAN BHAT, MD • W.H. WILSON TANG, MD

INTRODUCTION

Over the last 20 years the management of heart failure has shown major advancements not only in therapies but also in the availability and adoption of biomarkers that have helped significantly in the diagnosis and prognosis of heart failure. Before the development of biomarkers for heart failure, evaluation was more subjective, and prognostic biomarkers have added more objective assessments to help guide heart failure. Heart failure as a clinical entity continues to be associated with high mortality and recurrent hospitalizations.[1,2] Our discussion about cardiac biomarkers is going to be largely focused on heart failure with reduced ejection fraction (HFrEF) as opposed to heart failure with preserved ejection fraction (HFpEF) as most successful randomized controlled trials in the heart failure population have focused on the HFrEF population. In addition, there are still no proven therapies for HFpEF that improve mortality.[2]

The majority of heart failure biomarker studies used biomarkers to confirm or predict prognosis with a heart failure diagnosis. Clinically only the determination of left ventricular ejection fraction (LVEF) provides a reliable marker in selecting patients for guideline-directed medical therapies. We will focus on 4 major subtypes of biomarkers and their use in guiding heart failure management: (1) myocardial stress, (2) myocardial injury, (3) myocardial fibrosis, and (4) cardiorenal dysfunction (Fig. 9.1). It is important to emphasize that these biomarkers all describe the clinical consequences of heart failure rather than revealing the causes or triggers of heart failure. Hence their roles in guiding heart failure management have largely been confined to establishing the diagnosis of heart failure and assessing the clinical prognosis in patients with heart failure (and largely independent of individual drugs or interventions).

Biomarkers of Myocardial Stress

The most common and heavily used biomarker belongs to testing of circulating natriuretic peptides, B-type natriuretic peptide (BNP) and its prohormone fragment,

N-terminal pro-B-type natriuretic peptide (NT-pro-BNP; Fig. 9.2). BNP originates as a pre-prohormone, which is then processed to pro-BNP. Pro-BNP is then cleaved by the serine peptidase enzyme corin to produce biologically active BNP and inactive NT-pro-BNP. BNP is one of many substances that are degraded by neprilysin, which has recently become more clinically relevant with the results of clinical trials indicating potential benefits of neprilysin inhibition.[3] On average, NT-pro-BNP levels are approximately five to eight times higher than the corresponding BNP level.[4] Natriuretic peptides are primary counter-regulatory hormones produced in response to myocardial stress. Circulating natriuretic peptide assay levels may include a mix of NT-pro, BNP fragments, atrial natriuretic peptide (ANP), and C-type natriuretic peptide which have different levels of biological activity compared with BNP. ANP and BNP are both continuously released from the heart. Atrial stretch augments further ANP and BNP release. ANP is released mainly from the atria, whereas BNP is released by both tissues, but primarily the ventricle. Biologically, BNP specifically leads to an increase in natriuresis, vasodilation, and opposing effects of other neurohormonal systems. The levels of both these hormones are influenced by factors such as age, body mass index, and renal function. Specifically BNP levels in obese patients range 30%–40% lower than nonobese patients.[5] Race also plays an important role in the variability of the BNP assay with Asian and Black patients with heart failure having higher BNP levels than White and Hispanic patients.[6] Many prior trials have shown that BNP levels are elevated in patients with underlying heart failure, and stable levels are associated with stability in symptoms, even though a quarter of patients may present with levels lower than standard threshold for diagnosing heart failure.[2]

Natriuretic peptide testing is one of few biomarkers that have endorsements from clinical practice guidelines. In the latest 2017 American College of Cardiology Foundation (ACCF)/AHA guideline updates (Fig. 9.3), measuring of BNP or NT-pro-BNP level

Biomarkers in Cardiovascular Disease. DOI: 10.1016/B978-0-323-54835-9.00009-0

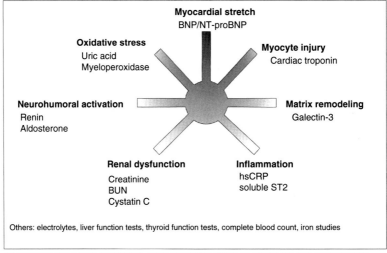

FIG. 9.1 Biomarkers of heart failure according to proposed underlying mechanisms. (Adapted from Braundwald E. Heart Failure. *JACC: Heart Failure.* 2013;1:120; with permission.)

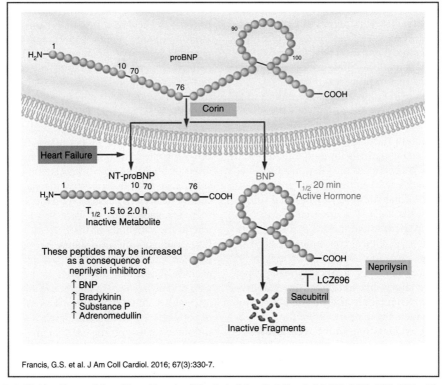

FIG. 9.2 Natriuretic peptides. (From Francis, GS, et al. *J Am Coll Cardiol*. 2016;67(3): 330-337; with permission.)

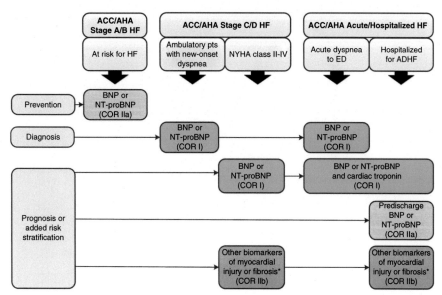

FIG. 9.3 2017 ACC/AHA/HFSA Focused Update of the 2013 ACCF/AHA Guideline for the management of acute heart failure with biomarker testing. (From Yancy CW, et al. *J Am Coll Cardiol*. 2017;70(6):776–803; with permission.)

*Other biomarkers of injury or fibrosis include soluble ST2 receptor, galectin-3, and high-sensitivity troponin.

received the highest level of recommendation (class I recommendation, level of evidence A) to establish prognosis or disease severity in chronic heart failure.[7] The guidelines also support measuring natriuretic peptide biomarkers in patients presenting with dyspnea to support or exclude a diagnosis of heart failure with the highest level of recommendation.[7] A new recommendation in the guidelines emphasizes that during a heart failure hospitalization, a predischarge natriuretic peptide level can be useful to establish a predischarge prognosis (class IIa recommendation, level of evidence B-NR).[7] The guidelines also suggest the additive benefit of using multiple biomarkers for risk stratification such as soluble suppression of tumorigenicity-2 (ST2) receptor, galectin-3 (Gal-3), and high-sensitivity cardiac troponin (cTn) in addition to NT-pro-BNP.

Several trials have examined the hypothesis that BNP-guided therapy, with serial measurements of BNP or NT-pro-BNP, can improve clinical outcomes in patients with established HFrEF. However, these randomized controlled trials have shown inconsistent results.[8–12] Notably, these clinical trials have been limited by significant heterogeneity in heart failure phenotype, variation in treatment strategies for targeted BNP levels, or the lack of consistent treatment protocol guidance. Specifically, the Guiding Evidence Based Therapy Using Biomarker Intensified Treatment in Heart Failure (GUIDE-IT) study which examined whether an NT-pro-BNP–guided

treatment strategy improved clinical outcomes versus usual care in high-risk patients with HFrEF was stopped for futility after a median of 15 months of follow-up.[13] The overall results were that routine NT-pro-BNP–guided therapy was not more effective than a usual care strategy in improving outcomes (Fig. 9.4). However, the study did have limitations as it did not exclude patients with known chronic kidney disease as it may not be realistic for these individuals to reach the target NT-pro-BNP as was directed in the GUIDE-IT protocol. In other words, there were individuals with persistently high NT-pro-BNP levels who were unable to reduce their heightened risk regardless of intention to treat, whereas others that had consistently low NT-pro-BNP levels that routine testing would not have reclassified their risks or changed their management.

The latest guidelines highlighted a new area of testing that may be more impactful to identify at-risk individuals for pre-emptive therapy to prevent heart failure. Two randomized clinical trials, NT-proBNP selected prevention of cardiac events in a population of diabetic patients without a history of cardiac disease (PONTIAC)[14] and The St Vincent's. Screening to Prevent Heart Failure (STOP-HF),[15] have demonstrated improvements in clinical outcomes with a strategy of using pre-emptive natriuretic peptide testing without overt symptoms or diagnosis of heart failure to identify high-risk patients for more aggressive heart failure–prevention strategies.

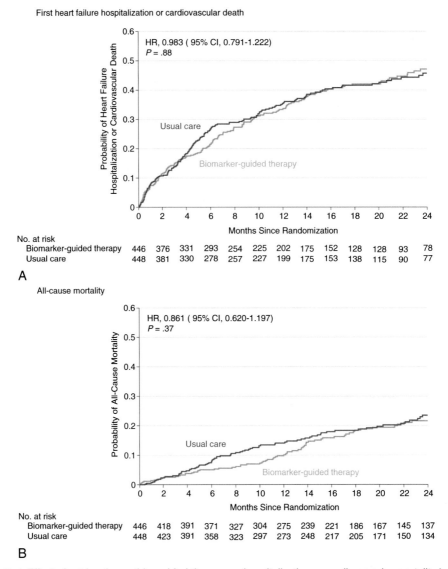

FIG. 9.4 Effect of natriuretic peptide–guided therapy on hospitalization or cardiovascular mortality in high-risk patients with heart failure and reduced ejection fraction. **(A)** First heart failure hospitalization or cardiocascular death. **(B)** All-cause mortality. (Felker GM, et al. *JAMA.* 2017;318(8):713; with permission.)

The overall result from these trials is that BNP should not be used alone and requires interpretation in the correct clinical context. Other cardiopulmonary disorders such as acute coronary syndrome (ACS), pulmonary hypertension, pulmonary embolism, renal dysfunction, advanced age, or arrhythmia are also associated with elevated BNP or NT-pro-BNP levels and hence potential cofounders when interpreting BNP or NT-pro-BNP levels.

Another newer biomarker for myocardial stress is ST2. This protein exists as both a soluble form (sST2) and a membrane-bound receptor form (ST2L).[16] Previous studies have shown that ST2 is associated with left ventricular strain, fibrosis, and ventricular remodeling.[16,17] Cardiac fibroblast stretching triggers ST2 gene expression.[18] Interleukin-33 (IL-33) has potential cardioprotective effects on the myocyte. IL-33 binds ST2L, which triggers antifibrotic, antiapoptic,

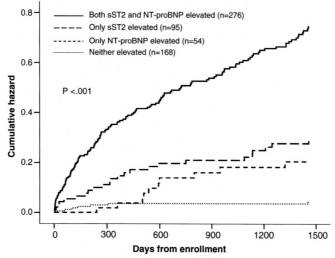

FIG. 9.5 Measurement of the interleukin family member ST2 in patients with acute dyspnea. (Results from the PRIDE study. Januzzi JL, et al. *J Am Coll Cardiol.* 2007;50(7):607–613; with permission.)

and antiremodeling effects.[17,19] However, high levels of sST2 block the cardioprotective effects because sST2 binds IL-33, which blocks binding to the ST2 receptor (STL2).[17] sST2 has prognostic value in chronic heart failure in the outpatient setting. This has been shown both independently and in addition to NT-pro-BNP and clinical risk scores.[20] Specifically, in patients with HFpEF, sST2 was more accurate than BNP or NT-pro-BNP in identifying severe diastolic dysfunction.[21] This suggests that the ST2 has a more specific role in following up HFpEF patients than BNP. Unlike natriuretic peptides, levels of sST2 are not affected by age, sex, body mass index, and valve disease.[22] The levels of sST2 positively correlate with increasing New York Heart Association class, worsening symptoms, and indicators of heart failure severity (norepinephrine levels, diastolic filling pressures, C-reactive protein (CRP), and BNP levels; Fig. 9.5).[22] Because of the predictive power of ST2, serial levels of sST2 to guide therapy could be used to guide therapy in both acute and chronic heart failure, in both HFpEF and HFrEF.[23,24]

sST2 has a possible role in helping to titrate guideline-directed therapy. In one study, sST2 levels in chronic heart failure patients fell after treatment with higher dose beta-blockers. Similarly, elevated sST2 concentrations (>35 ng/mL) can identify patients who may potentially benefit from higher doses of beta-blockers than those they are currently prescribed.[25] Another trial that showed the potential benefit of ST2 guided therapy was the Valsartan Heart Failure Trial (Val-Heft). In that study, treatment with valsartan reduced the rate of

increase in sST2 concentration compared with placebo. They also observed that an increase in sST2 was associated with adverse patient outcomes.[26] Treatment with a mineralocorticoid receptor antagonist (MRA) had a greater benefit among patients with acute heart failure exacerbations who had high sST2 concentrations.[27] The major limitation of these findings is the retrospective nature of these post hoc analyses from study data sets. Hence clinical guidelines regarding sST2 testing have received lower levels of supporting evidence and recommendations, and clinical adoption remains mixed.

There are emerging data to show the promise of sST2 testing in the acute decompensated heart failure setting. sST2 level was an independent predictor of prognosis regardless of LVEF and was a stronger predictor of prognosis than NT-pro-BNP, especially with serial assessment.[28,29] Whether the IL-33 or ST2 system could also be potential targets for future heart failure therapy remains a hot topic for future investigation.

Biomarkers of Myocardial Injury

The measure of myocardial injury in the modern era has been dominated by cTn. There are two principal cTns that are used clinically: (1) cardiac troponin I (cTnI) and (2) cardiac troponin T (cTnT). cTns have been widely adopted as the cardiac biomarker of choice for diagnosis and management of ACS. However, cTn is still an important biomarker for detection of myocardial injury in the setting of decompensated heart failure. Detecting cTn is useful in the diagnosis of ACS; however, the role of cTn levels in heart failure

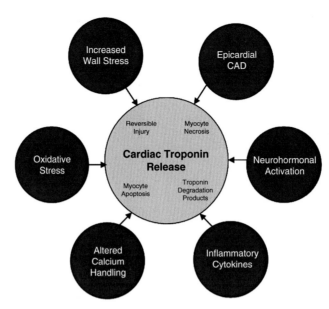

FIG. 9.6 Troponin elevation in heart failure: prevalence, mechanisms, and clinical implications. (Kociol RD, et al. *J AM Coll Cardiol*. 2010;56(14):1071–1078; with permission.)

is primarily risk stratification (class I recommendation, level of evidence in both acute and chronic heart failure; Fig. 9.6).[2] Elevated cTn concentrations have been showed to predict adverse outcomes in both acute and chronic heart failures.[2] In patients hospitalized with acute decompensated heart failure, those with elevated cTnI or cTnT had lower systolic blood pressures, lower ejection fraction, and higher rate of in-hospital mortality.[30] The underlying mechanism of cTn release in the setting of decompensated heart failure remains unclear as they do not follow the same trends as for ACS. The release of cTn is generally considered to be secondary to myocardial injury regardless of the mechanism (ischemia, necrosis, or apoptosis).[31] Quite a variety of factors influence the level of cTn elevation in heart failure, including differences in baseline characteristics in patient populations, clinical setting, and cTn assay used. In one study using a standard cTn assay, elevated cTn was detected in 25% of heart failure patients, and these patients had a poorer prognosis.[31]

In the era of high-sensitivity troponin assay (hs-cTn) the ability to detect myocardial injury in heart failure patients is even more sensitive. Using hs-cTn, elevated cTn can be detected in almost all patients with acute decompensated heart failure and the majority of patients with chronic heart failure.[32,33] Regardless of the assay used, elevated cTn is independently associated with adverse prognosis in patients with heart failure. It is always important to remember that ACS can be a trigger for acute heart failure. Interestingly, identifying those with detectable cTn using high-sensitivity assays has not contributed to incremental prognostic value for the patient cohorts over less sensitive assays at large as those detectable in the lower ranges have better outcomes to begin with (Grodin et al., AJM 2015). Owing to this, the 2013 ACCF/AHA guidelines recommend cTn measurements in all patients with acute heart failure to detect ACS and help determine treatment.[2]

With regard to cardiotoxicity, an increase in cTn over time (either due to chemotherapy or amyloidosis) indicates progression of cardiac dysfunction.[34,35] So far, there have not been any directed therapies that can reduce the rise of cTn in heart failure patients; however, early work has suggested that those with detectable cTnI and treated with open-label angiotensin-converting enzyme (ACE) inhibitors after cardiotoxic chemotherapy have less deterioration of cardiac function than those without them.[36]

Biomarkers of Myocardial Fibrosis

Inflammation has long been associated with heart failure, and available markers of inflammation such as CRP[37,38] and myeloperoxidase[39] have tracked prognosis. There are several biomarkers that correlate with myocardial fibrosis, but their history has been marked with assay variability and lack of specificity, and many of them have been restricted to research use only. Gal-3, a glycoprotein secreted by activated macrophages, has been touted as a biomarker for myocardial fibrosis.

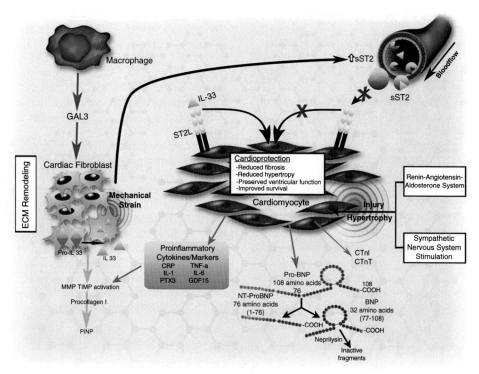

FIG. 9.7 Role of biomarkers for the prevention, assessment, and management of heart failure: a scientific statement from the American Heart Association. (Chow et al. *Circ* 2017;135; permission.)

Mechanistically, Gal-3 has been associated with various aspects of myocardial remodeling, including cell adhesion, inflammation, myocardial hypertrophy, fibroblast proliferation, and tissue fibrosis,[33,40] whereas direct Gal-3 infusion results in myocardial fibrosis in heart failure in a rat model.[41] In contrast, genetic disruption and pharmacological inhibition of Gal-3 in animal models prevent myocardial fibrosis, remodeling, and subsequent heart failure development.[42] Elevated Gal-3 levels have been associated with cardiac remodeling and poorer prognosis in patients with heart failure. Gal-3 has seen a higher predictive value in HFpEF patients than in HFrEF patients when predicting cardiac remodeling as assessed by diastolic echocardiographic parameters and poorer prognosis in terms of all-cause mortality and rehospitalization.[43-45] In experimental models, Gal-3 was associated with aldosterone-induced myocardial fibrosis; however, MRA treatment did not show any change in fibrosis when studied in chronic HFrEF patients.[46,47] The main benefit of measuring Gal-3 for risk stratification in heart failure patients depends on the diminishing propensity to recover myocardial function with increasing levels of Gal-3, likely due to increased amounts of fibrosis. For example, patient with low plasma Gal-3 levels have

shown clinical benefit when treated with rosuvastatin[48] or valsartan[49] for HFrEF. However, for HFrEF, patients with high Gal-3 level had worse outcomes, independent of treatment with guideline-directed therapy or NT-pro-BNP[44,50] (Fig. 9.7). One major caveat for the use of Gal-3 is that renal insufficiency affects Gal-3 levels and is a major confounder.[51,52] In fact, Gal-3 (also known as Mac2) is well known to be expressed in damaged renal tubules and macrophages, and elevated levels have been associated with progression of chronic kidney disease. Few studies, if any, have demonstrated any incremental value of Gal-3 testing above and beyond standard laboratory testing of creatinine and blood urea nitrogen (BUN) which are used to predict the progression of chronic kidney disease. In fact, when Gal-3 was compared with ST2, it was ST2 that was shown to be better in risk stratification and prognosis in patients with chronic heart failure in the outpatient setting.[53]

Biomarkers of Cardiorenal Dysfunction

Renal insufficiency is independently associated with poor prognosis in all phenotypes of heart failure.[54] The most basic renal function markers are BUN and creatinine levels. These are still widely used to measure renal function, but a wide variety of factors influence them, including sex, age, race, concurrent illness, and muscle mass. Cardiorenal syndrome (CRS) is a complex and serious condition that requires early identification and treatment. Therefore, BUN and creatinine may not reflect true renal function, and other candidate renal biomarkers are necessary. In fact, clinicians have yet to carefully define what aspects of "renal function" are relevant in different clinical settings—creatinine largely estimates filtration function and urea serves as a barometer of osmolyte balance, whereas many drugs and solutes rely on intact renal tubular function and their corresponding physiologic feedback to maintain salt and water balance that is critically important for heart failure (Fig. 9.8).

Cystatin C (CysC) is a cysteine protease inhibitor that is present in all tissue and produced at a constant rate, filtered freely, and neither secreted into the renal tubules or absorbed into the blood stream from the renal tubules. Given the abovementioned characteristics, it has been suggested as a newer and potentially more accurate replacement for creatinine to calculate glomerular filtration rate (GFR).[55] In a separate study, elevated CysC levels were associated with poor prognosis in both acute and chronic heart failure.[56] However, so far, CysC has been unable to differentiate between specific phenotype of CRS, so it has not been able to serve as a therapeutic target in heart failure.[56] Comparing various renal biomarkers in the setting of acute heart failure, the biomarker that has the strongest prognostic significance remains to be BUN.[57]

Another renal biomarker that is more specific for CRS is neutrophil gelatinase-associated lipocalin (NGAL), which is currently only available for clinical use in Europe and still undergoing clinical development in the United States. NGAL is a small protein found in neutrophil granules. After tubular kidney injury, both urine and plasma levels of NGAL are elevated and predict adverse prognosis in patients with heart failure. Specifically, the difference between the plasma and urinary NGAL levels is what helps identify CRS.[56] Even though urine NGAL levels are elevated in both patients with heart failure and acute kidney injury,

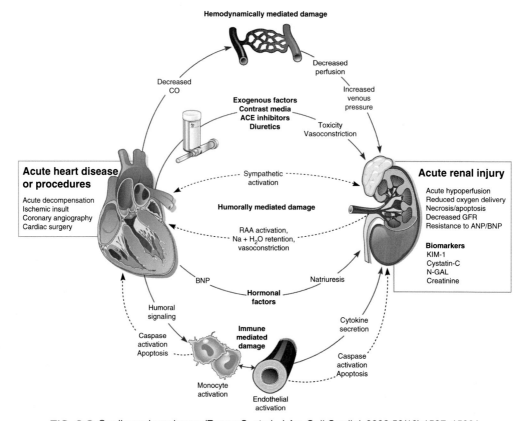

FIG. 9.8 Cardiorenal syndrome. (Ronco C, et al. *J Am Coll Cardiol.* 2008;52(19):1527–1539.)

the levels are lower in patients with heart failure than in patients with acute kidney injury.[58] Serum NGAL is associated with GFR and development of long-term renal dysfunction. Serum and urinary NGAL levels represent two different aspects of renal dysfunction and acute kidney injury.

There is a wealth of literature describing several novel acute kidney injury biomarkers such as N-acetyl-β-D-glucosaminidase (NAG) and kidney injury marker-1 (KIM-1). NAG is a lysosomal enzyme originating from the proximal tubular cells and indicates proximal tubular damage when present in urine. Urine NAG is associated with worsening renal function and mortality in patients with chronic heart failure.[56,59] NAG is limited in its ability to identify CRS as it is also increased in diabetes and hypertension, which are common comorbid conditions in heart failure patients.[56] On the other hand, KIM-1 is a glycoprotein expressed in the proximal renal tubule in kidney injury but not expressed in normal kidney tissue. KIM-1 levels were inversely associated with LVEF and directly associated with worsening congestive heart failure symptoms among patients with chronic heart failure without renal dysfunction.[60,61] Higher plasma KIM-1 levels are associated with poor prognosis and worsening renal function in the setting of acute heart failure; however, in a larger analysis, its prognostic value was lowered after covariate adjustments, with only 180-day mortality risk still remaining significant.[62] Theoretically, the abovementioned biomarkers for renal injury and CRS may be useful in certain subgroups of heart failure patients, although none of them have shown to be strongly predictive of acute or persistent renal injury in the setting of heart failure. This is in part due to the fact that unlike other nephrotoxic processes, the large majority of CRSs do not have overt tubular injury but largely exacerbated by raised renal sodium avidity and azotemia. Further research will help specify which subset of patients would benefit from serial biomarker measurement. Given that the different subsets of heart failure patients determined by the different biomarkers likely reflect differing underlying pathology, this could lead to more tailored therapeutics.

CONCLUSIONS

Cardiac biomarker–guided therapy offers more tailored therapy options given the wide heterogeneity seen in the heart failure phenotypes. It also potentially can prevent iatrogenic injury from inappropriate therapy. Currently the best prognostic indicators involve using multiple biomarkers in conjunction to help guide therapy and prognostication as opposed to being reliant on a single biomarker. In our own practice, we use serial NT-pro-BNP measurement as an outpatient procedure to help assess our patient's volume status and progression of heart failure. Going forward in the future, the specificity of biomarker-based therapy may help us identify individuals who would benefit from tailored therapy and provide novel targets for future drug development.

REFERENCES

1. Mozaffarian D, Benjamin EJ, Go AS, et al. Heart disease and stroke statistics-2015 update. *A Rep Am Heart Assoc*. 2015;131. https://doi.org/10.1161/CIR.0000000000000152.
2. Yancy CW, Jessup M, Bozkurt B, et al. 2013 ACCF/AHA guideline for the management of heart failure: executive summary: a report of the American college of cardiology foundation/American Heart Association task force on practice guidelines. *Circulation*. 2013;128(16):1810–1852. https://doi.org/10.1161/CIR.0b013e31829e8807.
3. McMurray JJV, Packer M, Desai AS, et al. Angiotensin-neprilysin inhibition versus enalapril in heart failure. *N Engl J Med*. 2014;371(11):993–1004. https://doi.org/10.1056/NEJMoa1409077.
4. Weber M, Hamm C. Role of B-type natriuretic peptide (BNP) and NT-proBNP in clinical routine. *Heart*. 2006;92(6):843–849. https://doi.org/10.1136/hrt.2005.071233.
5. Mehra MR, Uber PA, Park MH, et al. Obesity and suppressed B-type natriuretic peptide levels in heart failure. *J Am Coll Cardiol*. 2004;43(9):1590–1595. https://doi.org/10.1016/j.jacc.2003.10.066.
6. Krim SR, Vivo RP, Krim NR, et al. Racial/ethnic differences in b-type natriuretic peptide levels and their association with care and outcomes among patients hospitalized with heart failure: findings from get with the guidelines-heart failure. *JACC Hear Fail*. 2013;1(4):345–352. https://doi.org/10.1016/j.jchf.2013.04.008.
7. Yancy CW, Jessup M, Bozkurt B, et al. 2017 ACC/AHA/HFSA focused update of the 2013 ACCF/AHA guideline for the management of heart failure. *J Am Coll Cardiol*. 2017;70(6):776–803. https://doi.org/10.1016/j.jacc.2017.04.025.
8. Eurlings LWM, Van Pol PEJ, Kok WE, et al. Management of chronic heart failure guided by individual N-terminal ProB-type natriuretic peptide targets: results of the PRIMA (Can PRo-brain-natriuretic peptide guided therapy of chronic heart failure IMprove heart fAilure morbidity and mortality?). *Stud J Am Coll Cardiol*. 2010;56(25):2090–2100. https://doi.org/10.1016/j.jacc.2010.07.030.
9. Berger R, Moertl D, Peter S, et al. N-terminal pro-B-type natriuretic peptide-guided, intensive patient management in addition to multidisciplinary care in chronic heart failure. A 3-Arm, prospective, randomized pilot study. *J Am Coll Cardiol*. 2010;55(7):645–653. https://doi.org/10.1016/j.jacc.2009.08.078.

10. Persson H, Erntell H, Eriksson B, Johansson G, Swedberg K, Dahlström U. Improved pharmacological therapy of chronic heart failure in primary care: a randomized Study of NT-proBNP guided management of heart failure - SIGNAL-HF (Swedish intervention study - guidelines and NT-proBNP analysis in heart failure). *Eur J Heart Fail*. 2010;12(12):1300–1308. https://doi.org/10.1093/eurjhf/hfq169.

11. Januzzi JL, Rehman SU, Mohammed AA, et al. Use of amino-terminal ProB-type natriuretic peptide to guide outpatient therapy of patients with chronic left ventricular systolic dysfunction. *J Am Coll Cardiol*. 2011;58(18):1881–1889. https://doi.org/10.1016/j.jacc.2011.03.072.

12. B-type natriuretic peptide–guided heart failure therapy. *Arch Intern Med*. 2013;170(6):507–514.

13. Felker GM, Anstrom KJ, Adams KF, et al. Effect of natriuretic peptide–guided therapy on hospitalization or cardiovascular mortality in high-risk patients with heart failure and reduced ejection fraction. *JAMA*. 2017;318(8):713. https://doi.org/10.1001/jama.2017.10565.

14. Huelsmann M, Neuhold S, Resl M, et al. PONTIAC (NT-proBNP selected prevention of cardiac eveNts in a population of diabetic patients without A history of cardiac disease): a prospective randomized controlled trial. *J Am Coll Cardiol*. 2013;62(15):1365–1372. https://doi.org/10.1016/j.jacc.2013.05.069.

15. Ledwidge M, Gallagher J, Conlon C, et al. Natriuretic peptide–based screening and collaborative care for heart failure. *JAMA*. 2013;310(1):66. https://doi.org/10.1001/jama.2013.7588.

16. Weinberg EO, Shimpo M, Hurwitz S, ichi TS, Rouleau JL, Lee RT. Identification of serum soluble ST2 receptor as a novel heart failure biomarker. *Circulation*. 2003;107(5):721–726. https://doi.org/10.1161/01.CIR.0000047274.66749.FE.

17. Sanada S, Hakuno D, Higgins LJ, Schreiter ER, McKenzie ANJ, Lee RT. IL-33 and ST2 comprise a critical biomechanically induced and cardioprotective signaling system. *J Clin Invest*. 2007;117(6):1538–1549. https://doi.org/10.1172/JCI30634.

18. Weinberg EO, Shimpo M, De Keulenaer GW, et al. Expression and regulation of ST2, an interleukin-1 receptor family member, in cardiomyocytes and myocardial infarction. *Circulation*. 2002;106(23):2961–2966. https://doi.org/10.1161/01.CIR.0000038705.69871.D9.

19. Seki K, Sanada S, Kudinova AY, et al. Interleukin-33 prevents apoptosis and improves survival after experimental myocardial infarction through ST2 signaling. *Circ Hear Fail*. 2009;2(6):684–691. https://doi.org/10.1161/CIRCHEARTFAILURE.109.873240.

20. Ky B, French B, McCloskey K, et al. High-sensitivity ST2 for prediction of adverse outcomes in chronic heart failure. *Circ Hear Fail*. 2011;4(2):180–187. https://doi.org/10.1161/CIRCHEARTFAILURE.110.958223.

21. Wang YC, Yu CC, Chiu FC, et al. Soluble ST2 as a biomarker for detecting stable heart failure with a normal ejection fraction in hypertensive patients. *J Card Fail*. 2013;19(3):163–168. https://doi.org/10.1016/j.cardfail.2013.01.010.

22. Rehman SU, Mueller T, Januzzi JL. Characteristics of the novel interleukin family biomarker ST2 in patients with acute heart failure. *J Am Coll Cardiol*. 2008;52(18):1458–1465. https://doi.org/10.1016/j.jacc.2008.07.042.

23. Gaggin HK, Szymonifka J, Bhardwaj A, et al. Head-to-Head comparison of serial soluble ST2, growth differentiation factor-15, and highly-sensitive troponin T measurements in patients with chronic heart failure. *JACC Hear Fail*. 2014;2(1):65–72. https://doi.org/10.1016/j.jchf.2013.10.005.

24. Manzano-Fernández S, Januzzi JL, Pastor-Pérez FJ, et al. Serial monitoring of soluble interleukin family member ST2 in patients with acutely decompensated heart failure. *Cardiology*. 2012;122(3):158–166. https://doi.org/10.1159/000338800.

25. Gaggin HK, Motiwala S, Bhardwaj A, Parks KA, Januzzi JL. Soluble concentrations of the interleukin receptor family member ST2 and β-Blocker therapy in chronic heart failure. *Circ Hear Fail*. 2013;6(6):1209–1213. https://doi.org/10.1161/CIRCHEARTFAILURE.113.000457.

26. Anand IS, Rector TS, Kuskowski M, Snider J, Cohn JN. Prognostic value of soluble ST2 in the Valsartan heart failure trial. *Circ Hear Fail*. 2014;7(3):418–426. https://doi.org/10.1161/CIRCHEARTFAILURE.113.001036.

27. Maisel A, Xue Y, Van Veldhuisen DJ, et al. Effect of spironolactone on 30-day death and heart failure rehospitalization (from the COACH study). *Am J Cardiol*. 2014;114(5):737–742. https://doi.org/10.1016/j.amjcard.2014.05.062.

28. Januzzi JL, Peacock WF, Maisel AS, et al. Measurement of the interleukin family member ST2 in patients with acute dyspnea. Results from the PRIDE (Pro-Brain natriuretic peptide investigation of dyspnea in the Emergency Department) study. *J Am Coll Cardiol*. 2007;50(7):607–613. https://doi.org/10.1016/j.jacc.2007.05.014.

29. Tang WHW, Wu Y, Grodin JL, et al. Prognostic value of baseline and changes in circulating soluble ST2 levels and the effects of nesiritide in acute decompensated heart failure. *JACC Hear Fail*. 2016;4(1):68–77. https://doi.org/10.1016/j.jchf.2015.07.015.

30. Felker GM, Hasselblad V, Tang WHW, et al. Troponin I in acute decompensated heart failure: insights from the ASCEND-HF study. *Eur J Heart Fail*. 2012;14(11):1257–1264. https://doi.org/10.1093/eurjhf/hfs110.

31. Braunwald E. Heart failure. *JACC Hear Fail*. 2013;1(1):1–20. https://doi.org/10.1016/j.jchf.2012.10.002.

32. Xue Y, Clopton P, Peacock WF, Maisel AS. Serial changes in high-sensitive troponin i predict outcome in patients with decompensated heart failure. *Eur J Heart Fail*. 2011;13(1):37–42. https://doi.org/10.1093/eurjhf/hfq210.

33. De Boer RA, Daniels LB, Maisel AS, Januzzi JL. State of the art: newer biomarkers in heart failure. *Eur J Heart Fail*. 2015;17(6):559–569. https://doi.org/10.1002/ejhf.273.

34. Cardinale D, Sandri MT, Colombo A, et al. Prognostic value of troponin I in cardiac risk stratification of cancer patients undergoing high-dose chemotherapy. *Circulation.* 2004;109(22):2749–2754. https://doi.org/10.1161/01.CIR. 0000130926.51766.CC.

35. Ky B, Putt M, Sawaya H, et al. Early increases in multiple biomarkers predict subsequent cardiotoxicity in patients with breast cancer treated with doxorubicin, taxanes, and trastuzumab. *J Am Coll Cardiol.* 2014;63(8):809–816. https://doi.org/10.1016/j.jacc.2013.10.061.

36. Cardinale D, Colombo A, Sandri MT, et al. Prevention of high-dose chemotherapy-induced cardiotoxicity in high-risk patients by angiotensin-converting enzyme inhibition. *Circulation.* 2006;114(23):2474–2481. https://doi.org/10.1161/CIRCULATIONAHA.106.635144.

37. Kalogeropoulos AP, Tang WHW, Hsu A, et al. High-sensitivity C-reactive protein in acute heart failure: insights from the ASCEND-HF trial. *J Card Fail.* 2014;20(5): 319–326. https://doi.org/10.1016/j.cardfail.2014.02.002.

38. Tang WHW, Shrestha K, Van Lente F, et al. Usefulness of C-reactive protein and left ventricular diastolic performance for prognosis in patients with left ventricular systolic heart failure. *Am J Cardiol.* 2008;101(3):370–373. https://doi.org/10.1016/j.amjcard.2007.08.038.

39. Tang WHW, Wu Y, Nicholls SJ, Hazen SL. Plasma myeloperoxidase predicts incident cardiovascular risks in stable patients undergoing medical management for coronary artery disease. *Clin Chem.* 2011;57(1):33–39. https://doi.org/10.1373/clinchem.2010.152827.

40. Yang R-Y, Rabinovich GA, Liu F-T. Galectins: structure, function and therapeutic potential. *Expert Rev Mol Med.* 2008;10:e17. https://doi.org/10.1017/S1462399408000719.

41. Sharma UC, Pokharel S, Van Brakel TJ, et al. Galectin-3 marks activated macrophages in failure-prone hypertrophied hearts and contributes to cardiac dysfunction. *Circulation.* 2004;110(19):3121–3128. https://doi.org/10.1161/01.CIR.0000147181.65298.4D.

42. Yu L, Ruifrok WPT, Meissner M, et al. Genetic and pharmacological inhibition of galectin-3 prevents cardiac remodeling by interfering with myocardial fibrogenesis. *Circ Hear Fail.* 2013;6(1):107–117. https://doi.org/10.1161/CIRCHEARTFAILURE.112.971168.

43. de Boer RA, Lok DJA, Jaarsma T, et al. Predictive value of plasma galectin-3 levels in heart failure with reduced and preserved ejection fraction. *Ann Med.* 2011;43(1):60–68. https://doi.org/10.3109/07853890.2010.538080.

44. Edelmann F, Holzendorf V, Wachter R, et al. Galectin-3 in patients with heart failure with preserved ejection fraction: results from the Aldo-DHF trial. *Eur J Heart Fail.* 2015;17(2):214–223. https://doi.org/10.1002/ejhf.203.

45. Shah RV, Chen-Tournoux AA, Picard MH, Van Kimmenade RRJ, Januzzi JL. Galectin-3, cardiac structure and function, and long-term mortality in patients with acutely decompensated heart failure. *Eur J Heart Fail.* 2010;12(8):826–832. https://doi.org/10.1093/eurjhf/hfq091.

46. Calvier L, Miana M, Reboul P, et al. Galectin-3 mediates aldosterone-induced vascular fibrosis. *Arterioscler Thromb Vasc Biol.* 2013;33(1):67–75. https://doi.org/10.1161/ATVBAHA.112.300569.

47. Gandhi PU, Motiwala SR, Belcher AM, et al. Galectin-3 and mineralocorticoid receptor antagonist use in patients with chronic heart failure due to left ventricular systolic dysfunction. *Am Heart J.* 2015;169(3):404–411.e3. https://doi.org/10.1016/j.ahj.2014.12.012.

48. Gullestad L, Ueland T, Kjekshus J, et al. Galectin-3 predicts response to statin therapy in the controlled rosuvastatin multinational trial in heart failure (CORONA). *Eur Heart J.* 2012;33(18):2290–2296. https://doi.org/10.1093/eurheartj/ehs077.

49. Anand IS, Rector TS, Kuskowski M, Adourian A, Muntendam P, Cohn JN. Baseline and serial measurements of galectin-3 in patients with heart failure: relationship to prognosis and effect of treatment with valsartan in the Val-HeFT. *Eur J Heart Fail.* 2013;15(5):511–518. https://doi.org/10.1093/eurjhf/hfs205.

50. AbouEzzeddine OF, Haines P, Stevens S, et al. Galectin-3 in heart failure with preserved ejection fraction. A RELAX trial substudy (phosphodiesterase-5 inhibition to improve clinical status and exercise capacity in diastolic heart failure). *JACC Hear Fail.* 2015;3(3):245–252. https://doi.org/10.1016/j.jchf.2014.10.009.

51. Gopal DM, Kommineni M, Ayalon N, et al. Relationship of plasma galectin-3 to renal function in patients with heart failure: effects of clinical status, pathophysiology of heart failure, and presence or absence of heart failure. *J Am Heart Assoc.* 2012;1(5). https://doi.org/10.1161/JAHA.112.000760.

52. Tang WHW, Shrestha K, Shao Z, et al. Usefulness of plasma galectin-3 levels in systolic heart failure to predict renal insufficiency and survival. *Am J Cardiol.* 2011;108(3):385–390. https://doi.org/10.1016/j.amjcard.2011.03.056.

53. Bayes-Genis A, De Antonio M, Vila J, et al. Head-to-head comparison of 2 myocardial fibrosis biomarkers for long-term heart failure risk stratification: ST2 versus galectin-3. *J Am Coll Cardiol.* 2014;63(2):158–166. https://doi.org/10.1016/j.jacc.2013.07.087.

54. Damman K, Testani JM. The kidney in heart failure: an update. *Eur Heart J.* 2015;36(23):1437–1444. https://doi.org/10.1093/eurheartj/ehv010.

55. Shlipak MG, Matsushita K, Ärnlöv J, et al. Cystatin C versus creatinine in determining risk based on kidney function. *N Engl J Med.* 2013;369(10):932–943. https://doi.org/10.1056/NEJMoa1214234.

56. Brisco MA, Testani JM. Novel renal biomarkers to assess cardiorenal syndrome. *Curr Heart Fail Rep.* 2014;11(4):485–499. https://doi.org/10.1007/s11897-014-0226-4.

57. Tang WHW, Dupont M, Hernandez AF, et al. Comparative assessment of short-term adverse events in acute heart failure with cystatin C and other estimates of renal function: results from the ASCEND-HF trial. *JACC Hear Fail.* 2015;3(1):40–49. https://doi.org/10.1016/j.jchf.2014.06.014.

58. Dupont M, Shrestha K, Singh D, et al. Lack of significant renal tubular injury despite acute kidney injury in acute decompensated heart failure. *Eur J Heart Fail.* 2012;14(6): 597–604. https://doi.org/10.1093/eurjhf/hfs039.

59. Damman K, Masson S, Hillege HL, et al. Clinical outcome of renal tubular damage in chronic heart failure. *Eur Heart J.* 2011;32(21):2705–2712. https://doi.org/10.1093/eurheartj/ehr190.

60. Damman K, Van Veldhuisen DJ, Navis G, et al. Tubular damage in chronic systolic heart failure is associated with reduced survival independent of glomerular filtration rate. *Heart.* 2010;96(16):1297–1302. https://doi.org/10.1136/hrt.2010.194878.

61. Emmens JE, ter Maaten JM, Matsue Y, et al. Plasma kidney injury molecule-1 in heart failure: renal mechanisms and clinical outcome. *Eur J Heart Fail.* 2016;18(6). https://doi.org/10.1002/ejhf.426.

62. Grodin JL, Perez AL, Wu Y, et al. Circulating kidney injury Molecule-1 levels in acute heart failure. Insights from the ASCEND-HF trial (acute study of clinical effectiveness of nesiritide in decompensated heart failure). *JACC Hear Fail.* 2015;3(10):777–785. https://doi.org/10.1016/j.jchf.2015.06.006.

CHAPTER 10

Cardiac Biomarkers in Acute Myocardial Infarction

MAHMOUD ALLAHHAM, MD • MOHITA SINGH, MD • HANI JNEID, MD

CARDIAC BIOMARKERS IN ACUTE CORONARY SYNDROME

Acute myocardial infarction (AMI) is defined by the presence of myocardial necrosis in the clinical setting of acute myocardial ischemia as supported by history, physical examination, electrocardiograph (ECG) findings, and biochemical markers of myocardial necrosis. However, given the advances including the development of highly sensitive and specific myocardial tissue biomarkers and the improvement in management of patients with myocardial infarction (MI), we are able to both detect very minute levels of myocardial injury and/or abort myocardial injury and necrosis very early after its onset. Given the wide array of biomarkers available with varying degrees of sensitivity and specificity, this chapter aims to provide an overview of the role of contemporary and emerging biomarkers in patients with acute coronary syndrome (ACS) and AMI. We focus particularly on patients with non-ST elevation myocardial infarction given this syndrome will depend to a larger extent on risk stratification and diagnostic assays to dictate in-hospital treatment. Although cardiac biomarkers play an important role in patients with ST-elevation myocardial infarction, they are less likely to influence in-hospital treatment strategies, especially the need for emergent reperfusion. Reperfusion therapy, whether percutaneous coronary intervention (PCI) or fibrinolytic, should not await the result of cardiac biomarker measurements.

HISTORICAL BIOMARKERS

Aspartate transaminase (AST) was the first biomarker used in the diagnosis of AMI and was widely used in the 1960s and incorporated into the World Health Organization definition of AMI. However, AST is not specific for cardiac muscle. Two additional cardiac biomarkers emerged by 1970s: (1) lactate dehydrogenase (LDH) and (2) creatine kinase (CK). Neither is specific for cardiac muscle, but CK is more specific than LDH in the context of AMI, especially in patients having other comorbidities. Myoglobin, a small globular oxygen-carrying protein found in heart and striated skeletal muscle, rises after acute myocardial injury and became a useful biomarker in the differential diagnosis of suspected AMI. In the era of high-sensitivity cardiac troponin (hs-cTn), myoglobin is no longer needed as an early marker of myocardial necrosis.

Advancements in electrophoresis allowed the detection of cardiac-specific isoenzymes of CK and LDH. These assays played an important role in the diagnosis of AMI for 2 decades; however, the lack of specificity and the high rate of false-positive results limited their usefulness.

Cardiac Troponins

In the late 1990s a sensitive and reliable radioimmunoassay was developed to detect serum troponin. Troponin T and I isoforms, known as cardiac troponins (cTn), are highly specific and sensitive to cardiac myocytes. Troponin is a component of the contractile apparatus within skeletal and cardiac myocytes. The sensitivity for detecting an AMI with troponin T and I approaches 100% when sampled 6–12 h after AMI onset.

From a clinical standpoint, cardiac troponin T and I appear to have equal clinical use. Numerous studies demonstrate that troponins appear in the serum 4–10 h after the onset of AMI. Troponin levels peak at 12–48 h but remain elevated for 4–10 days. The plasma half-life of cTn is around 2 h. Several properties inherent to cardiac troponins confer significant advantage to their diagnostic use. Troponin I and troponin T subunits are virtually exclusive to the myocardium, where they occur in high concentrations. In the setting of myocardial necrosis, cardiac troponins are swiftly released into the blood stream, and this release tends to be proportionate to the magnitude of the myocardial damage. Although the precise mechanism by which troponin is eliminated from the body remains unclear, it is hypothesized that troponin is cleared, at least partially, by the reticuloendothelial system.

Biomarkers in Cardiovascular Disease. https://doi.org/10.1016/B978-0-323-54835-9.00010-7

It is important to remember that elevated troponins are markers of myocardial necrosis which can be caused by multiple disease processes other than coronary pathology. There are numerous intracardiac diseases than can cause troponin elevation, including myocarditis, pericarditis, acute exacerbation of heart failure, cardiac trauma, and tachyarrhythmias. In addition, many extra-cardiac disease processes can lead to demand ischemia and myocardial necrosis, such as sepsis, pulmonary embolism, and drug toxicity, among many others. Because troponin is renally cleared, patients with chronic kidney disease can have persistently elevated troponins or a baseline troponin elevation. As mentioned earlier, serial changes in troponin (greater than 20%) are generally more concerning for coronary disease and thus help distinguish acute MI from noncoronary causes of troponin elevation.[1]

Patients with myocardial ischemia can have persistently elevated troponins for up to 14 days after presentation.[1] Before the development of high-sensitivity troponin assays, this posed a significant challenge to diagnosing reinfarction in patients with recent acute MI. Historically, it was a common practice to use creatine kinase-muscle/brain (CK-MB) for the diagnosis of suspected reinfarction given its quick clearance (generally within 48h). However, modern high-sensitivity troponin assays made it possible to detect serial changes in a timely manner. Even though the use of troponin assays to diagnose reinfarction has not been extensively studied, it is suggested that a serial increase in troponin of greater than 20% using a high-sensitivity assay is suggestive of reinfarction. This is one area that requires further investigation.

Definition of Myocardial Infarction

According to the Third Universal Definition of MI Task Force, AMI can be subclassified into five different types. Type 1 MI is a spontaneous MI resulting from an atherosclerotic plaque disruption (e.g., rupture, ulceration, erosion dissection) and a superimposed intraluminal thrombus. This ultimately results in acute reduction in myocardial blood flow and myocardial necrosis. However, 5%–20% of patients with type 1 MI, particularly women, may have non-obstructive coronary artery disease (CAD) on angiography,[2] a term recently recognized as MI with non-obstructive coronary artery disease (MINOCA).

Type 2 MI is an MI secondary to myocardial oxygen demand-supply imbalance, irrespective of the presence or absence of obstructive CAD. Myocardial necrosis may result from coronary vasospasm, endothelial dysfunction or direct toxic effects of endogenous or exogenous high circulation catecholamine levels, and other etiologies. The disparity in myocardial oxygen supply and demand may occur in the presence of fixed underlying atherosclerotic disease.

Type 3 MI describes patients who present with sudden cardiac death and symptoms suggestive of possible MI as suggested by history or ECG changes but die before biomarkers can be obtained. Type 4 MI and type 5 MI describe MIs associated with revascularization procedures. They refer to myocardial injury or infarction incurred during instrumentation of the heart either during PCI or coronary artery bypass grafting (CABG), respectively. An updated document summarizing a new universal definition of MI is currently underway and is expected to be released in late 2018 (Table 10.1).

The writing group for the 2012 Third Universal definition of MI emphasized the importance of using only troponin as a biomarker to diagnose MI. Only in the absence of cardiac troponins it is recommended to use CK-MB.

There are two components of troponin abnormalities for the diagnosis of AMI as defined by the 2012 Third Universal Definition of MI: (1) absolute elevation and (2) serial changes. The absolute elevation is defined as a troponin measurement above the 99th percentile of the upper reference level of the particular assay being used. In addition to at least 1 value above the 99th percentile, a serial change of more than 20% in either direction is required to make the diagnosis of

TABLE 10.1
Third Universal Definition of MI Classifications

MI Type	Definition	Examples
1	Atherosclerotic plaque disruption and a superimposed intraluminal thrombus	Rupture, ulceration, and erosion dissection
2	Myocardial oxygen demand-supply imbalance	Coronary vasospasm and endothelial dysfunction
3	Death occurs before biomarkers are obtained	Sudden death with typical history and/or ECG changes
4	MI associated with PCI or stent thrombosis	IST
5	MI associated with cardiac surgery	CABG

Adapted with modification from Thygesen K, Alpert JS, Jaffe AS, et al. Third universal definition of myocardial infarction. *Circulation*. 2012;126:2020–2035.

acute MI. In cases that fail to meet the first criteria of absolute troponin elevation >99% of the upper reference level, a serial change greater than 3 standard deviations is required to make the diagnosis of acute MI.[2]

When comparing the diagnostic value using the 99th percentile cutoff to that of serial changes in troponins, it has been shown that that the latter has higher specificity.[3] This is to be expected considering that several non-MI disease processes can cause a consistently elevated troponin, whereas they are less likely to cause a significant serial change compared with acute MI. Furthermore, it has been shown that using absolute values for the serial change in troponins (i.e., in ng/dL) yielded higher specificity for acute MI than relative changes (i.e., percent change from initial troponin).[3]

The underlying theme is that there should be evidence of myocardial necrosis as documented by elevations in cardiac biomarkers. There are increasing numbers of biomarkers available that both increase the diagnostic yield and risk stratification of patients who present with AMI. Given the multitude of options available, there is a lack of consensus even among the leading experts regarding the choice of optimal biomarkers in patients with suspected AMI. We will therefore summarize the current recommendations from the guidelines by the European Society of Cardiology (ESC) and American Heart Association (AHA)/American College of Cardiology (ACC) and then highlight the differences and similarities in the two guidelines so that clinicians can make informed decisions in these patients.

A Summary of Recommendations by the Various Societies: Issues and Controversies

The writing group of the 2015 ESC guideline recommended the use of biomarkers in all patients with suspected Non-ST elevation acute coronary syndrome (NSTE-ACS). Overall, the guidelines recommended using hs-cTn preferentially over CK and its MB isozyme, as well as contemporary cardiac troponin assays. Per the guideline, high-sensitivity assays were preferred because they had a higher negative predictive value and led to earlier detection of acute MI (specifically about 4% absolute and 20% relative increase in the detection of type I MI and twofold increase in detection of type 2 MI).[4] The guidelines also acknowledge a correlation between the levels of high-sensitivity troponin and the quantitative cardiomyocyte damage so that higher levels of troponins suggest a higher likelihood of MI. For example, elevations greater than 4 times the upper limit of normal have greater than 90% positive predictive value for type I MI, but a three- to four-time increase will only have a 50%–60% positive predictive value.[4]

Furthermore, the guidelines bring attention to the fact that dynamic changes in biomarkers or rising levels of high-sensitivity troponin are much more suggestive of acute MI as it is common for individuals in a general population to have detectable levels of cardiac troponins measured with a high-sensitivity assay. However, they did note that currently there was no clear evidence that the diagnostic accuracy gained by the high-sensitivity troponin translated to identification of a clinically relevant and previously misidentified population. Of note, the authors counseled against attributing elevated cardiac troponins to impaired clearance in patients with renal dysfunction and also noted the possibility of aortic dissection and pulmonary embolism in a patient who presents with chest pain and elevated cardiac troponin.[4]

The writing group of the AHA/ACC 2014 guideline for non–ST-elevation ACS took a somewhat similar approach, but with slight differences.[1] At the time of the publication of the ACC/AHA NSTE-ACS guideline, hs-cTn assays were not available in the United States. The writing group argued that the development of contemporary cardiac biomarkers with high sensitivity and specificity, namely troponin I and troponin T, made these biomarkers the mainstay diagnostic strategy for ACS.[1] The modern assays are reliable, fast, and relatively inexpensive, making them an attractive diagnostic modality. The AHA/ACC 2014 guidelines recommend measuring troponins at presentation and 3–6 h after the onset of symptoms in patients with suspected ACS (LOE: A). This interval of measurement allows for identification of any significant upward or downward trend which would be consistent with ACS. If the time of symptoms onset is unclear as it is often the case, the guidelines recommend establishing the time of presentation as the time of onset and trending the troponins accordingly (LOE: A). Furthermore, in patients whose clinical picture or EKG findings are highly concerning for ACS but whose initial troponins are within normal limits, the guidelines recommend trending the troponins beyond the aforementioned 6 hours after onset of symptoms (LOE: A).[1] When comparing the diagnostic value using the 99th percentile cutoff to that of serial changes in troponins, it has been shown that the latter has higher specificity.[3]

It is worth noting that different assays of contemporary troponins have varying reference ranges, and thus, troponin measurements should be interpreted according to the predefined reference values specific to the particular assay being used. Furthermore, time to positivity can vary with different assays. Most modern assays turn positive within the first 2–4 h after initial onset of symptoms, but some may take up to 12 h.[1] It is thus reasonable to measure troponins beyond the initial 6 h in high-risk patients as suggested by the guidelines, even though the modern assays allow us to confirm or rule out acute MI within 6 h in the majority of patients.[1]

In emergency departments (EDs), the use of point-of-care (POC) troponin assays is commonplace as they provide nearly instantaneous results that can aid in efficient triage of patients presenting with cardiac symptoms. Hospitals with higher POC assay utilization were found to have shorter ED wait times, and patients with positive POC troponins were more likely to receive early anti-ischemic therapies.[5] Although these point-of-care assays do serve a role in the ED setting, they have been shown to be significantly less sensitive than formal troponin assays performed in the laboratory.[6] Furthermore, laboratory assays undergo consistent standardization which is vital for reliable results. It is thus recommended that POC assays be used judiciously given their inferior sensitivity compared their laboratory counterparts.

Notably, before the development of troponin assays, CK-MB was the primary biomarker used in the diagnosis of acute MI. Modern troponin assays are significantly more sensitive and specific for myocardial necrosis than CK-MB, rendering the latter's diagnostic utility in this era to be largely unnecessary.[7–9] There may be limited use for CK-MB in estimating the size of MI and possibly detecting MIs after PCI, but there is significant controversy in that regard, and the guidelines do not recommend its use for either purpose.[1]

Myoglobin was another commonly used biomarker for diagnosing acute MI. It is a small ubiquitous molecule that is swiftly released into the blood stream from damaged myocytes. Its small size and rapid release made it a useful biomarker for early detection of MI. However, with the advent of high-sensitivity troponin assays, troponin elevations can now be detected faster than myoglobin, thus myoglobin is no longer needed for early detection.[10]

In addition to the significant diagnostic use of cardiac troponins, they also provide notable prognostic value. The AHA/ACC 2014 guideline recommends the use of the conventional troponin assays for short- and long-term prognostication (LOE: B). Furthermore, the guidelines recommend remeasuring troponin once on day 3 or 4 in patients with MI as an "index of infarct size and dynamics of necrosis" (LOE: B).[1] When compared to initial EKG and predischarge stress test, troponin elevation was found to provide greater prognostic assessment.[3] In one study, the degree of elevation in both peak and single-point troponin values strongly correlated with infarct size measured using cardiac magnetic resonance imaging.[11] Both absolute troponin elevation and serial troponin increase of >30% were

found to be predictive of cardiac events and death and thus serve a major role in risk stratification of patients after MI.[12] In addition to prognostic value after acute MI, cardiac troponins can play a significant role in guiding management. Patients with elevated troponin benefit from early revascularization and intensive management.[1] For example, a sub-study from the Platelet Inhibition and Patient Outcomes (PLATO) trial demonstrated that elevated high-sensitivity cardiac troponin T (hs-TnT) levels are associated with substantial benefits from ticagrelor treatment (compared to clopidogrel), which were observed in invasively and noninvasively managed patients.[13] On the other hand, there was no apparent benefit of ticagrelor over clopidogrel among subjects with normal hs-TnT levels.[13]

The AHA/ACC 2014 guidelines recommend using B type natriuretic peptide (BNP) for prognostic purposes (LOE: B).[1] Even though its diagnostic use is negligible compared to troponin, BNP can be a valuable prognostic tool as it was found to predict mortality more accurately than troponin in patients presenting with acute chest pain.[14] In addition to its value in predicting mortality, BNP elevation in the first few days after the onset of symptoms was found to be predictive of recurrence of MI and new or worsening heart failure at 10 months.[15] Furthermore, elevated BNP was found to be useful in predicting high risk for mortality in cohorts with normal troponins and should thus be used to risk-stratify patients thought to be of low risk because of normal troponins (Table 10.2).[16]

TABLE 10.2
AHA/ACC 2014 Versus ESC 2015 Guidelines Recommendations on Biomarkers

Biomarker	AHA/ACC 2014	ESC 2015
Troponin	Recommended contemporary troponin for diagnosis and prognosis	Recommended high-sensitivity troponin for diagnosis and prognosis
CK-MB	Not recommended	Recommended to assess timing of MI
Copeptin	Not addressed	Recommended when troponin not available
Myoglobin	Not recommended	Not addressed
BNP	Recommended for prognostic use	Not addressed

The hs-cTn Assays

After the inception of the initial first-generation assays, fifth-generation hs-cTn assays have now been developed and used widely. The recent approval by the FDA of the hs-cTn assays have ushered a new era. The hs-cTn assays have increased diagnostic accuracy in patients with AMI compared with the contemporary sensitive troponin and are also superior to conventional cardiac biomarkers. Many hospitals now have replaced conventional cTn tests with hs-cTn T and I assays, which can detect troponin at concentrations 10- to 100-fold lower than conventional assays. Although hs-cTn assays are very sensitive, they are less specific for AMI when using the 99th percentile as a single cutoff level.

Rapid rule-in and rule-out diagnostic strategies for patients with chest pain in the ED are now available and help clinicians risk-stratify patients and enable discharge with very low risk. In principle, this improves assessment and makes ED care more cost-effective. Notably, the hs-cTn assays also maintain high diagnostic accuracy in patients with renal dysfunction (especially when higher optimal cutoff levels are used).

However, it is important to note that troponin elevation can occur secondary to etiologies other than myocyte injury and necrosis (e.g., apoptosis, normal cell turnover). There is a risk of misinterpretation of elevated troponin results; in some series, nearly 15% of patients presenting with elevated hs-cTn and chest pain did not have real ACS. The ESC guidelines recommend using hs-Tn algorithms such as the 3-h algorithm. It is, however, important to note that these hs-cTn algorithms should always be used in conjunction with clinical assessment including a good history taking, a physical examination, 12-lead ECG, and possibly additional cardiac testing.

Additional Biomarkers of Cardiac Injury

Myoglobin and LDH should no longer be used for the evaluation of patients with ACS or AMI. There are mixed data regarding the use of copeptin, which is the C-terminal portion of the arginine vasopressin precursor peptide that is secreted from the pituitary gland early in the course of AMI. Some data point to its use in identifying a subgroup of low-risk patients presenting to the ED with suspected AMI who can possibly be discharged home safely. Given that copeptin is a marker of stress, it should be elevated at the onset of MI and can be used when troponin or high-sensitivity troponin are not available. However, in the presence of the rapid rule-out hs-cTn assays, copeptin is unlikely to add a significant incremental value. Heart-type fatty acid–binding protein is a low-molecular-weight protein that behaves similarly to myoglobin in its kinetics and release but is a potentially more specific test to the heart. It is not currently approved for clinical use in the United States.

Overall, we do not currently recommend the routine use of copeptin or other unproven novel biomarkers in patients with ACS or AMI.

CONCLUSIONS

The novel cardiac biomarkers have become more sensitive in recent decades. The currently used hs-cTn assays are highly valuable for diagnosing AMI. Various rule-in and rule-out algorithms have been proposed using different time points and cutoff values, which help with rapid triaging and decision-making in patients with suspected AMI.

DISCLOSURES

The authors have no disclosures and no relations with industry.

REFERENCES

1. Amsterdam EA, Wenger NK, Brindis RG, ACC/AHA Task Force Members, et al. 2014 AHA/ACC guideline for the management of patients with non-ST-elevation acute coronary syndromes: a report of the American College of Cardiology/American heart association Task Force on practice guidelines. *Circulation*. 2014;130:e344–e426.
2. Thygesen K, Alpert JS, Jaffe AS, Simoons MS, Chaitman BR, White HD. Third universal definition of myocardial infarction. *Circulation*. 2012;126:2020–2035.
3. Apple FS, Smith SW, Pearce LA, et al. Delta changes for optimizing clinical specificity and 60-day risk of adverse events in patients presenting with symptoms suggestive of acute coronary syndrome utilizing the ADVIA Centaur TnI-Ultra assay. *Clin Biochem*. 2012;45:711–713.
4. Roffi M, Patrono C, et al. 2015 ESC guidelines for the management of acute coronary syndromes in patients presenting without persistent st-segment elevation Task Force for the management of acute coronary syndromes in patients presenting without persistent st-segment elevation of the European Society of Cardiology (ESC). *Eur Heart J*. 2016;37:267–315.
5. Takakuwa KM, Ou FS, Peterson ED, et al. The usage patterns of cardiac bedside markers employing point-of-care testing for troponin in non-ST-segment elevation acute coronary syndrome: results from CRUSADE. *Clin Cardiol*. 2009;32:498–505.
6. Venge P, Ohberg C, Flodin M, et al. Early and late outcome prediction of death in the emergency room setting by point-of-care and laboratory assays of cardiac troponin I. *Am Heart J*. 2010;160:835–841.

7. Volz KA, McGillicuddy DC, Horowitz GL, et al. Creatine kinase-MB does not add additional benefit to a negative troponin in the evaluation of chest pain. *Am J Emerg Med.* 2012;30:188–190.

8. Newby LK, Roe MT, Chen AY, et al. Frequency and clinical implications of discordant creatine kinase-MB and troponin measurements in acute coronary syndromes. *J Am Coll Cardiol.* 2006;47:312–318.

9. Kavsak PA, MacRae AR, Newman AM, et al. Effects of contemporary troponin assay sensitivity on the utility of the early markers myoglobin and CKMB isoforms in evaluating patients with possible acute myocardial infarction. *Clin Chim Acta.* 2007;380:213–216.

10. Eggers KM, Oldgren J, Nordenskjold A, et al. Diagnostic value of serial measurement of cardiac markers in patients with chest pain: limited value of adding myoglobin to troponin I for exclusion of myocardial infarction. *Am Heart J.* 2004;148:574–581.

11. Giannitsis E, Steen H, Kurz K, et al. Cardiac magnetic resonance imaging study for quantification of infarct size comparing directly serial versus single time-point measurements of cardiac troponin T. *J Am Coll Cardiol.* 2008;51:307–314.

12. Apple FS, Pearce LA, Smith SW, et al. Role of monitoring changes in sensitive cardiac troponin I assay results for early diagnosis of myocardial infarction and prediction of risk of adverse events. *Clin Chem.* 2009;55:930–937.

13. Wallentin L, Lindholm D, Siegbahn A, et al. PLATO study group. Biomarkers in relation to the effects of ticagrelor in comparison with clopidogrel in non-ST-elevation acute coronary syndrome patients managed with or without in-hospital revascularization: a substudy from the Prospective Randomized Platelet Inhibition and Patient Outcomes (PLATO) trial. *Circulation.* 2014;129(3): 293–303.

14. Haaf P, Reichlin T, Corson N, et al. B-type natriuretic peptide in the early diagnosis and risk stratification of acute chest pain. *Am J Med.* 2011;124:444–452.

15. De Lemos JA, Morrow DA, Bentley JH, et al. The prognostic value of B-type natriuretic peptide in patients with acute coronary syndromes. *N Engl J Med.* 2001;345:1014–1021.

16. Weber M, Bazzino O, Navarro Estrada JL, et al. N-terminal B-type natriuretic peptide assessment provides incremental prognostic information in patients with acute coronary syndromes and normal troponin T values upon admission. *J Am Coll Cardiol.* 2008;51:1188–1195.

CHAPTER 11

Biomarkers to Assist in the Evaluation of Chest Pain: A Practical Guide

NAVDEEP SEKHON, MD • W. FRANK PEACOCK, MD, FACEP, FACC

CASE PRESENTATION

You are working in a small emergency department (ED) with a medical student when a 55-year-old male presents with undifferentiated chest pain that started yesterday. As the medical student presents the patient to you, the student states that she wants to order a myoglobin, creatinine kinase MB isoenzyme (CK-MB), and troponin times three. While you are educating her on the proper use of cardiac biomarkers, she wonders aloud why so many patients with chest pain are admitted to the hospital despite the fact that they have normal biomarkers and nonischemic electrocardiograms (EKGs). You suddenly realize that this teaching moment is going to take a little longer and dive into the evidence …

INTRODUCTION

Chest pain is a common medical complaint. In 2013 over 6 million patients visited the ED for evaluation of chest pain.[1] A shared concern for these patients is that they may be having an acute myocardial infarction (AMI). Even after evaluation in the ED, it is estimated that up to 3% of patients with AMI are erroneously discharged home.[2-4] This potentially high rate of missed AMI causes much apprehension among clinicians, which is compounded by the fact that missed AMIs are the third most common cause of successful malpractice claims against ED clinicians.[5]

Electrocardiograms (ECGs) are an essential component of the workup for suspected acute coronary syndrome (ACS); however, it is only diagnostic in the 2% of patients in whom an ST-elevation myocardial infarction (STEMI) is identified.[3] For the other 98% of patients with suspected ACS, further investigation is needed.

To help clinicians evaluate the patient presenting with suspected ACS but a nondiagnostic ECG, biomarkers have been developed to help risk stratify those individuals who have the possibility of AMI. In this chapter, we will discuss the use of cardiac biomarkers in the risk

stratification of patients presenting with chest pain to the ED and will pay particular attention to the use of risk stratification scores to help disposition patients.

INDIVIDUAL CARDIAC MARKERS AND THEIR USE IN THE EVALUATION OF CHEST PAIN

The Ideal Cardiac Marker

Before we discuss the individual cardiac markers, it is important to understand what an ideal cardiac marker would do. This helps to assess the limitations of the cardiac markers that are currently available and in clinical use.

An ideal cardiac marker would appear early in the serum after the onset of the AMI, and the test result could be obtained quickly.[6] This allows for clinicians to make the diagnosis rapidly. Another trait that would be helpful is that it would be specific for ruling in and sensitive for ruling out AMI, thus limiting the number of false-positive and negative results as the marker would only be positive in AMI and not during other processes that cause death of cardiac myocytes.[7,8] Additional characteristics of an ideal cardiac marker would be that it would be of low cost, reproducible, and reliable. Unfortunately, none of the current cardiac markers meet all of the abovementioned traits of the ideal cardiac marker, which makes the role of a clinician in history and physical examination so important.

Myoglobin

Myoglobin is one of the classic cardiac markers that have been used to evaluate patients for possible AMI. Its benefits are that it can become positive (abnormal) within 1 h after myocardial necrosis and can clear within 24 h after the event.[9,10] Unfortunately, myoglobin is not specific for the death of cardiac myocytes, and levels can be elevated in renal disease as well as damage to skeletal muscle. Serum myoglobin is both less sensitive and less specific for the diagnosis of AMI

Biomarkers in Cardiovascular Disease. https://doi.org/10.1016/B978-0-323-54835-9.00011-9

than troponins.[11,12] This has led to most clinicians stop using myoglobin in the evaluation of chest pain. In fact, neither the American Heart Association (AHA)[13,14] nor the third Universal Definition of Myocardial Infarction[15] recommend the routine use of myoglobin for the evaluation of patient with suspected ACS.

Creatinine Kinase and CK-MB

Creatinine kinase and CK-MB are additional traditional cardiac markers that have been used for the evaluation of acute chest pain. Their use has fallen out of favor secondary to the fact that they have been found to be both less sensitive and specific for the diagnosis of AMI than the cardiac troponins.[11,16] Similar to myoglobin, neither the AHA [13,14] nor the third Universal Definition of Myocardial Infarction[15] support the use of CK-MB for the diagnosis of AMI. Historically, it was also argued that CK-MB was useful in infarct sizing and identifying reinfarction given its more rapid rise. These considerations are outdated as treatment decisions are not directed by the size of the infarction, and troponin detection with the newer highly sensitive troponin assays occurs with the same temporal relation to cardiac necrosis as CK-MB.

Cardiac Troponin I and T

Troponin is a structural protein that is a component of the thin filaments in a sarcomere and is made up of three components, namely, troponin C, I, and T. It is present in all muscle cells. Troponin C does not have a cardiac specific form, making its use in the evaluation for ACS limited. However, cardiac troponins I and T have myocardial specific forms, which is thus elevated only in the setting of cardiac myocyte cell necrosis. This unique feature provides a highly specific test for cardiac cellular injury that is the basis for the definition of myocardial infarction.

Defining Normal

Assay development requires the determination of a "normal" cutpoint found within a population of individuals who do not suffer from the disease the assay is designed to define. As with all cardiac markers, this is performed by its measurement in at least 1000 individuals without known coronary artery disease (CAD). As a matter of convention, the 99th percentile troponin value is defined as the upper reference level (URL). In addition, the coefficient of variation should be less than 10% at the 99th percentile, which helps to explain the interinstitutional difference in cardiac troponin cutoff levels. For the diagnosis of myocardial injury, any cardiac troponin above the URL which occurs in <1% of the normal population serves as the definition of abnormal. Because of the critical role of the myocardium in meeting the metabolic needs of the corpus, troponin concentrations exceeding the URL are almost always associated with an increased risk of short-term mortality.

Cardiac troponins are now the single and most important cardiac marker for the acute evaluation of chest pain. They are now part of the definition of AMI, which may be stratified into 5 categories depending on the underlying pathology and the actual amount of troponin elevation.

Troponins and Universal Classification of Myocardial Infarction

A type 1 AMI is caused by atherosclerotic plaque rupture, ulceration, fissuring, or dissection that results in thrombus in the coronary arteries, thereby resulting in myocardial ischemia.[17] This is the type of myocardial infarction that most clinicians worry about when they think of ACS and which may require early intervention by cardiology.

A type 1 AMI is defined as the detection of a rise or fall of cardiac troponins with at least one level above the 99th percentile reference limit in conjunction with:
- ischemic symptoms
- new/presumed ST changes or new/presumed Left Bundle Branch Block
- new pathological Q waves
- evidence of new loss of viable myocardium on cardiac imaging
- evidence of intracoronary thrombus on angiography or autopsy[17]

Even though the sensitivity and specificity of troponins are superior to those of CK-MB and myoglobin in the diagnosis of ACS, there are a variety of conditions that may result in non–type I AMI troponin elevations. In the ED, these are most common due to a mismatch in oxygen need and delivery to the myocardium (e.g., cocaine use resulting in coronary artery vasospasm, tachycardia, and hypertension). It is important to know that a positive troponin demonstrates that there is myocardial necrosis. An elevated troponin however does not identify the etiology of necrosis, and a thorough history, physical, and further diagnostic testing is needed to identify the etiology of the myocardial necrosis.

A type 2 AMI is defined as myocardial infarction due to ischemia, which is caused from oxygen supply-demand mismatch in the myocardium, not from a ruptured plaque. It is commonly the result of an oxygen delivery supply-demand mismatch to the myocardium, although direct myocardial injury (e.g., a gun-shot

TABLE 11.1
Causes of Elevated Cardiac Troponins[1,189]

Acute coronary syndrome	Drug toxicity	Post PCI
Trauma (contusion, pacing)	Apical ballooning syndrome	Pulmonary embolism
Heart failure (acute and chronic)	Coronary vasospasm	Severe pulmonary hypertension
Hypertensive emergency	Myocarditis	Arrhythmias
Hypotension	Endocarditis	Severe anemia
Renal failure	Sarcoid	Coronary vasculitis
Stroke	Subarachnoid hemorrhage	

PCI, percutaneous coronary intervention.

wound) may also result in a troponin elevation. For a type 2 AMI, the focus is on discovering the underlying etiology. Whereas a type I AMI requires ultimately a cardiac catheterization, anticoagulation, and antiplatelet therapy, the treatment of a type 2 AMI may include similar approaches but also requires diagnostic and therapeutic interventions directed at discovering and treating at the underlying cause. A list of conditions that may cause elevated troponins are listed in Table 11.1.[15]

Myocardial necrosis, as identified by an elevated troponin, regardless of etiology, is always associated with increased adverse risks for the patient. Even with patients who do end up having an elevated troponin that is not from ACS, it is always an independent predictor for mortality.[20]

Given that there are a variety of causes for an elevated troponin, a thorough history and physical examination is necessary to ensure that there is no alternative reason for the troponin elevation before making the diagnosis of a non–ST-elevation myocardial infarction (NSTEMI). Interestingly, the specificity of cardiac troponins for mortality is higher than its specificity for ACS.

Ruling out AMI

Of the estimated 10.2 million annual US Emergency Department presentations for suspected ACS,[21] it is estimated that approximately 80% will ultimately be found to have a noncardiac etiology. Thus, a triage process is needed, whereby the physician must determine which patients do not have ACS. Although low-risk

patients may be immediately discharged (i.e., a patient with clearly obvious zoster (shingles) as the etiology for their chest pain) and high-risk patients immediately transferred to the cardiac catheterization laboratory (e.g., STEMI), the majority of the remainder must undergo additional testing. If the initial ECG is nondiagnostic and the initial troponin is below the URL, what is the appropriate diagnostic strategy?

Some physicians support a "1 and done" strategy of troponin testing in patients presenting with suspected ACS. The logic of this approach is that in patients with constant symptoms for >6 h, a rising troponin due to the presence of an ACS would have been detectable by the time of troponin measurement. Although this may be true in selected patients,[22] it is not without risk. The clinical presentation must be carefully considered, and its subjective characteristics be weighed assiduously by the physician. When the slightest doubt exists, a second troponin measurement 3–6 h later is the preferred strategy to rule out AMI according to the Universal Definition of Myocardial Infarction.[17]

Large trials have demonstrated that the sensitivity for this strategy depends on the initially detected troponin, and it may be acceptably high with specific assays and cut points. However, this begs the question of what is an acceptably high sensitivity to rule out AMI, and is this appropriate to use for discharge? The crux of the previous question is what the acceptable miss rate is for AMI. As we create algorithms that are more sensitive, the expense is the specificity which causes more patients who do not have an AMI to undergo additional testing, radiation, and intervention. These are not without risk. Although no clear definition is to be found in guidelines, a consensus definition in the emergency physician community generally defines a reasonable sensitivity of 99% for adverse cardiac events.[23] It is this sensitivity at which risks of hospitalization and unnecessary testing are balanced by the risks of misdiagnosis of ACS.

Timing of Serial Troponins

In the setting of a myocardial infarction of sufficient size as to be detectable by biomarker testing, cardiac troponin is generally believed to be elevated 2–4 h after symptom onset. Consideration of symptom onset timing is germane because if a patient presents with 1 h of chest pain, the cardiac troponin may be negative even in the setting of an ongoing AMI. Thus, in someone with acute chest pain, repeating the troponin measurement can be helpful. The most recent AHA guidelines on this topic recommend repeating the troponin measurement between 3 and 6 h after the initial troponin measurement for acute chest pain.[14,24,25]

There are caveats to this strategy. Although negative higher sensitivity troponin assays (only recently available in the United States) are associated with very low 30-day adverse cardiac event rates and thus are effective at excluding the presence of AMI or ACS, these are not universally available in the United States. The majority of cardiac troponin assays currently used may not be sensitive enough to exclude an ACS and may lead to clinicians admitting these patients for additional testing if they are at high risk.

Troponins can be elevated for protracted periods, i.e., 5–10 and 5–14 days for troponin I and T, respectively. This allows cardiac troponins to be used to detect AMIs that occurred for up to 2 weeks in the past and even longer in patients with diminished renal function.[19,26,27]

High-Sensitivity Troponins

Although only recently approved by the US Food and Drug Administration, high-sensitivity troponins (hs-Tn) have been used internationally for nearly a decade and will change our approach to the undifferentiated chest pain patient. The hs-Tn differs from the earlier generation troponins in that they can detect serum troponins at a far lower level (typically at least 10-fold increases in sensitivity). For the clinician who is evaluating the patient with acute chest pain, this is helpful as it would make the test more sensitive for detecting an AMI. To be defined as a high-sensitivity troponin, one has to be able to detect troponin levels in at least 50% of healthy individuals in the population of interest.[28]

Recent studies suggest that with the use of hs-Tn, clinicians can rapidly rule out ACS and identify a low-risk population that would not benefit from provocative testing and could be rapidly discharged from the emergency center. There is evidence that in patients who present to the ED with suspected ACS, an undetectable initial hs-Tn makes it highly unlikely that the symptoms are cardiac in origin (sensitivities from studies range from 96.3% to 100%).[29–31] Higher sensitivities for ruling out AMI are seen by considering the 1-h hs-Tn data, with an undetectable initial hs-Tn ruling out AMI (sensitivities, 96.7%–100%).[31,32] In addition, studies show that between 26.5%[29] and 61%[31] of patients could be rapidly ruled out from having an AMI using hs-Tn and safely discharged from the hospital.[29] These data show the promise of hs-Tn in the evaluation of acute chest pain, but one must consider that negative hs-Tn does not preclude high-risk CAD, for which additional workup may be indicated.

So it is clear that the hs-Tn has the ability to identify a low-risk population that does not require any additional cardiac testing. However, it also has the possibility to increase downstream testing as more patients will have a troponin level above the URL, but not have a clear type I AMI. The elevated, but not a type I AMI, troponin level may encourage providers to do more provocative in testing (example stress testing) to ensure that patients do not have any underlying obstructive CAD,[33] and hence how this affects safety and costs of care will need to be determined. It should be noted that the use of the hs-Tn can reduce the ED length of stay for patients with chest pain by 9.1%.[34]

Point-of-Care Troponins

When the point-of-care troponins were introduced clinically, there was great excitement about how they can reduce the length of ED stays by reducing laboratory turn-around times and thereby helping with cost-savings by decreasing the emergency center length of stay.[35] This may have been true earlier when the sensitivity of laboratory and that of point-of-care troponins were similar.[36–40] However, in recent years the level at which troponins can be reliably detected using laboratory-based troponins have improved at a faster rate than that of point-of-care assays. How the features of costs, low-level detection, time-dependent operational pressures, individual patient risk stratification, and their intersection in the clinical environment are adjudicated for the point-of-care troponins remain to be determined.

Brain Natriuretic Peptide

Though brain natriuretic peptide (BNP) was initially developed to assess congestive heart failure, there is evidence to suggest that an elevated BNP in the context of an AMI does have prognostic value. An elevated BNP in a patient with AMI has been shown to portend increased mortality within 7 days, a tighter culprit lesion, and an increased likelihood of the involvement of left anterior descending coronary artery.[41] Although BNP does provide prognostic information and can corroborate an underlying cardiac pathology, as a single marker, it is not sensitive or specific enough to make the diagnosis of AMI and should not be used as such.

RISK STRATIFICATION SCORES AND ACS

As cardiac troponins may not be sufficiently sensitive to exclude ACS in selected patients, the clinician is confronted with the issue of what to do with a suspected ACS patient with a "negative" (less <99th percentile) troponin. Classically, the next step in the workup is provocative cardiac testing (i.e., treadmill stress test, nuclear, echocardiogram, or magnetic resonance imaging [MRI]-based stress test, and coronary computed tomographic angiography [CCTA]). It is up to the clinician to choose which patients would benefit from these tests. To aid the clinician, risk stratification rules have been developed to help decide which patients could benefit from further testing and which patients can be safely discharged home. Currently, for low-risk suspected ACS patients who are admitted to the hospital, less than 5% of patients have a positive workup.[42] This is an obvious area for improvement and could provide great savings to the health-care system as well as save patients from unnecessary testing, radiation, and interventions. Thus there has been much interest in the development of risk stratification scores to help guide clinicians.

Traditional Risk Stratification Rules

For patients with unstable angina/NSTEMI, multiple risk stratification tools have been developed to assess the risk for major adverse coronary events (MACE; which include death, revascularization, and AMI). This helps the provider decide which patients necessitate further interventions and the level of care that can best suit the patient.

Thrombolysis in Myocardial Infarction Score

The Thrombolysis in Myocardial Infarction (TIMI) score was one of the first risk stratification scores to be used. It was developed to assess a patient's risk for MACE after being diagnosed with unstable angina/NSTEMI to determine which patients would benefit from early invasive therapy. It is important to note that it was not initially developed to assess which patients can be safely discharged without further workup (Table 11.2).

The TIMI score has been validated in the ED to assess the risk stratification for MACE within 30 days of presentation by Pollack et al.[44] The rate of 30-day MACE is presented in Table 11.3.

Although the TIMI score provides risk stratification for patients with suspected ACS, even a low TIMI score does not equate to the absence of risk, as patients who had a TIMI score of 0 still had a 2.1% risk of a MACE in 30 days, and those with a TIMI score of 1 had a risk of 5%. To further improve the sensitivity of the TIMI score, a strategy of an accelerated diagnostic protocol (ADP) was developed.

In one ADP that included an undetectable high-sensitivity cardiac troponin T (hs-TnT) or cardiac troponin I (cTnI) at 0 and 2 h, no ischemic changes on EKG and a TIMI score of 0 were met in 12.3% of patients who were discharged with a 30-day sensitivity for MACE of 99.2%.[45] This first study was followed by the 2-Hour Accelerated Diagnostic Protocol to Assess Patients With Chest Pain Symptoms Using Contemporary Troponins as the Only Biomarker (ADAPT) trial which used the same strategy of a negative cTnI at 0 and 2 h, a nonischemic EKG and a TIMI score of zero, but applied a higher sensitivity troponin and identified 20% of patients as low

risk with a sensitivity of 99.7%.[46] Cullen et al. repeated the ADP protocol using high-sensitivity cardiac troponin I (hs-TnI) and a TIMI of 0 or 1 and successfully identified 38.6% of patients as low risk with a sensitivity of 99.2%.[47] Ultimately, the ADP strategy shows that using a higher sensitivity troponin helps identify patients as low risk who do not require further intervention and allows clinicians to safely send more patients home.

Other traditional risk stratification rules such as the Global Registry of Acute Coronary Events (GRACE) score and the Platelet Glycoprotein IIb/IIIa in Unstable Angina: Receptor Suppression Using Integrilin Therapy (PURSUIT) score are rarely used now with the advent of newer risk scores that have been shown to be superior and more sensitive.

TABLE 11.2
TIMI Score[43]

Criteria	Value
Age ≥ 65 years	+1
≥3 CAD risk factors[a]	+1
Known CAD (stenosis > 50%)	+1
Acetylsalicylic acid use in past 7 days	+1
Severe angina (≥2 episodes in 24 h)	+1
EKG ST changes ≥ 0.5 mm	+1
Positive cardiac marker	+1

[a]CAD risk factors: family history of CAD, hypertension, hypercholesterolemia, diabetes, and history of tobacco abuse.

TABLE 11.3
Rate of MACE with TIMI Score[44]

RATES OF MACE ASSOCIATED WITH THE TIMI SCORE TO AN UNSELECTED EMERGENCY DEPARTMENT POPULATION	
Number of TIMI Risk Factors	**Rate of MACE in 30 Days (%)**
0	2.1
1	5
2	10.1
3	19.5
4	22.1
5	39.2
6	45
7	100

HEART Score

To further assess which patients presenting acutely with chest pain can be safely sent home without provocative testing or cardiac imaging, the History, EKG, Age, Risk Factors and Troponin (HEART) score was developed. The criteria for this score are listed in Table 11.4.

Using the HEART score, patients with a score less than or equal to 3 are considered low risk and safe for discharge home without further testing. Multiple studies show that the HEART score is superior to the TIMI score in recognizing a low-risk cohort that can be safely discharged from the ED without further testing.[49,50] Applying hs-Tns, as opposed to the cTns used in the earlier studies, the HEART score becomes more sensitive for identifying a low-risk population that is not in need of further evaluation. Santi et al. evaluated 1378 patients using hs-TnT and were able to send home 37.2% of patients with no MACE at 180 days.[51] A modified HEART score with a normal hs-TnT was able to safely discharge patients with a sensitivity of 99.8%.[52]

There are some drawbacks to the HEART score. First, the patient's history is highly weighted and is subjective in its interpretation, allowing for large practice variation. In addition, the HEART score may identify certain patients as low risk that most clinicians would not feel are low risk. According to the HEART score, if you have an isolated positive troponin with some ECG changes, they should be classified as low risk. How the subjective parameters of the HEART score impact its overall use is unclear. In a recent large prospective randomized, stepped-wedge, observational trial applying the HEART score in 3648 patients, across 9 Dutch hospitals, no difference in early discharge, readmissions, repeat ED visits, or outpatient visits was found compared with standard care. Standard care was defined as usual ED care including EKGs, X-rays, laboratory testing, and clinical decision rules without the use of the HEART score.[53]

ED Assessment of Chest Pain Score Accelerated Diagnostic Pathway

Another risk stratification rule that has been developed to help discharge chest pain patients from the ED is the Emergency Department Assessment of Chest Pain Score (EDACS). The EDACS score is given in Table 11.5.

TABLE 11.4
The HEART Score[48]

History	Slightly suspicious	0
	Moderately suspicious	1
	Highly suspicious	2
EKG	Normal	0
	Nonspecific repolarization disturbance	1
	Significant ST depression	2
Age	<45	0
	45–65	1
	>65	2
Risk factors[a]	No known risk factors	0
	1–2 risk factors	1
	≥3 risk factors	2
Initial troponin	Normal	0
	1–2 times normal limit	1
	>2 times the normal limit	2

[a]Risk factors: hypertension, hypercholesterolemia, diabetes mellitus, obesity (BMI > 30 kg/m²), smoking (within the past 3 months), positive family history (parent or sibling with CAD before the age of 65 years), and atherosclerotic disease.

TABLE 11.5
EDACS Score[54]

Age (years)		18–45	+2
		46–50	+4
		51–55	+6
		56–60	+8
		61–65	+10
		66–70	+12
		71–75	+14
		76–80	+16
		81–85	+18
		86+	+20
Gender		Male	+5=6
		Female	0
Aged 18–50 years and known CAD or more than 3 risk factors			+4
Signs and symptoms	Diaphoresis		+3
	Radiates to arm or shoulder		+5
	Pain occurred or worse with inspiration		−4
	Pain is reproduced by palpation		−6

EDACS defines a low-risk cohort as having a score less than 16. Applying EDACS to an ADP of a nondiagnostic ECG and negative 0 and 2-h cTn's safely identified patients who can be discharged home without further workup. The initial validation study showed that 41.6% of patients were identified as low risk with sensitivity for 30-day MACE being 100% (95% confidence interval [CI], 94.2%–100%).[54]

The recent ICare-ACS study, a prospective step-wedge design observational trial of 31,332 patients, demonstrated an increase in safe 6-h ED discharge rate (odds ratio [OR], 2.4; 95% CI, 2.3–2.6), a decrease in the median (interquartile range) ED length of stay by 2.9 h, and no change in 30-day MACE between EDACS and standard therapy control groups (0.52 vs. 0.44%; P = .96). In fact, no adverse event occurred in any patient for whom the pathways were correctly followed.[55]

An issue with the EDACS score is that it is heavily weighted by age. Regardless of this, in one prospective trial, it has been directly compared to the HEART score and found to be equally sensitive, but with the ability to safely send more patients home.[56] The EDACS score has also been evaluated with hs-TnI in 2017 and showed that with hs-TnI, 41.6% of patients were safely risk stratified for discharge.[57]

Comparison of the Risk Scores

The EDACS, HEART, and TIMI scores can all be used to risk stratify the patient for suspected ACS. A table of their respective components is shown in Fig. 11.1.

A key difference between EDACS and the HEART score is that the EDACS score heavily weights the age of the patient, whereas the HEART score weighs more heavily the clinician's gestalt of the patient's clinical history.

Greenslade et al. completed a study comparing the HEART and the EDACS score with 0- and 2-h hs-Tn. The study demonstrated that both the HEART score and the EDACS score performed well in ruling out AMI, with similar sensitivities of 97.9% (95% CI, 92.7%–99.7%). This study did note that the EDACS score was able to rule out more patients (62.5%) than the HEART score (49.8%).[58]

Singer et al. did a prospective evaluation also comparing the EDACS and HEART scores using the cTns that were available in the United States (not hs-Tn). Using the EDACS and HEART scores, they had to use a lower cutoff to ensure greater than 99% sensitivity for ruling out AMI. The lower cutoff was less than or equal to 11 for the EDACS score and less than or equal to two for the HEART score. Using the traditional cutoffs, the EDACS and HEART scores were not significantly different. Interestingly, the C-Statistic was better for the EDACS score.[56]

General Approach in Risk Stratification for ACS

All patients who present to the ED with chest pain require an EKG if ACS is suspected. If the EKG shows no evidence of an STEMI, the patient should then receive two troponins at 0 and 2 or 3 h after arrival. If the troponins are negative, the EKG nonischemic, and have a low risk score, the patient can be safely ruled out for

---

Suspected ACS Risk Scores

- Use criteria
  - EDACS:
    - Is to be used with accelerated diagnostic pathway (any diagnostic ECG change or elevated 0 and 2 hour troponin excludes use)
    - Age >17 and symptoms consistent with ACS
    - Normal vital signs
    - No ongoing chest pain or crescendo angina
  - HEART
    - Age >20 and symptoms consistent with ACS
    - No new ECG changes or ST elevation >1mm
    - No hypotension
    - No life expectancy <1 year
    - No other illness requiring hospitalization
  - TIMI
    - No entry criteria

Characteristic	EDACS	HEART	TIMI
Age	X	X	X
Sex	X		
>1 angina event today			X
Gestalt of history risk		X	
Risk Factors	X	X	X
Aspirin in week prior			X
Diaphoresis	X		
Radiation	X		
Pleuritic	X		
Reproducible	X		
ST changes		X	X
Positive Marker			
Troponin elevation		x	X

FIG. 11.1 Characteristics used in the EDACS, HEART, and TIMI scores.

Approach to Suspected Acute Myocardial Infarction

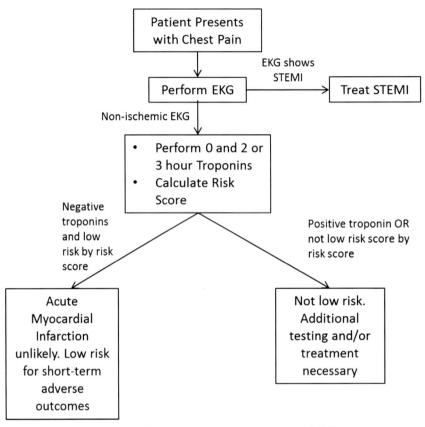

FIG. 11.2 Algorithm for approach to suspected AMI.

AMI. If there is still continued concern for ACS, provocative testing may be indicated either in hospital or in the outpatient setting (Fig. 11.2).

PROVOCATIVE TESTING AND CORONARY COMPUTED TOMOGRAPHY

Even if a patient's troponins do not become positive during their evaluation in the ED, there is still the fear that the patient may have obstructive CAD that may result in a near-term myocardial infarction or death. To obviate this fear, many patients will receive additional functional or anatomic testing to evaluate for inducible ischemia. Although the timing of when this should occur relative to a patient's presentation is controversial, common methods include the exercise treadmill test (ETT), the stress echocardiogram (SE), and myocardial perfusion imaging (MPI), coronary calcium scoring, and CCTA.

Exercise Treadmill Test

The ETT is carried out by having a patient raise his/her heart rate to 85% of their maximal heart rate, usually done with a treadmill or an exercise bike. During exercise, the ECG is monitored to assess for dynamic EKG changes. As the results are defined by ST segment changes, an eligible patient must have normal ST segments at baseline. This requirement results in a subset of patients who cannot receive an ETT due to abnormal ST segments and includes ST and T wave changes at resting EKG, left ventricular hypertrophy, left bundle branch block, and digoxin effect. Other exclusions include the inability to mount a heart rate response secondary to poor exercise reserve and the use of beta-blockers.[59] A positive test has significant ST segment depression. Interestingly, inability to tolerate the exercise has a poor prognostic value.[60]

The sensitivity and specificity of the ETT for detection are low for significant CAD, with sensitivities as low as 70% and specificities close to 75%.[61–63] However, it is relatively inexpensive and does have some prognostic value which encourages its continued use.[64]

In low-risk patients, ETT has limited use. When a test with a poor specificity and sensitivity is used in a population with a low pretest probability of disease, most positives will be false and cause unnecessary downstream testing. For example, in a study of 1027 patients under the age of 40 years, 4 individuals had positive stress tests, with no evidence of obstructive disease on downstream testing.[65] Most of the benefit of an ETT is in the intermediate-risk patient to help guide further management.[63,66]

Stress Echocardiography

The SE allows the clinician to get real-time anatomic and physiologic information by using echocardiography in conjunction with chemically or exercise-induced stress. The clinician can look for evidence of inducible wall motion abnormalities which helps drive downstream care and risk stratifies a cohort that is able to be discharged without further testing.[67] A study of 9000 patients showed that a normal SE was associated with an annual myocardial infarction or death risk of less than 1%.[68] Another study showed that in low-risk patients presenting to the ED, the SE had a negative predictive value of 98.6% for cardiac events.[69] These studies suggest that a normal SE is reassuring in a patient who presents with acute chest pain.

MYOCARDIAL PERFUSION IMAGING

MPI makes use of compounds such as technetium-99m sestamibi, technetium-99m tetrofosmin, and thallium to identify areas of myocardial ischemia. These compounds are rapidly taken up by viable myocardium and slowly by ischemic myocardium. Their uptake can be imaged during stress and at rest. An abnormal test is defined as a fixed myocardial defect or evidence of reversible ischemia.[70] A meta-analysis of 14 studies showed that a normal MPI test had a 1-year risk of death or AMI of 0%–1.8%[70–72] compared with an abnormal stress MPI test which had a 1-year event rate between 7% and 30%.[70]

There is some controversy regarding the supremacy of MPI versus a stress echocardiography. A recent 2016 review of a database of 48,202 patients compared the outcomes for MPI versus stress echocardiography. The authors reported no change in revascularization and death, between MPI and stress echo, but did show decreased testing and interventions in the SE group.[73]

Coronary Computed Tomographic Angiography

CCTA is another manner to risk stratify patients who present with suspected ACS. The CCTA is an anatomic test, which assesses for the presence of plaques, but it is not a functional test. This means that the CCTA can assess for obstructive CAD, but not for cardiac ischemia. Thus a positive CCTA usually will require further downstream testing. This means the CCTA has limited use in patients with known CAD as it will inevitably show evidence of CAD. In addition, high-risk patients generally do not benefit from CCTA as their pretest probability of underlying CAD is already high, so these patients will likely have CAD and would likely need functional testing to help further risk stratify.[74,75]

Contraindications to CCTA include:
- creatinine greater than 1.5 mg/dL
- allergy to iodinated contrast agent
- pregnancy
- contraindications to beta-blocker (e.g., active asthma)
- irregular heart rate such as atrial fibrillation due to the gating required
- uncontrolled tachycardia heart rates need to be close to 60–70 bpm for the test
- weight > 150 kg.[76]

A benefit of the CCTA is that it can rapidly rule out a low-risk subset of patients who can then be discharged from the hospital. The American College of Radiology Imaging Network-PA Trial looked at 1370 patients randomized to either standard stress or CCTA. They showed that 49.6% of CCTA patients could be discharged home from the ED, whereas the standard stress arm sent home 22.7%. Also the CCTA patients were discharged from the ED 6 h faster than the standard stress arm and that none with <50% lesion on CCTA had an AMI or was dead within 30 days.[77]

Another suspected ACS CCTA study was the Rule Out Myocardial Infarction using Computer Assisted Tomography-II Trial. This was a randomized controlled trial of 1000 patients comparing CCTA to standard evaluation. There was no difference in the 28-day cardiovascular events or costs. However, the rate of discharge from the ED was higher in the CCTA group (47% vs. 12%), and the length of stay was decreased by 7.6 h.[78] CCTA is able to rapidly identify a large cohort of low-risk patients that can be safely discharged. However, they receive more average radiation exposure,[75,79] downstream testing, and invasive testing, but without a decrease in AMI and interventions compared with standard care. Finally, in a study by Hulten et al., patients who received CCTA, as opposed to standard stress testing, received coronary angiography at a rate of 8.4% versus 6.3% and revascularization at a rate of 4.6% versus 2.6%.[80] Recently, efforts are being made to combine CCTA with positron emission tomography scans which will allow the combined functional and anatomical assessment, and the study of its value will be of interest.

Coronary Artery Calcium Scoring

Coronary artery calcium scoring uses computed tomography to identify calcified plaque and attempts to risk stratify patients for the presence of significant CAD.[81] The thought behind coronary artery calcium scoring is that patients with a low total coronary artery calcium load would be at low risk for ACS. For patients presenting with a chest pain to the ED, few studies have been carried out assessing its use. Chaikriangkrai et al. completed a meta-analysis of seven studies involving 3556 patients and found that 60% were identified as having a coronary artery calcium score of 0. Having a coronary artery calcium score of 0, in conjunction with a nondiagnostic EKG and a negative troponin, had a sensitivity of 96% and a specificity of 60% for MACEs in a year.[82] Further research is needed to define the role of coronary artery calcium scoring for the patient with emergent chest pain.

Controversies in Provocative/CCTA Testing

The provocative testing of low- and intermediate-risk patients has been encouraged by the AHA in their Guidelines for the Management of non-ST Segment Elevation Myocardial Infarction and ACS s.[14] However, this recommendation is controversial. The underlying theory behind provocative testing for low- and intermediate-risk patients is that having inducible ischemia has a negative prognostic value (which has not been proven) and that these patients would benefit from coronary revascularization. That being said, there is yet to be a convincing study that shows that coronary revascularization improves outcome in the troponin-negative patient. In fact, there have been multiple studies that demonstrate that coronary revascularization has no effect on outcomes in the troponin-negative patient compared with medical management.[83–85]

All of the provocative testing methods and CCTA have relatively low specificities. This is challenging as in a low-risk patient population, large numbers of patients may undergo unnecessary interventions because of the high rate of false positives. A study by Hartsell et al., of 1276 patients, reiterates this point. They showed that the false-positive rate for MPI, stress echocardiography, and CCTA are 75%, 66.7%, and 42.9%, respectively.[86] This underlies the importance of using risk stratification rules such as the HEART and EDACS scores to ensure that the patient does not receive unnecessary testing, intervention, and radiation with only negligible benefit.

THE ROLE OF CARDIAC MARKERS IN THE EVALUATION OF NON-ACS ETIOLOGIES OF CHEST PAIN

Biomarkers have the greatest use in the evaluations of suspected ACS. However, the patient with acute chest pain may be suffering from other life-threatening etiologies. We will discuss the role of cardiac markers in the evaluation of non-ACS etiologies of chest pain.

The Role of Cardiac Markers in the Evaluation for Pulmonary Embolism (PE)

Pulmonary embolism is a life-threatening cause of chest pain for the patient with acute chest pain. The diagnosis is often challenging because classically thought signs/symptoms are not sensitive or specific. To aid in the evaluation for pulmonary embolism, risk scores have been developed such as the Well's Score[87] and the PERC score[88] to help risk stratify patients and drive further diagnostic testing such a D-dimer. The diagnosis is usually made using imaging strategies such as computed tomography or ventilation-perfusion (VQ) scan.

The role of cardiac markers for the diagnosis of pulmonary embolism is limited. Troponins are neither a sensitive or specific marker for pulmonary embolism. For example, one study found that only 16.6% of 627 patients with an acute pulmonary embolism had an elevated cTnI.[89] However, it should be noted that in the patient with an acute pulmonary embolism, elevated troponins are associated with worse clinical outcomes (mortality, hypotension, right ventricular dysfunction, intubation, and shock) and may serve as a negative prognostic factor.[89–91]

The Role of Cardiac Markers in the Evaluation for Myocarditis

Myocarditis is the inflammation of the myocardium and can be caused by a variety of etiologies. The most common etiologies are viral, toxins, and autoimmune. The classic patient presentation is a patient with chest pain, arrhythmias, and heart failure.

Diagnosis is challenging. The gold standard for definitive diagnosis is an endomyocardial biopsy, which is an invasive test. Recently, cardiac MRI has gained a more prominent role in the diagnosis of myocarditis.[92]

The role of cardiac markers in the evaluation for myocarditis is limited. Troponin elevations are not specific or sensitive for the diagnosis of myocarditis.[93] However, having a positive troponin does increase the likelihood of myocarditis, but further testing is need to confirm the diagnosis. Interestingly, the presence and degree of elevation of troponin levels do not seem to affect long-term outcomes for the patient with myocarditis.[94,95]

The Role of Cardiac Markers in the Diagnosis of Aortic Dissection

An aortic dissection occurs when blood penetrates the intima of the aorta, shearing it off the vessel wall from the underlying media. It is a life-threatening emergency. It commonly presents as a tearing chest pain that radiates to the back. Underlying risk factors include hypertension, Marfan syndrome, advanced age, and smoking.

It is important to have a high index of suspicion as patients with aortic dissection often present atypically. Diagnosis is commonly made with computed tomographic angiography of the chest which demonstrates the defect in the aortic wall. Other possible diagnostic imaging modalities include MRI and transesophageal echocardiogram.

The role of cardiac biomarkers in the diagnosis of aortic dissection is limited. However, there is evidence that having an elevated troponin is associated with death in the patient having an acute aortic dissection.[96,97] The only biomarker that has shown promise to be sensitive as a screen for aortic dissection is the D-dimer. A meta-analysis of four studies (1557 patients) showed that in low-risk patients a negative D-dimer (<0.50 μg/mL) had a sensitivity of 98.0% (95% CI, 96.3%–99.1%).[98] Further studies are needed to assess the use of D-dimer to preclude acute aortic dissection.

CONCLUSION

In summary, cardiac markers play a crucial rule in the approach to the undifferentiated chest pain patient. The most important cardiac marker is the cardiac troponin, and it should be used to help risk stratify the patient for ACS. However, even a negative troponin does not preclude the presence of obstructive CAD and 30-day MACEs. Risk stratification rules such as the HEART and EDACS Accelerated Diagnostic Pathway scores have been developed to help decide which patients can benefit from further testing such as ETT, MPI, stress echocardiography, and CCTA.

REFERENCES

1. National Hospital Ambulatory Medical Care Survey: 2013 emergency department summary tables. In: *Center for Disease Control and Prevention*. 2013.
2. Schull MJ, Vermeulen MJ, Stukel TA. The risk of missed diagnosis of acute myocardial infarction associated with emergency department volume. *Ann Emerg Med*. 2006;48(6):647–655.
3. Pope JH, Aufderheide TP, Ruthazer R, et al. Missed diagnoses of acute cardiac ischemia in the emergency department. *N Engl J Med*. 2000;342(16):1163–1170.
4. Christenson J, Innes G, McKnight D, et al. Safety and efficiency of emergency department assessment of chest discomfort. *CMAJ*. 2004;170(12):1803–1807.
5. Kachalia A, Gandhi TK, Puopolo AL, et al. Missed and delayed diagnoses in the emergency department: a study of closed malpractice claims from 4 liability insurers. *Ann Emerg Med*. 2007;49(2):196–205.
6. Wu AH, Apple FS, Gibler WB, Jesse RL, Warshaw MM, Valdes R. National Academy of Clinical Biochemistry Standards of Laboratory Practice: recommendations for the use of cardiac markers in coronary artery diseases. *Clin Chem*. 1999;45(7):1104–1121.
7. Adams JE, Abendschein DR, Jaffe AS. Biochemical markers of myocardial injury. Is MB creatine kinase the choice for the 1990s? *Circulation*. 1993;88(2):750–763.
8. Apple F, Preese L, Panteghini M, Vaidya H, Bodor G, Wu A. Markers for myocardial injury. *J Clin Immunoassay*. 1994;Vol. 17:6–48.
9. Jaffe AS, Babuin L, Apple FS. Biomarkers in acute cardiac disease: the present and the future. *J Am Coll Cardiol*. 2006;48(1):1–11.
10. Gilkeson G, Stone MJ, Waterman M, et al. Detection of myoglobin by radioimmunoassay in human sera: its usefulness and limitations as an emergency room screening test for acute myocardial infarction. *Am Heart J*. 1978;95(1):70–77.
11. Stone MJ, Willerson JT, Gomez-Sanchez CE, Waterman MR. Radioimmunoassay of myoglobin in human serum. Results in patients with acute myocardial infarction. *J Clin Invest*. 1975;56(5):1334–1339.
12. Eggers KM, Oldgren J, Nordenskjöld A, Lindahl B. Diagnostic value of serial measurement of cardiac markers in patients with chest pain: limited value of adding myoglobin to troponin I for exclusion of myocardial infarction. *Am Heart J*. 2004;148(4):574–581.
13. Dagnone E, Collier C, Pickett W, et al. Chest pain with nondiagnostic electrocardiogram in the emergency department: a randomized controlled trial of two cardiac marker regimens. *CMAJ*. 2000;162(11):1561–1566.

14. Kavsak PA, MacRae AR, Newman AM, et al. Effects of contemporary troponin assay sensitivity on the utility of the early markers myoglobin and CKMB isoforms in evaluating patients with possible acute myocardial infarction. *Clin Chim Acta.* 2007;380(1-2):213–216.

15. Amsterdam EA, Wenger NK, Brindis RG, et al. 2014 AHA/ACC Guideline for the Management of Patients with Non-ST-Elevation Acute Coronary Syndromes: a report of the American College of Cardiology/American Heart Association Task Force on Practice Guidelines. *J Am Coll Cardiol.* 2014;64(24):e139–e228.

16. Thygesen K, Alpert JS, Jaffe AS, et al. Third universal definition of myocardial infarction. *Glob Heart.* 2012;7(4):275–295.

17. Anderson JL, Adams CD, Antman EM, et al. 2012 ACCF/AHA focused update incorporated into the ACCF/AHA 2007 guidelines for the management of patients with unstable angina/non-ST-elevation myocardial infarction: a report of the American College of Cardiology Foundation/American Heart Association Task Force on Practice Guidelines. *Circulation.* 2013;127(23):e663–828.

18. Thygesen K, Alpert JS, Jaffe AS, et al. Third universal definition of myocardial infarction. *Circulation.* 2012;126(16):2020–2035.

19. Thygesen K, Mair J, Katus H, et al. Recommendations for the use of cardiac troponin measurement in acute cardiac care. *Eur Heart J.* 2010;31(18):2197–2204.

20. Ammann P, Maggiorini M, Bertel O, et al. Troponin as a risk factor for mortality in critically ill patients without acute coronary syndromes. *J Am Coll Cardiol.* 2003;41(11):2004–2009.

21. National Hospital Ambulatory Medical Care Survey. *Emergency Department Summary Tables;* 2014. Prevention CfDCa, ed. https://www.cdc.gov/nchs/data/nhamcs/web_tables/2014_ed_web_tables.pdf2014.

22. Zhelev Z, Hyde C, Youngman E, et al. Diagnostic accuracy of single baseline measurement of Elecsys Troponin T high-sensitive assay for diagnosis of acute myocardial infarction in emergency department: systematic review and meta-analysis. *BMJ.* 2015;350:h15.

23. Than M, Herbert M, Flaws D, et al. What is an acceptable risk of major adverse cardiac event in chest pain patients soon after discharge from the Emergency Department?: a clinical survey. *Int J Cardiol.* 2013;166(3):752–754.

24. Collinson P. Detecting cardiac events - state-of-the-art. *Ann Clin Biochem.* 2015;52(Pt 6):702–704.

25. Keller T, Zeller T, Ojeda F, et al. Serial changes in highly sensitive troponin I assay and early diagnosis of myocardial infarction. *JAMA.* 2011;306(24):2684–2693.

26. Apple FS, Murakami MM. Cardiac troponin and creatine kinase MB monitoring during in-hospital myocardial re-infarction. *Clin Chem.* 2005;51(2):460–463.

27. Fridén V, Starnberg K, Muslimovic A, et al. Clearance of cardiac troponin T with and without kidney function. *Clin Biochem.* 2017;50(9):468–474.

28. Apple FS, Collinson PO. Biomarkers ITFoCAoC. Analytical characteristics of high-sensitivity cardiac troponin assays. *Clin Chem.* 2012;58(1):54–61.

29. Bandstein N, Ljung R, Johansson M, Holzmann MJ. Undetectable high-sensitivity cardiac troponin T level in the emergency department and risk of myocardial infarction. *J Am Coll Cardiol.* 2014;63(23):2569–2578.

30. Rubini Giménez M, Hoeller R, Reichlin T, et al. Rapid rule out of acute myocardial infarction using undetectable levels of high-sensitivity cardiac troponin. *Int J Cardiol.* 2013;168(4):3896–3901.

31. Reichlin T, Schindler C, Drexler B, et al. One-hour rule-out and rule-in of acute myocardial infarction using high-sensitivity cardiac troponin T. *Arch Intern Med.* 2012;172(16):1211–1218.

32. Mueller C, Giannitsis E, Christ M, et al. Multicenter evaluation of a 0-hour/1-hour algorithm in the diagnosis of myocardial infarction with high-sensitivity cardiac troponin T. *Ann Emerg Med.* 2016;68(1):76–87.e74.

33. Shah AS, Anand A, Sandoval Y, et al. High-sensitivity cardiac troponin I at presentation in patients with suspected acute coronary syndrome: a cohort study. *Lancet.* 2015;386(10012):2481–2488.

34. Peck D, Knott J, Lefkovits J. Clinical impact of a high-sensitivity troponin assay introduction on patients presenting to the emergency department. *Emerg Med Australas.* 2016;28(3):273–278.

35. Singer AJ, Ardise J, Gulla J, Cangro J. Point-of-care testing reduces length of stay in emergency department chest pain patients. *Ann Emerg Med.* 2005;45(6):587–591.

36. Collinson P, Goodacre S, Gaze D, Gray A, Team RR. Very early diagnosis of chest pain by point-of-care testing: comparison of the diagnostic efficiency of a panel of cardiac biomarkers compared with troponin measurement alone in the RATPAC trial. *Heart.* 2012;98(4):312–318.

37. Loten C, Attia J, Hullick C, Marley J, McElduff P. Point of care troponin decreases time in the emergency department for patients with possible acute coronary syndrome: a randomised controlled trial. *Emerg Med J.* 2010;27(3):194–198.

38. Ryan RJ, Lindsell CJ, Hollander JE, et al. A multicenter randomized controlled trial comparing central laboratory and point-of-care cardiac marker testing strategies: the Disposition Impacted by Serial Point of Care Markers in Acute Coronary Syndromes (DISPO-ACS) trial. *Ann Emerg Med.* 2009;53(3):321–328.

39. Renaud B, Maison P, Ngako A, et al. Impact of point-of-care testing in the emergency department evaluation and treatment of patients with suspected acute coronary syndromes. *Acad Emerg Med.* 2008;15(3):216–224.

40. Collinson PO, John C, Lynch S, et al. A prospective randomized controlled trial of point-of-care testing on the coronary care unit. *Ann Clin Biochem.* 2004;41(Pt 5):397–404.

41. Morrow DA, de Lemos JA, Sabatine MS, et al. Evaluation of B-type natriuretic peptide for risk assessment in unstable angina/non-ST-elevation myocardial infarction: B-type natriuretic peptide and prognosis in TACTICS-TIMI 18. *J Am Coll Cardiol.* 2003;41(8):1264–1272.

42. Winchester DE, Brandt J, Schmidt C, Allen B, Payton T, Amsterdam EA. Diagnostic yield of routine noninvasive cardiovascular testing in low-risk acute chest pain patients. *Am J Cardiol.* 2015;116(2):204–207.

43. Antman EM, Cohen M, Bernink PJ, et al. The TIMI risk score for unstable angina/non-ST elevation MI: a method for prognostication and therapeutic decision making. *JAMA*. 2000;284(7):835–842.

44. Pollack CV, Sites FD, Shofer FS, Sease KL, Hollander JE. Application of the TIMI risk score for unstable angina and non-ST elevation acute coronary syndrome to an unselected emergency department chest pain population. *Acad Emerg Med*. 2006;13(1):13–18.

45. Aldous SJ, Richards MA, Cullen L, Troughton R, Than M. A new improved accelerated diagnostic protocol safely identifies low-risk patients with chest pain in the emergency department. *Acad Emerg Med*. 2012;19(5):510–516.

46. Than M, Cullen L, Aldous S, et al. 2-Hour accelerated diagnostic protocol to assess patients with chest pain symptoms using contemporary troponins as the only biomarker: the ADAPT trial. *J Am Coll Cardiol*. 2012;59(23):2091–2098.

47. Cullen L, Mueller C, Parsonage WA, et al. Validation of high-sensitivity troponin I in a 2-hour diagnostic strategy to assess 30-day outcomes in emergency department patients with possible acute coronary syndrome. *J Am Coll Cardiol*. 2013;62(14):1242–1249.

48. Six AJ, Backus BE, Kelder JC. Chest pain in the emergency room: value of the HEART score. *Neth Heart J*. 2008;16(6):191–196.

49. Sun BC, Laurie A, Fu R, et al. Comparison of the HEART and TIMI risk scores for suspected acute coronary syndrome in the emergency department. *Crit Pathw Cardiol*. 2016;15(1):1–5.

50. Poldervaart JM, Langedijk M, Backus BE, et al. Comparison of the GRACE, HEART and TIMI score to predict major adverse cardiac events in chest pain patients at the emergency department. *Int J Cardiol*. 2017;227:656–661.

51. Santi L, Farina G, Gramenzi A, et al. The HEART score with high-sensitive troponin T at presentation: ruling out patients with chest pain in the emergency room. *Intern Emerg Med*. 2017;12(3):357–364.

52. McCord J, Cabrera R, Lindahl B, et al. Prognostic utility of a modified HEART score in chest pain patients in the emergency department. *Circ Cardiovasc Qual Outcomes*. 2017;10(2).

53. Poldervaart JM, Reitsma JB, Backus BE, et al. Effect of using the heart score in patients with chest pain in the emergency department: a stepped-wedge, cluster randomized trial. *Ann Intern Med*. 2017;166(10):689–697.

54. Flaws D, Than M, Scheuermeyer FX, et al. External validation of the emergency department assessment of chest pain score accelerated diagnostic pathway (EDACS-ADP). *Emerg Med J*. 2016;33(9):618–625.

55. Than MP, Pickering JW, Dryden JM, et al. Icare-acs (improving care processes for patients with suspected acute coronary syndrome): a study of cross-system implementation of a national clinical pathway. *Circulation*. 2017.

56. Singer AJ, Than MP, Smith S, et al. Missed myocardial infarctions in ED patients prospectively categorized as low risk by established risk scores. *Am J Emerg Med*. 2017;35(5):704–709.

57. Than MP, Pickering JW, Aldous SJ, et al. Effectiveness of EDACS versus ADAPT accelerated diagnostic pathways for chest pain: a pragmatic randomized controlled trial embedded within practice. *Ann Emerg Med*. 2016;68(1):93–102.e101.

58. Greenslade JH, Carlton EW, Van Hise C, et al. Diagnostic accuracy of a new high-sensitivity troponin I assay and five accelerated diagnostic pathways for ruling out acute myocardial infarction and acute coronary syndrome. *Ann Emerg Med*. 2018;71(4):439–451.e433.

59. Polanczyk CA, Johnson PA, Hartley LH, Walls RM, Shaykevich S, Lee TH. Clinical correlates and prognostic significance of early negative exercise tolerance test in patients with acute chest pain seen in the hospital emergency department. *Am J Cardiol*. 1998;81(3):288–292.

60. Hill J, Timmis A. Exercise tolerance testing. *BMJ*. 2002;324(7345):1084–1087.

61. Roberts R, Graff LG. Economic issues in observation unit medicine. *Emerg Med Clin North Am*. 2001;19(1):19–33.

62. Patterson RE, Eisner RL, Horowitz SF. Comparison of cost-effectiveness and utility of exercise ECG, single photon emission computed tomography, positron emission tomography, and coronary angiography for diagnosis of coronary artery disease. *Circulation*. 1995;91(1):54–65.

63. Gibbons RJ, Balady GJ, Bricker JT, et al. ACC/AHA 2002 guideline update for exercise testing: summary article. A report of the American College of Cardiology/American Heart Association Task Force on practice guidelines (committee to update the 1997 exercise testing guidelines). *J Am Coll Cardiol*. 2002;40(8):1531–1540.

64. Amsterdam EA, Kirk JD, Diercks DB, Lewis WR, Turnipseed SD. Immediate exercise testing to evaluate low-risk patients presenting to the emergency department with chest pain. *J Am Coll Cardiol*. 2002;40(2):251–256.

65. Scott AC, Bilesky J, Lamanna A, et al. Limited utility of exercise stress testing in the evaluation of suspected acute coronary syndrome in patients aged less than 40 years with intermediate risk features. *Emerg Med Australas*. 2014;26(2):170–176.

66. Greenslade JH, Parsonage W, Ho A, et al. Utility of routine exercise stress testing among intermediate risk chest pain patients attending an emergency department. *Heart Lung Circ*. 2015;24(9):879–884.

67. Chandra A, Rudraiah L, Zalenski RJ. Stress testing for risk stratification of patients with low to moderate probability of acute cardiac ischemia. *Emerg Med Clin North Am*. 2001;19(1):87–103.

68. Metz LD, Beattie M, Hom R, Redberg RF, Grady D, Fleischmann KE. The prognostic value of normal exercise myocardial perfusion imaging and exercise echocardiography: a meta-analysis. *J Am Coll Cardiol*. 2007;49(2):227–237.

69. Lerakis S, Aznaouridis K, Synetos A, et al. Predictive value of normal dobutamine stress echocardiogram in patients with low-risk acute chest pain. *Int J Cardiol*. 2010;144(2):289–291.

70. Iskander S, Iskandrian AE. Risk assessment using single-photon emission computed tomographic technetium-99m sestamibi imaging. *J Am Coll Cardiol*. 1998;32(1):57–62.

71. Brown KA, Altland E, Rowen M. Prognostic value of normal technetium-99m-sestamibi cardiac imaging. *J Nucl Med.* 1994;35(4):554–557.

72. Berman DS, Hachamovitch R, Kiat H, et al. Incremental value of prognostic testing in patients with known or suspected ischemic heart disease: a basis for optimal utilization of exercise technetium-99m sestamibi myocardial perfusion single-photon emission computed tomography. *J Am Coll Cardiol.* 1995;26(3):639–647.

73. Davies R, Liu G, Sciamanna C, Davidson WR, Leslie DL, Foy AJ. Comparison of the effectiveness of stress echocardiography versus myocardial perfusion imaging in patients presenting to the emergency department with low-risk chest pain. *Am J Cardiol.* 2016;118(12):1786–1791.

74. Bittencourt MS, Hulten EA, Veeranna V, Blankstein R. Coronary computed tomography angiography in the evaluation of chest pain of suspected cardiac origin. *Circulation.* 2016;133(20):1963–1968.

75. Radecki RP. CT coronary angiography: new risks for low-risk chest pain. *Emerg Med J.* 2013;30(10):856–857.

76. Galperin-Aizenberg M, Cook TS, Hollander JE, Litt HI. Cardiac CT angiography in the emergency department. *AJR Am J Roentgenol.* 2015;204(3):463–474.

77. Litt HI, Gatsonis C, Snyder B, et al. CT angiography for safe discharge of patients with possible acute coronary syndromes. *N Engl J Med.* 2012;366(15):1393–1403.

78. Hoffmann U, Truong QA, Schoenfeld DA, et al. Coronary CT angiography versus standard evaluation in acute chest pain. *N Engl J Med.* 2012;367(4):299–308.

79. Henzlova M, Savino J, Levine E, et al. Comparative effectiveness of coronary CT angiography versus stress testing using high-efficiency spect myocardial perfusion imaging and stress-only imaging in the emergency department. *J Am Coll Cardiol.* 2013;61.

80. Hulten E, Pickett C, Bittencourt MS, et al. Outcomes after coronary computed tomography angiography in the emergency department: a systematic review and meta-analysis of randomized, controlled trials. *J Am Coll Cardiol.* 2013;61(8):880–892.

81. Neves PO, Andrade J, Monção H. Coronary artery calcium score: current status. *Radiol Bras.* 2017;50(3):182–189.

82. Chaikriangkrai K, Palamaner Subash Shantha G, Jhun HY, et al. Prognostic value of coronary artery calcium score in acute chest pain patients without known coronary artery disease: systematic review and meta-analysis. *Ann Emerg Med.* 2016;68(6):659–670.

83. Hoenig MR, Aroney CN, Scott IA. Early invasive versus conservative strategies for unstable angina and non-ST elevation myocardial infarction in the stent era. *Cochrane Database Syst Rev.* 2010;(3):CD004815.

84. Stergiopoulos K, Brown DL. Initial coronary stent implantation with medical therapy vs medical therapy alone for stable coronary artery disease: meta-analysis of randomized controlled trials. *Arch Intern Med.* 2012;172(4):312–319.

85. Stergiopoulos K, Boden WE, Hartigan P, et al. Percutaneous coronary intervention outcomes in patients with stable obstructive coronary artery disease and myocardial ischemia: a collaborative meta-analysis of contemporary randomized clinical trials. *JAMA Intern Med.* 2014;174(2):232–240.

86. Hartsell S, Dorais J, Preston R, et al. False-positive rates of provocative cardiac testing in chest pain patients admitted to an emergency department observation unit. *Crit Pathw Cardiol.* 2014;13(3):104–108.

87. Kline JA, Mitchell AM, Kabrhel C, Richman PB, Courtney DM. Clinical criteria to prevent unnecessary diagnostic testing in emergency department patients with suspected pulmonary embolism. *J Thromb Haemost.* 2004;2(8):1247–1255.

88. Kline JA, Courtney DM, Kabrhel C, et al. Prospective multicenter evaluation of the pulmonary embolism rule-out criteria. *J Thromb Haemost.* 2008;6(5):772–780.

89. Ghaffari S, Sepehrvand N, Pourafkari L, et al. Factors associated with elevated cardiac troponin levels in patients with acute pulmonary thromboembolism. *J Crit Care.* 2018;44:383–387.

90. Aksay E, Yanturali S, Kiyan S. Can elevated troponin I levels predict complicated clinical course and inhospital mortality in patients with acute pulmonary embolism? *Am J Emerg Med.* 2007;25(2):138–143.

91. Mehta NJ, Jani K, Khan IA. Clinical usefulness and prognostic value of elevated cardiac troponin I levels in acute pulmonary embolism. *Am Heart J.* 2003;145(5):821–825.

92. Janardhanan R. Myocarditis with very high troponins: risk stratification by cardiac magnetic resonance. *J Thorac Dis.* 2016;8(10):E1333–E1336.

93. Smith SC, Ladenson JH, Mason JW, Jaffe AS. Elevations of cardiac troponin I associated with myocarditis. Experimental and clinical correlates. *Circulation.* 1997;95(1):163–168.

94. Kobayashi D, Aggarwal S, Kheiwa A, Shah N. Myopericarditis in children: elevated troponin I level does not predict outcome. *Pediatr Cardiol.* 2012;33(7):1040–1045.

95. Imazio M, Brucato A, Barbieri A, et al. Good prognosis for pericarditis with and without myocardial involvement: results from a multicenter, prospective cohort study. *Circulation.* 2013;128(1):42–49.

96. Li ZD, Liu Y, Zhu J, et al. Risk factors of pre-operational aortic rupture in acute and subacute Stanford type A aortic dissection patients. *J Thorac Dis.* 2017;9(12):4979–4987.

97. Vrsalovic M. Prognostic effect of cardiac troponin elevation in acute aortic dissection: a meta-analysis. *Int J Cardiol.* 2016;214:277–278.

98. Asha SE, Miers JW. A systematic review and meta-analysis of D-dimer as a rule-out test for suspected acute aortic dissection. *Ann Emerg Med.* 2015;66(4):368–378.

CHAPTER 12

Biomarkers in Shortness of Breath

ANNA MARIE CHANG, MD, MSCE • MORGAN OAKLAND, MD

OVERVIEW OF DYSPNEA

Dyspnea, which makes up for 3.7-million ED visits in a given year, is one of the most chief common complaints for older adults.[1] Dyspnea is believed to be caused by a combination of mechanisms. There is a wide range of causes of dyspnea including various cardiac, pulmonary, neuromuscular, psychiatric, and metabolic etiologies. The American Thoracic Society defined dyspnea as "a term to characterize a subjective experience of breathing discomfort." Acute myocardial infarction (AMI), PE, and congestive heart failure (CHF) are all potentially life-threatening diagnoses that can present as dyspnea in isolation or in combination with a myriad of symptoms. Because of the mortality associated with these conditions, rapid diagnosis is essential for patient care to improve time to medical intervention. Over the latter half of the 20th century, much effort was put into biomarker research and assay development to fill this void. Currently biomarkers are used not only to guide diagnosis of these high-mortality conditions but have also been shown to have prognostic value. Biomarker assays for these disease processes tend to be highly sensitive but nonspecific, yielding positive results for a variety of reasons unrelated to the condition it was designed to diagnose. Consequently, risk stratification is necessary to facilitate biomarker use, highlighting the importance of a thorough history and physical examination in an effort to prevent unnecessary testing and interventions, which come with their own set of risks. Present-day research is focusing on improving assays of existing biomarker and the development of biomarker use for other potential diagnoses, all of which will be discussed in this chapter.

WORKUP OF DYSPNEA IN THE ED

A methodical, focused history and physical examination will frequently narrow down to an otherwise daunting differential diagnosis in the dyspneic patient. Therefore the initial clinical evaluation of a patient with shortness of breath is extremely important. The evaluation begins with assessing and managing the patient's airway, breathing, and circulation. This approach is standard in emergency medicine and reflects the focus on triage and prioritization of the most life-threatening problems. It is useful to obtain cardiac rhythm, vital signs, and pulse oximetry. A febrile, tachycardic patient needs to be examined for pneumonia, whereas a profoundly hypertensive patient may be suffering from flash pulmonary edema. Given the multiple life-threatening causes of shortness of breath, early Intravenous (IV) access and cardiopulmonary monitoring is frequently warranted in dyspneic patients.

Although there are many causes of dyspnea, a good history will often greatly narrow the differential. Key historical features include associated symptoms (pain, fever, and cough), time and circumstances of onset (trauma, exertion, position, or medication adherence), prior episodes or chronic diagnoses, and a thorough description of symptoms. Chronic conditions such as asthma, chronic obstructive pulmonary disease (COPD), deep vein thrombosis, coronary artery disease, human immunodeficiency virus (HIV), and malignancy are helpful in guiding one's workup. Usage of prescribed medications or recreational drugs along with a history of prior respiratory support, trauma, surgery, or immobility can also provide hints to a particular etiology. Many patients suffer from chronic dyspnea as a result of heart failure, asthma, COPD, or other chronic diseases. They will often be able to compare symptoms to prior episodes or elicit a history of medication nonadherence or specific triggers. In acute shortness of breath a history of recent immobilization, travel, or leg swelling will warrant a workup for venous thromboembolism, whereas a patient with exertional dyspnea and radiating chest pain would be more susceptible for angina. Acutely ill or noncommunicative patients may be unable to provide a history, and thus, examination and diagnostic testing become more crucial in forming a diagnosis and treatment plan.

After the initial evaluation of the airway, breathing, and circulation, a more detailed physical examination

Biomarkers in Cardiovascular Disease. https://doi.org/10.1016/B978-0-323-54835-9.00012-0

can be helpful in management and diagnosis. Repeat physical examinations throughout the treatment are also often warranted. Serial examination allows providers to determine the clinical course and informs diagnosis, treatment, and disposition. Lung auscultation aids in evaluating pneumonia, heart failure, pneumothorax, asthma, and COPD. Focal crackles increases the suspicion for pneumonia, whereas bibasilar crackles may be more suggestive of CHF. Unilaterally absent or decreased breath sounds may represent a pneumothorax, pleural effusion, or obstructive plug in the bronchus. Volume status and cardiac examination may lead to the diagnosis of valvular disease, heart failure, tamponade, or shock. Signs of heart failure as the cause of dyspnea include volume overload as documented by jugular venous distension, rales at the lung bases, dependent edema, and evidence of end-organ dysfunction. On the other hand, underdistended veins along with dry skin and mucous membranes may indicate sepsis, neoplasm, or failure to thrive as the etiology of dyspnea. When warranted by history or clinical suspicion, full exposure, extremity checks, trauma evaluation, neurologic examination, airway visualization, and abdominal examination may also be useful.

Once the patient is stable, a more thorough history may provide clues to the etiology of shortness of breath. Description of the onset, frequency, intensity, duration, and alleviating or exacerbating factors are important.

Upon first encounter with a dyspneic patient, several physical signs can signify impending respiratory failure or a particularly deadly etiology. Accessory muscle use, stridor, diaphoresis, pallor, cyanosis, and lethargy are all concerning signs and warrant emergent intervention. The pulmonary examination can provide significant insight to the etiology. Audible wheezes, stridor, diminished breath sounds, and crackles all highlight underlying disease processes and are useful in the evaluation of dyspnea. Cardiac examination, similarly, can narrow down the differential diagnosis as muffled heart sounds, arrhythmias, murmurs, and extra heart sounds are potentially diagnostic in the setting of dyspnea.

Several imaging studies are frequently indicated in the dyspneic patient. At the bedside, we can perform lung and cardiac ultrasound and nasopharyngeal laryngoscopy. Bedside echocardiography gives us limited but extremely valuable information. Septal flattening is concerning for PE. Decreased ejection fraction along with a distended intravenous fluids (IVF) may indicate heart failure as the diagnosis. A significant pericardial or pleural effusion will be evident on bedside echocardiography. Segmental wall motion abnormalities enable us to diagnose AMI when prior information is available.

This examination can even be repeated throughout a patient's course to evaluate for worsening wall motion abnormalities. Serial inferior vena cava measurements and respiratory variation is a well-described method for evaluating fluid responsiveness in dyspneic or septic patients. Minimal training is required for emergency physicians and health-care providers to learn these skills, and they are extremely important in managing the dyspneic patient. Formal echocardiography or Doppler sonography may be useful in certain patients. The most common imaging study in shortness of breath is the chest X-ray that helps in many diagnoses including heart failure, pneumothorax, pneumonia, and obstructive disease. Computerized tomography (CT) scan is also useful in diagnosing more subtle pneumonias and pneumothoraces, chronic lung pathology, and PE. Ventilation perfusion scanning may be required for evaluating for PE in patients with renal failure or contrast allergy.

In addition to history, physical examination, and imaging, many laboratory studies are high yielding in the evaluation or shortness of breath. It would be inappropriate to consider biomarkers in the absence of a good history and physical examination as described previously. When supplemented with history, physical examination, and imaging, the vast majority of patients will benefit from laboratory biomarker evaluation. Several common tests including blood count, metabolic profile, troponin, BNP, and arterial blood gas that are part of the emergency physician's initial evaluation are performed.

In the rest of this chapter, we will discuss the diagnostic biomarkers that may be an adjunct to diagnosing the patient's cause of shortness of breath.

TROPONIN

Standard cardiac troponin (cTn) assays have been in use since the late 1990s and are the gold standard for the diagnosis of acute coronary syndrome but can be elevated due to a variety of noncoronary causes of cardiac ischemia, including hypoxia, PE, sepsis, and CHF. It is useful in detecting possible cardiac causes of dyspnea. In converse, it may be elevated in noncardiac conditions that may cause myocardial ischemia. Troponin is one of the protein complexes that make up thin filaments in myocytes and play a significant role in regulating muscle contractions by facilitating the interaction between actin and myosin filaments. cTn consists of three subunits, troponin C, troponin I, and troponin-T. Troponin C is present in skeletal myocytes and is therefore nonspecific, whereas troponin I and troponin-T are highly specific to cardiac myocytes. Myocardial injury results in leaking of troponin I and troponin-T into the blood within 3–4 hours of cardiac insult. The concentration of cTn T or I is necessary to aid in the early diagnosis of AMI. The Universal Definition recommends that cTn are useful in the detection of myocardial necrosis and that detection of a rise/and or fall is "essential to the diagnosis of AMI."[2] These assays quantify the amount of cardiomyocyte necrosis, and thus, the higher the level is, the more cell death has occurred. An increased cTn concentration is defined as a value exceeding the 99th percentile of a normal reference population (upper reference limit [URL]). This discriminatory 99th percentile is designated as the decision level for the diagnosis of myocardial infarction and must be determined for each specific assay with appropriate quality control in each laboratory and can be found in the package inserts. The United States Food and Drug Administration cleared the first fifth-generation troponin-T, which has been used in Europe in other regions for over 5 years.[3,4] By expert consensus, a high-sensitivity assay is defined so that they detect a level in >50% of apparently healthy subjects, and they have a coefficient of variation of <10% at the 99th percentile URL of the assay. Any troponin elevation is associated with increased morbidity and mortality risk, no matter the condition or chronicity, and thus, the emergency physician should never disregard an elevation and call it a "troponin leak." Any detectable troponin is always worse than no troponin, and higher levels of troponin always portend a worse prognosis than lower levels of troponin. In PE a rise in troponin levels has been associated with an increase in overall mortality, major clinical events, and recurrence of PE during the hospital stay.[5–7] Increases in troponin in both sepsis[8,9] and CHF suggest myocardial injury and have also been shown to be associated with worsening short-[10,11] and long-term[12,13] prognosis.

B-type Natriuretic Peptide

BNP has many uses in the assessment of dyspneic patients with and without underlying left ventricular dysfunction. This hormone is produced in the heart and released by the cardiac ventricles. Production of BNP occurs when pro-BNP is cleaved. BNP is released in response to volume overload or increased cardiac wall stress. The half life of BNP is 20 min on average, and it is primarily excreted through the kidney. Therefore levels will be elevated in renal failure patients. Physiologic effects of BNP include promotion of diuresis and natriuresis, as well as reduction in blood pressure. Long-term effects of BNP include reduced cardiac

remodeling and hypertrophy.[14] BNP is a particularly helpful biomarker in the diagnosis of heart failure in the emergent setting.

The Breathing Not Properly trial[15] was a large multinational, prospective study validating BNP as a diagnostic tool in CHF. This study enrolled 1586 patients presenting to EDs with dyspnea in whom BNP was measured. Seven hundred and forty four patients (47%) were eventually diagnosed with an acute exacerbation of CHF. Cardiologists blinded to the BNP results subsequently diagnosed the patients with the presence or absence of CHF. Patients with a diagnosis of acute CHF had mean (±standard deviation) BNP levels of 675 ± 450 pg per milliliter, whereas those without CHF had BNP levels of 110 ± 225 pg per milliliter. This study concluded that BNP was more useful than any other biomarker, history or physical exam finding in the diagnosis of CHF. A value of 100 pg per milliliter or more for BNP was the strongest independent predictor of CHF, with an odds ratio of 29.60. When clinical suspicion for CHF exists in the dyspneic ED patient, the American College of Cardiology,[16] American Heart Association, and the Heart Failure Society of America all recommend BNP testing when available.[17]

With a basis of strong evidence linking elevated BNP to heart failure, recent research is focusing on other uses of this biomarker. One recent meta-analysis[18] found an association between predischarge BNP threshold and readmission. The average discharge threshold for BNP was set at 250 pg/mL or the equivalent value of amino-terminal probrain-type natriuretic peptide (NT-pro-BNP) or an absolute reduction of at least 30% and concluded that these discharge thresholds reduced both mortality and readmission rate. Unfortunately the findings in this study were of low strength which significantly limits our ability to apply these results clinically. In addition, using BNP to guide heart failure treatment has not been shown to be effective.[19,20]

Aside from heart failure, many pathologies including pulmonary hypertension,[21,22] PE,[23] myocardial infarction,[24,25] endocarditis, renal failure, and sepsis can lead to elevated BNP. Conversely, levels are relatively lower in men, young patients, and those who are obese.[26,27] Although high levels of BNP are useful in diagnosing CHF as the etiology of dyspnea, it is important to not rely on mildly elevated levels in ruling out other serious causes of acute dyspnea.

As previously mentioned, levels are elevated in renal failure patients given reduced glomerular filtration rate. Other factors may further lead to elevation of BNP in renal failure patients including volume overload and underlying cardiac disease. This biomarker is therefore not considered useful in the evaluation of heart failure in the renal failure patients. A randomized comparison study[28] compared BNP testing in patients with and without renal failure. This study enrolled 452 patients presenting to the hospital with dyspnea. Two hundred and forty had known underlying renal failure and 212 did not. Patients were randomly sorted into BNP testing or no BNP testing groups. Overall the study noted a 7-day reduction in hospital stay for patients when BNP testing was used in subjects without renal failure. An absolute cost reduction was also noted. Unfortunately, this association was not found in renal failure patients. The study concluded that BNP testing is not useful in renal failure patients.

D-DIMER

PE is another potentially life-threatening condition on the differential diagnosis of an acutely dyspneic patient. D-dimer is a product of fibrin degradation that has served as the biomarker of choice in evaluating for pulmonary emboli and other types of venous thromboembolism. Plasmin, the primary enzyme in fibrinolysis, creates a variety of monomers and multimers during the break down of the fibrin matrix, but it is the cleavage at the D fragment site of cross-linked fibrin that results in D-dimer formation.[29] The D-dimer fragment consists of two D domains and 1 E domain and is quantified by D-dimer assays in a variety of ways. The most common quantification method involves measurement by enzyme-linked immunosorbent assay (ELISA).[30] D-dimer assays are great for ruling out PE in a dyspneic patient but have very poor specificity due to the fact that any activation of the coagulation cascade including trauma, disseminated intravascular coagulation surgery, infection, pregnancy, liver disease, and malignancy can all cause elevated D-dimer levels.

Current use of the D-dimer assay relies on clinical gestalt and risk stratification with clinical prediction guides such as the Pulmonary Embolism Rule out Criteria (PERC),[31] Well's criteria,[32] and revised Geneva score.[33,34] Low-risk and PERC-negative patients do not need further testing. Patients at moderate risk or low risk but PERC-positive may undergo D-dimer testing. On the other hand, diagnostic imaging is recommended for patients at high risk for PE, and D-dimer testing should be deferred. Modern ELISA test kits and ELISA-derived D-dimer assays have a sensitivity of >95% and a specificity of about 40%.[35] However, positive predictive values for D-dimer assays decrease in the aforementioned conditions that activate the clotting cascade and elevate D-dimer levels. Recent studies have focused mostly on attempting to standardize D-dimer in these populations that tend to have baseline elevation in D-dimer.[36,37]

PROCALCITONIN

Procalcitonin is the peptide precursor to calcitonin. Normal levels vary by laboratory but are very low in the healthy patient. The level of procalcitonin rises in response to a proinflammatory stimulus and is significantly increased in bacterial infections. Viral infections, however, will not lead to elevation. The lack of viral response is thought to result from the virus-stimulated synthesis of α-interferon by macrophages, which, in turn, inhibits tumor necrosis factor synthesis. In a large literature review referencing over 40 years of publications related to the use of the biomarker procalcitonin, the conclusion was made that this biomarker remains useful for the evaluation of processes causing systemic inflammation including sepsis and infectious or inflammatory processes[38] while cautioning us on the many limitations of its references including the insufficient sensitivity and specificity of this assay and the broad range of subjects and clinical settings used throughout the referenced literature.

Studies have indicated that procalcitonin has a limited but valuable role in our management of shortness of breath. The Biomarkers in Acute Heart Failure (BACH) trial was a prospective, international study of 1641 ED patients with shortness of breath. Procalcitonin was more accurate (area under the curve [AUC], 72.3%) than any other individual clinical variable for the diagnosis of pneumonia in all patients, especially in those with obstructive lung disease and in those with acute heart failure (AHF). The combination of physician gestalt for pneumonia with procalcitonin values increased the accuracy to >86% for the diagnosis of pneumonia in all patients.[39] Procalcitonin may also be helpful to evaluate whether antibiotics are necessary in patients with pneumonia.[40] In patients with final diagnoses of pneumonia or acute exacerbation of obstructive pulmonary disease, the use of procalcitonin significantly reduced overall exposure to antibiotics by reducing the number of patients in whom antibiotics were initiated, as well as the duration of antibiotic use. The adjusted relative risk of antibiotic exposure in this study was 0.49 (95% confidence interval [CI], 0.44–0.55; $P < .0001$). Patient outcomes were not compromised by reducing antibiotic exposure, and the outcomes measured were similar in both the procalcitonin and control groups. Therefore procalcitonin continues to be used to guide antibiotic use in patients with acute lower respiratory tract infections. Schuetz et al. randomized patients to a procalcitonin-based algorithm for antibiotic use versus usual care. Over 1300 patients were randomized, and the rate of overall adverse outcomes including death, intensive care unit admission, disease-specific complications, or recurrent infection was similar in the procalcitonin and control groups (15.4% [n = 103] vs. 18.9% [n = 130]). The mean duration of antibiotics exposure was lower in the procalcitonin group (5.7 vs. 8.7 days), and there were fewer antibiotic-associated adverse effects (19.8% [n = 133]) in the procalcitonion group than in the control group (28.1% [n = 193]).[41]

Compared to other markers such as C-reactive protein (CRP), procalcitonin may be a better diagnostic tool for infants with a bacterial infection. Among the 2047 infants included in a prospective cohort study of French pediatric EDs, 139 (6.8%) were diagnosed as having a serious bacterial infection and 21 (1.0%) as having an invasive bacterial infection (IBI). Using a cutoff value of 0.3 ng/mL for procalcitonin (PCT) and 20 mg/L for CRP, negative likelihood ratios were 0.3 (95% CI, 0.2–0.5) for identifying serious bacterial infections and 0.1 (95% CI, 0.03–0.4) and 0.3 (95% CI, 0.2–0.7) for identifying IBIs.[42] Therefore when used with other indicators including white blood cell count, urinalysis, and CRP, procalcitonin can help us identify and exclude serious bacterial infections in children. For these reasons, this biomarker is becoming increasingly available in pediatric hospitals.

Procalcitonin is still frequently used but is no longer part of the routine evaluation of the dyspneic patient in the ED because of its insufficient sensitivity and specificity especially in certain populations. It is unreliable in patients with significant immunocompromise or concomitant pathology. In neutropenic patients, levels will be falsely low. Conversely, levels can be elevated secondary to nonbacterial disease including renal failure, cancer, shock, trauma, and surgery.

Research efforts continue to search for appropriate uses for procalcitonin. Many studies have indicated a strong correlation with serious bacterial infections and significant morbidity and mortality. However, the sensitivity and specificity is generally too low to make this a reliable test to determine whether or not to give antibiotics to the dyspneic ED patient. A recent multicenter prospective trial indicated that procalcitonin measurements at admission and at 72 h correlated with survival at both 30 and 90 days after discharge.[43] Further research in this area may lead us to use this biomarker in triage and prognostication of dyspneic ED patients.

NOVEL BIOMARKERS

Although troponin, BNP, and D-dimer are helpful in the evaluation of shortness of breath, novel biomarkers are constantly being evaluated to help improve the diagnosis of patients with shortness of breath. Adrenomedullin (ADM) and atrial natriuretic peptide (ANP) are biomarkers that participate in volume regulation and are associated with hypervolemic states. ANP acts on the kidneys to facilitate elimination of water and sodium in response to volume overload, hypernatremia, renin angiotensin aldosterone system activation, and sympathetic stimulation. ADM is a potent vasodilator found in numerous tissues throughout the body that is stimulated by volume overload and increased cardiac pressures.

The BACH study group also studied midregional pro–atrial natriuretic peptide (MR-pro-ANP) and midregional proadrenomedullin (MR-pro-ADM). They used a cutoff of ≥120 pmol/L for MR-pro-ANP and found that at this level, it was noninferior to BNP for AHF and had moderate ability to accurately predict 90-day survival for heart failure patients.[44] In addition, the group found that pro-ADM was useful in predicting 90-day all-case mortality.[45] Ongoing research continues to tease out the prognostic value of these biomarkers as adjuncts rather than as sole biomarkers for initial evaluation and diagnosis.

The suppression of tumorigenicity (ST2) gene, a member of the interleukin-1 receptor family, has been shown to be upregulated in a model of heart failure and was elevated in a cohort of 599 patients with shortness of breath in the ED in the Pro-Brain Natriuretic Peptide Investigation of Dyspnea in the Emergency Department study. The investigators determined that although NT-pro-BNP was better for the diagnosis of AHF, ST2 was a strong predictor of death at 1 year.[46]

Dieplinger et al. measured 10 established and novel biomarkers in 251 ED patients with shortness of breath. The biomarkers evaluated in this work included BNP, midregional pro-A-type natriuretic peptide (MR-pro-ANP), midregional proadrenomedullin (MR-pro-ADM), the C-terminal part of the arginine vasopressin prohormone (copeptin), the C-terminal endothelin-1 precursor fragment, the soluble isoform of the interleukin-1 receptor family member ST2 (sST2), chromogranin A (CgA), adiponectin, proguanylin, and prouroguanylin. The group analyzed these biomarkers and found that MR-pro-ANP (relative risk (RR), 1.6; 95% CI, 1.1–2.2; P = .008), sST2 (RR, 1.7; 95% CI, 1.3–2.3; P < .001), and CgA (RR, 1.5; 95% CI, 1.2–1.9, P < .001) were independently associated with 1-year mortality[47] but did not discuss if they were useful in the diagnosis of various causes of shortness of breath. In patients diagnosed with heart failure, the group found that MR-pro-ANP was elevated.[48]

Multimarker Panels

Singer et al.[50] analyzed the incremental benefit of a point-of-care biomarker panel to evaluate shortness of breath in the ED. In 301 patients, they evaluated a multimarker panel including troponin, myoglobin, creatinine kinase-myocardial band isoenzyme, D-dimer, and BNP and found that this panel did not improve the diagnosis of acute cardiopulmonary conditions. On the other hand, Travaglino et al. evaluated 501 patients with shortness of breath for 30- and 90-day mortality and readmission using a combination of procalcitonin, MR-pro-ADM, and MR-pro-ANP. Using these multimarker panels, the AUC was 0.73 for 30-day mortality, which suggests that they may be moderately useful.[43] Eurlings et al. evaluated the prognostic ability of a multimarker panel to evaluate shortness of breath in the ED. The group evaluated a panel including NT-pro-BNP, high-sensitivity troponin-T, cystatin C, CRP, and galectin-3 in over 600 patients. The group found that high-sensitivity CRP (hs-CRP), high-sensitivity cTnT (hs-cTnT), Cyst-C, and NT-pro-BNP were independent predictors of 90-day mortality, and increased number of elevated biomarkers was associated with poor outcomes. The group developed a risk score incorporating age ≥75 years, systolic blood pressure <110 mm Hg, history of heart failure, dyspnea New York Heart Association functional class IV, hs-cTnT≥0.04 μg/L, hs-CRP≥25 mg/L, and Cys-C≥1.125 mg/L and had an AUC of 0.85 (95% CI, 0.81 to 0.89).[49]

CONCLUSION

Technologic advancements have led to widespread use of biomarkers in medicine. Improved sensitivity of assays has improved diagnosis of major causes of dyspnea, however, at the expense of specificity. Troponin and BNP are the most validated biomarkers to evaluate for cardiac etiologies of shortness of breath. D-dimer may be useful in the ruling out PE. Procalcitonin may be less useful in the diagnosis and prognosis of pneumonia in adults. Multimarker panels are a promising step in the right direction toward combating this dilemma and the unnecessary interventions that have come as a result. Future research on subsets of populations that are most affected by these "false positives" will be crucial in improving efficiency and overall patient care. The development of new biomarkers will inevitably present unique challenges of their own as application becomes more widespread, but the potential of expanding biomarker use to other relevant causes of dyspnea is an exciting prospect (Table 12.1).

TABLE 12.1
Diagnosis and Related Biomarker

Disorder	Additional History	Physical Examination	Biomarker
Acute coronary syndrome	Chest pain or palpitations	Cyanosis, crackles, edema, JVD Jugular venous distension, Hepatojugular reflux, paroxysmal nocturnal dyspnea, oral contraceptive pill, murmurs, S3 or S4, HJR, hypertension	Troponin
Congestive heart failure	Orthopnea, PND, edema	Cyanosis, crackles, edema, JVD, murmurs, S3 or S4, HJR, hypertension	BNP
COPD exacerbation	Worsening dyspnea, increased sputum volume or purulence	Wheezing, prolonged expiratory phase	
Asthma	History of asthma or allergies, chest tightness	Wheezing, prolonged expiratory phase	
Pneumonia	Fever, cough, sputum production	Fever, decreased breath sounds, crackles	Procalcitonin
Pulmonary embolism	Pleuritic chest pain, lower extremity pain and swelling, long travel, OCP use, previous history	Leg swelling	D-dimer

REFERENCES

1. Pines JM, Mullins PM, Cooper JK, Feng LB, Roth KE. National trends in emergency department use, care patterns, and quality of care of older adults in the United States. *J Am Geriatr Soc.* 2013;61(1):12–17. https://doi.org/10.1111/jgs.12072.

2. Thygesen K, Alpert JS, Jaffe AS, et al. Third universal definition of myocardial infarction. *J Am Coll Cardiol.* 2012;60(16): 1581–1598. https://doi.org/10.1016/j.jacc.2012.08.001.

3. Sherwood MW, Kristin Newby L. High-sensitivity troponin assays: evidence, indications, and reasonable use. *J Am Heart Assoc.* 2014;3(1):e000403. https://doi.org/10.1161/JAHA.113.000403.

4. *Next-Generation Troponin Test Cleared by FDA.* January 19, 2017. https://www.medpagetoday.com/Cardiology/MyocardialInfarction/62620.

5. Becattini C, Vedovati MC, Agnelli G. Prognostic value of troponins in acute pulmonary embolism: a meta-analysis. *Circulation.* 2007;116(4):427–433. https://doi.org/10.1161/CIRCULATIONAHA.106.680421.

6. Kilinc G, Dogan OT, Berk S, Epozturk K, Ozsahin SL, Akkurt I. Significance of serum cardiac troponin I levels in pulmonary embolism. *J Thorac Dis.* 2012;4(6):588–593. https://doi.org/10.3978/j.issn.2072-1439.2012.10.13.

7. Meyer T, Binder L, Hruska N, Luthe H, Buchwald AB. Cardiac troponin I elevation in acute pulmonary embolism is associated with right ventricular dysfunction. *J Am Coll Cardiol.* 2000;36(5):1632–1636. https://doi.org/10.1016/S0735-1097(00)00905-0.

8. Sheyin O, Davies O, Duan W, Perez X. The prognostic significance of troponin elevation in patients with sepsis: a meta-analysis. *J Acute Crit Care Heart Lung.* 2015;44(1): 75–81. https://doi.org/10.1016/j.hrtlng.2014.10.002.

9. Zochios V, Valchanov K. Raised cardiac troponin in intensive care patients with sepsis, in the absence of angiographically documented coronary artery disease: a systematic review. *J Intensive Care Soc.* 2015;16(1):52–57. https://doi.org/10.1177/1751143714555303.

10. Nishio Y, Sato Y, Taniguchi R, et al. Cardiac troponin T vs other biochemical markers in patients with congestive heart failure. *Circ J.* 2007;71(5):631–635.

11. Jacob J, Martín-Sanchez FJ, Herrero P, Miró O, Llorens P. Miembros del grupo ICA-SEMES. [Prognostic value of troponin in patients with acute heart failure attended in Spanish Emergency Departments: TROP-ICA study (TROPonin in acute heart failure)]. *Med Clin Barc.* 2013;140(4):145–151. https://doi.org/10.1016/j.medcli.2012.06.029.

12. Demir M, Kanadasi M, Akpinar O, et al. Cardiac troponin T as a prognostic marker in patients with heart failure: a 3-year outcome study. *Angiology.* 2007;58(5):603–609. https://doi.org/10.1177/0003319707307344.

13. Ishii J, Cui W, Kitagawa F, et al. Prognostic value of combination of cardiac troponin T and B-type natriuretic peptide after initiation of treatment in patients with chronic heart failure. *Clin Chem.* 2003;49(12):2020–2026. https://doi.org/10.1373/clinchem.2003.021311.

14. Essential biochemistry and physiology of (NT-pro)BNP - Hall. *Eur J Heart Fail.* 2004. Wiley Online Library. http://onlinelibrary.wiley.com/doi/10.1016/j.ejheart.2003.12.015/full.

15. Maisel AS, Krishnaswamy P, Nowak RM, et al. Rapid measurement of B-type natriuretic peptide in the emergency diagnosis of heart failure. *N Engl J Med.* 2002;347(3): 161–167. https://doi.org/10.1056/NEJMoa020233.

16. Cardiac Biomarkers and Heart Failure, American College of Cardiology. https://www.acc.org/%2flatest-in-cardiology%2farticles%2f2015%2f02%2f09%2f13%2f00%2fcardiac-biomarkers-and-heart-failure.

17. Chow SL, Maisel AS, Anand I, et al. Cardiology O behalf of the AHACPC of the C on C, sciences C on BC, young C on CD in the, nursing C on C and S, Council on cardiopulmonary CC, prevention C on E and, Biology C on FG and T, Research and C on Q of C and O. Role of biomarkers for the prevention, assessment, and management of heart failure: a Scientific Statement from the American heart association. *Circulation.* January 2017:CIR.0000000000000490. https://doi.org/10.1161/CIR.0000000000000490.

18. McQuade CN, Mizus M, Wald JW, Goldberg L, Jessup M, Umscheid CA. Brain-type natriuretic peptide and amino-terminal pro-brain-type natriuretic peptide discharge thresholds for acute decompensated heart failure: a systematic review. *Ann Intern Med.* 2017;166(3):180–190. https://doi.org/10.7326/M16-1468.

19. Felker GM, Anstrom KJ, Adams KF, et al. Effect of natriuretic peptide-guided therapy on hospitalization or cardiovascular mortality in high-risk patients with heart failure and reduced ejection fraction: a randomized clinical trial. *JAMA.* 2017;318(8):713–720. https://doi.org/10.1001/jama.2017.10565.

20. Pfisterer M, Buser P, Rickli H, et al. TIME-CHF investigators. BNP-guided vs symptom-guided heart failure therapy: the trial of intensified vs standard medical therapy in elderly patients with congestive heart failure (TIME-CHF) randomized trial. *JAMA.* 2009;301(4):383–392. https://doi.org/10.1001/jama.2009.2.

21. Yap LB, Ashrafian H, Mukerjee D, Coghlan JG, Timms PM. The natriuretic peptides and their role in disorders of right heart dysfunction and pulmonary hypertension. *Clin Biochem.* 2004;37(10):847–856. https://doi.org/10.1016/j.clinbiochem.2004.06.002.

22. Nagaya N, Nishikimi T, Okano Y, et al. Plasma brain natriuretic peptide levels increase in proportion to the extent of right ventricular dysfunction in pulmonary hypertension. *J Am Coll Cardiol.* 1998;31(1):202–208.

23. Bajaj A, Rathor P, Sehgal V, et al. Prognostic value of biomarkers in acute non-massive pulmonary embolism: a systematic review and meta-analysis. *Lung.* 2015;193(5):639–651. https://doi.org/10.1007/s00408-015-9752-4.

24. Darbar D, Davidson NC, Gillespie N, et al. Diagnostic value of B-Type natriuretic peptide concentrations in patients with acute myocardial infarction. *Am J Cardiol.* 1996;78(3):284–287. https://doi.org/10.1016/S0002-9149(96)00278-0.

25. Mayr A, Mair J, Schocke M, et al. Predictive value of NT-pro BNP after acute myocardial infarction: relation with acute and chronic infarct size and myocardial function. *Int J Cardiol.* 2011;147(1):118–123. https://doi.org/10.1016/j.ijcard.2009.09.537.

26. Mehra MR, Uber PA, Park MH, et al. Obesity and suppressed B-type natriuretic peptide levels in heart failure. *J Am Coll Cardiol.* 2004;43(9):1590–1595. https://doi.org/10.1016/j.jacc.2003.10.066.

27. Wang TJ, Larson MG, Levy D, et al. Impact of obesity on plasma natriuretic peptide levels. *Circulation.* 2004;109(5):594–600. https://doi.org/10.1161/01.CIR.0000112582.16683.EA.

28. Mueller C, Laule-Kilian K, Scholer A, et al. B-type natriuretic peptide for acute dyspnea in patients with kidney disease: insights from a randomized comparison. *Kidney Int.* 2005;67(1):278–284. https://doi.org/10.1111/j.1523-1755.2005.00079.x.

29. Goldhaber SZ, Vaughan DE, Tumeh SS, Loscalzo J. Utility of cross-linked fibrin degradation products in the diagnosis of pulmonary embolism. *Am Heart J.* 1988;116(2 Pt 1):505–508.

30. Ginsberg JS, Brill-Edwards PA, Demers C, Donovan D, Panju A. D-dimer in patients with clinically suspected pulmonary embolism. *Chest.* 1993;104(6):1679–1684.

31. Kline JA, Courtney DM, Kabrhel C, et al. Prospective multicenter evaluation of the pulmonary embolism rule-out criteria. *J Thromb Haemost.* 2008;6(5):772–780. https://doi.org/10.1111/j.1538-7836.2008.02944.x.

32. Wolf SJ, McCubbin TR, Feldhaus KM, Faragher JP, Adcock DM. Prospective validation of Wells Criteria in the evaluation of patients with suspected pulmonary embolism. *Ann Emerg Med.* 2004;44(5):503–510. https://doi.org/10.1016/S0196064404003385.

33. Le Gal G, Righini M, Roy P-M, et al. Prediction of pulmonary embolism in the emergency department: the revised Geneva score. *Ann Intern Med.* 2006;144(3):165–171.

34. Penaloza A, Verschuren F, Meyer G, et al. Comparison of the unstructured clinician gestalt, the wells score, and the revised Geneva score to estimate pretest probability for suspected pulmonary embolism. *Ann Emerg Med.* 2013;62(2):117–124.e2. https://doi.org/10.1016/j.annemergmed.2012.11.002.

35. Stein PD, Hull RD, Patel KC, et al. D-dimer for the exclusion of acute venous thrombosis and pulmonary embolism: a systematic review. *Ann Intern Med.* 2004;140(8):589–602.

36. Schouten HJ, Geersing GJ, Koek HL, et al. Diagnostic accuracy of conventional or age adjusted D-dimer cut-off values in older patients with suspected venous thromboembolism: systematic review and meta-analysis. *BMJ.* 2013;346:f2492.

37. Righini M, Van Es J, Den Exter PL, et al. Age-adjusted D-dimer cutoff levels to rule out pulmonary embolism: the ADJUST-PE study. *JAMA.* 2014;311(11):1117–1124. https://doi.org/10.1001/jama.2014.2135.

38. Becker KL, Snider R, Nylen ES. Procalcitonin assay in systemic inflammation, infection, and sepsis: clinical utility and limitations. *Crit Care Med.* 2008;36(3):941–952. https://doi.org/10.1097/CCM.0B013E318165BABB.

39. Maisel A, Neath S-X, Landsberg J, et al. Use of procalcitonin for the diagnosis of pneumonia in patients presenting with a chief complaint of dyspnoea: results from the BACH (Biomarkers in Acute Heart Failure) trial. *Eur J Heart Fail.* 2012;14(3):278–286. https://doi.org/10.1093/eurjhf/hfr177.

40. Christ-Crain M, Jaccard-Stolz D, Bingisser R, et al. Effect of procalcitonin-guided treatment on antibiotic use and outcome in lower respiratory tract infections: cluster-randomised, single-blinded intervention trial. *Lancet.* 2004;363(9409):600–607. https://doi.org/10.1016/S0140-6736(04)15591-8.

41. Schuetz P, Christ-Crain M, Thomann R, et al. Group for the PS. Effect of procalcitonin-based guidelines vs standard guidelines on antibiotic use in lower respiratory tract infections: the ProHOSP randomized controlled trial. *JAMA.* 2009;302(10):1059–1066. https://doi.org/10.1001/jama.2009.1297.

42. Milcent K, Faesch S, Guen CG-L, et al. Use of procalcitonin assays to predict serious bacterial infection in young febrile infants. *JAMA Pediatr.* 2016;170(1):62–69. https://doi.org/10.1001/jamapediatrics.2015.3210.

43. Travaglino F, Russo V, De Berardinis B, et al. Thirty and ninety days mortality predictive value of admission and in-hospital procalcitonin and mid-regional pro-adrenomedullin testing in patients with dyspnea. Results from the VERyfing DYspnea trial. *Am J Emerg Med.* 2014;32(4):334–341. https://doi.org/10.1016/j.ajem.2013.12.045.

44. Maisel A, Mueller C, Nowak R, et al. Mid-region pro-hormone markers for diagnosis and prognosis in acute dyspnea: results from the BACH (biomarkers in acute heart failure) trial. *J Am Coll Cardiol.* 2010;55(19):2062–2076. https://doi.org/10.1016/j.jacc.2010.02.025.

45. Maisel A, Mueller C, Nowak RM, et al. Midregion pro-hormone adrenomedullin and prognosis in patients presenting with acute dyspnea: results from the BACH (biomarkers in acute heart failure) trial. *J Am Coll Cardiol.* 2011;58(10):1057–1067. https://doi.org/10.1016/j.jacc.2011.06.006.

46. Januzzi JL, Peacock WF, Maisel AS, et al. Measurement of the interleukin family member ST2 in patients with acute dyspnea: results from the PRIDE (Pro-Brain natriuretic peptide investigation of dyspnea in the emergency department) study. *J Am Coll Cardiol.* 2007;50(7):607–613. https://doi.org/10.1016/j.jacc.2007.05.014.

47. Dieplinger B, Gegenhuber A, Kaar G, Poelz W, Haltmayer M, Mueller T. Prognostic value of established and novel biomarkers in patients with shortness of breath attending an emergency department. *Clin Biochem.* 2010;43(9):714–719. https://doi.org/10.1016/j.clinbiochem.2010.02.002.

48. Dieplinger B, Gegenhuber A, Haltmayer M, Mueller T. Evaluation of novel biomarkers for the diagnosis of acute destabilised heart failure in patients with shortness of breath. *Heart.* 2009;95(18):1508–1513. https://doi.org/10.1136/hrt.2009.170696.

49. Eurlings LW, Sanders-van Wijk S, van Kimmenade R, et al. Multimarker strategy for short-term risk assessment in patients with dyspnea in the emergency department: the MARKED (multi mARKer emergency dyspnea)-risk score. *J Am Coll Cardiol.* 2012;60(17):1668–1677. https://doi.org/10.1016/j.jacc.2012.06.040.

50. Singer AJ, Thode HC, Green GB, et al. The incremental benefit of a shortness–of–breath biomarker panel in Emergency Department Patients with Dyspnea. *Acad Emerg Med.* 2016;16(6):448–494. https://doi.org/10.1111/j.1553-2712.2009.00415.

CHAPTER 13

Biomarkers for Antiplatelet Therapy

RAZVAN T. DADU, MD, PHD • NEAL S. KLEIMAN, MD

INTRODUCTION

Antiplatelet therapies in addition to aspirin are mostly used to prevent stent thrombosis (ST) and recurrent myocardial infarction (MI) in patients with recent acute coronary syndrome (ACS) or who have undergone percutaneous coronary intervention (PCI) for stable coronary artery disease (CAD).[1-4] A P2Y12 antagonist such as clopidogrel, prasugrel, and ticagrelor is typically used in combination with aspirin in this patient population.[3,4] Cangrelor is another available intravenous antiplatelet drug that is primarily used during PCI. In this chapter we will focus on biomarkers used to assess the efficacy of oral antiplatelet therapies.

P2Y12 antagonists act by inhibiting adenosine diphosphonate (ADP)-mediated platelet activation. ADP is released from alpha storage granules after platelet activation and binds P2Y12 receptor in the part that resides outside the cell. Once ADP and P2Y12 form disulphide bonds, the outer part of the receptors undergoes inward conformational changes.[5] P2Y12 receptor is coupled with $G_{\alpha l2}$ and $G_{\beta\gamma}$. Activation of P2Y12 receptor results in activation of $G_{\alpha l2}$, which is responsible for activation of phosphoinositide-3-kinase and inhibition of adenylyl cyclase which results in decreased cyclic adenosine monophosphate levels within the platelet.[6-10] This sequence of intracellular events promotes alpha and dense granule release, activation of integrin (GPIIb-IIa), amplification of platelet aggregation, and stabilization of platelet aggregate.[10] All three commercially available drugs, clopidogrel, ticagrelor, and prasugrel, have the common mechanism of action of preventing ADP from binding P2Y12 with the final result being the inhibition of platelet activation. Clopidogrel and prasugrel are thienopyridines that are selective and irreversible inhibitors of P2Y12.[11] Both are prodrugs that require hepatic oxidation by cytochrome P450 to form active metabolites.[11] To become biologically active, clopidogrel must be metabolized in the liver by members of the cytochrome P450 family in two sequential steps.[8] The enzymes CYP3A4, CYP3A5, CYP2C9, and CYP1A2 are involved in one step, and enzymes CYP2B6 and CYP2C19 are involved in both the steps.[12]

Cytochrome P450 2C19 (CYP2C19) is located in hepatocellular endoplasmic reticulum. It is part of the cytochrome P450 mixed-function oxidase system and is encoded by the CYP2C19 gene located on chromosome 10 arm q24. The active metabolites of clopidogrel and prasugrel are equally potent; however, the active metabolite for prasugrel is more efficiently generated, and its plasma concentration after a therapeutic dose is higher.[11,13,14] Ticagrelor on the other hand is a reversible P2Y12 antagonist that does not require further modification to become active.[15,16] The onset of action after a loading dose occurs within 30 minutes for prasugrel and ticagrelor, whereas for clopidogrel, the onset occurs between 2 and 6 hours after administration, depending on the loading dose [11,15] (Table 13.1). Prasugrel[17] and ticagrelor[18] have been shown in randomized clinical trials to be superior to clopidogrel in preventing CVD events. Therefore current guidelines support their preferential use over clopidogrel in patients with ACS treated with PCI (class IIa).[17] However, clopidogrel remains a widely prescribed drug due to lesser risk of bleeding and its availability in generic formulation.[18,19] Currently clopidogrel is the only P2Y12 antagonist that has an indication in patients who have undergone coronary stent placement for stable ischemic heart disease.

A subgroup of patients that continue to suffer from adverse cardiovascular events despite appropriate therapy with antiplatelet drugs prompted a good deal of further research in this area.[8,20,21] Observations were first reported by Gurbel et al. of a widely variable response of platelet aggregation to standard clopidogrel dosing.[22] Multiple mechanisms were found to be involved in the variability of the response to clopidogrel treatment (Table 13.2).[8] Several attempts were made to identify biomarkers that can help assess platelet function (typically by measuring the degree of platelet reactivity [PR]) and quantify a patient's response to antiplatelet therapy.[23-27,29,30] In addition to PR, the presence of genetic variants of enzymes involved in clopidogrel metabolism was also studied as possible markers to identify individuals who were less likely to respond to clopidogrel.[31,32] CYP2C19 genetic variants

Biomarkers in Cardiovascular Disease. https://doi.org/10.1016/B978-0-323-54835-9.00013-2

TABLE 13.1
Pharmacology of Oral P2Y12 Inhibitors

	Clopidogrel	Prasugrel	Ticagrelor
Receptor	Irreversible	Irreversible	Reversible
Prodrug	Yes	Yes	No
Activation/liver metabolism	Prodrug/variable liver metabolism	Prodrug/predictable liver metabolism	Active drug/no liver metabolism
Dosing	Load: 300–600 mg oral; maintenance: 75 mg daily	Loading: 60 mg orally; maintenance: 10 mg daily	Loading: 180 mg orally; maintenance: 90 mg twice a day
Onset of action after loading dose	2–6 h	30 min	30 min
Duration of effect	3–10 days	7–10 days	3–5 days
Plasma half-life	30–60 min	30–60 min	6–12 h
CYP drug interaction	CYP2C19	No	CYP3A
Clinical use	ACS (invasively and noninvasively managed), stable CAD, PCI, PAD, and ischemic stroke	ACS undergoing PCI	ACS (invasive or noninvasively managed) or history of MI

ACS, acute coronary syndrome; *CAD*, coronary artery disease; *CYP*, cytochrome P450; *MI*, myocardial infarction; *PAD*. peripheral arterial disease; *PCI*, percutaneous coronary intervention.

TABLE 13.2
Factors Contributing to Clopidogrel Response Variability

Genetic factors	Polymorphism of CYP
	Polymorphism of GPIa
	Polymorphism P2Y12
	Polymorphism GPIIIa
Clinical factors	Poor compliance
	Under dosing
	Poor absorption
	Drug-drug interactions
	Acute coronary syndrome
	Diabetes
	Elevated body mass index
Cellular factor	Accelerated plated turnover
	Reduced CYP3A metabolic activity
	Increased ADP exposure
	Upregulation of the P2Y12 pathway
	Upregulation of the P2Y1 pathway
	Upregulation of P2Y-independent pathway

showed a strong association with poor response, likely due to the fact that it is involved in both the metabolism steps of clopidogrel.[12] In the gene encoding for CYP2C19 a single nucleotide polymorphism 681G-A (rs4244285) in exon 5, mapped to the long arm of chromosome 10 (10q24.1–q24.3), that encodes for a cryptic splice variant resulted in no enzyme activity in vivo.[33] There are several genetic variants of the CYP2C19 with different penetrance in general population which are summarized in Table 13.3.

Several techniques are available for measuring platelet function. Light transmittance aggregometry (LTA) is an older technique that was associated with significant methodological variability, which prevented the development of a uniform definition of poor responders to clopidogrel. More recently, other methods such as Multiplate Analyzer (F.Hoffman–La Roche Ltd, Basel, Switzerland), Biocytex, Asnieres, France, and Platelet Function Analysis (PFA 100) (Siemens Healthineers) were developed and have been successful in measuring PR. Vasodilator-stimulated phosphoprotein-phosphorylation (Diagnostica Stago) is another platelet function test that is more specific to the P2Y12 pathway and is associated with less variability than LTA.[34] "VerifyNow" P2Y12 Assay [Accumetrics, San Diego, California] is a point-of-care assay that measures platelet aggregation in whole blood by performing turbidimetric measurement of

TABLE 13.3
CYP2C19 Variants

CYP2C19		
Variant Effect Allelic Frequency Frequency in general population		
*2 Loss of function/co-dominant	15%	25%
*3 Loss of function	<1%	Very rare
*4 Loss of function/recessive	1%	2%
*5 Loss of function	<1%	Very rare
*6 Loss of function	<1%	Very rare

agglutination of platelets to fibrinogen-coated microbeds. This assay is also specific to P2Y12 pathway.[35]

Two point-of-care assays for CYP2C19 genotyping are currently available: (1) the Spartan RX (Spartan Bioscience, Inc., Ontario, Canada) and (2) the VERIGENE (Luminex Corporation, Austin, TX) assays. These tests are capable of identifying the two most common loss of-function alleles (CYP2C19*2 and *3) and gain of-function allele (CYP2C19*17).[31] Other tests such as Affymetrix Targeted Human drug-metabolizing enzymes and transporters 1.0 Assay (Affymetrix) or oligonucleotide ligation assay (SNPlex; Applied Biosystems) has been used in clinical trials.[36,37] Different studies reported good reproducibility of CYP2C19 genotyping methods and high levels of interassay agreement.[38,39]

PLATELET REACTIVITY

PR and CVD Risk Prediction

Multiple studies have investigated the association between PR and subsequent cardiovascular events in patients with CAD treated with antiplatelet therapy either as part of a post-PCI regimen or as a part of medical therapy[40-43] and have in general shown that PR does not add incremental predictive value in patients with CAD who are medically managed. Therefore its role as a risk marker in this patient population is less defined and will not be discussed in this chapter.[25,44]

The Assessment of Dual AntiPlatelet Therapy With Drug Eluting Stents (ADAPT-DES) trial evaluated the association between high PR and definite or probable ST in 8583 patients who received PCI for ACS or stable CAD.[40] In this trial a 2- to 3-fold increased risk of ST in univariate (hazard ratio [HR], 3.00; 95% confidence interval [CI], 1.39–6.49) and after multivariate analysis (HR, 2.49; 95% CI, 1.43–4.31) was shown. A PR>208 was also associated with increased 1-year MI incidence,

but not with 1-year mortality.[40] Similar findings are reported by Park et al. showing that a PR>235 platelet reactivity units (PRU) was independently associated with a composite endpoint of death MI, ST, and stroke in patients undergoing PCI for ACS (HR, 2.03; 95% CI, 1.30–3.18).[42] Finally a large meta-analysis by Brar et al. showed that PR in the highest quartile was associated with increased death, MI, and ST (HR, 2.62; 95% CI, 1.78–3.87; P<.001) compared with the first quartile. In the same meta-analysis a PR>230 was an independent predictor of the composite outcome as well as individual outcomes of death and stroke.[43] In addition to these clinical endpoints, several other studies have shown a positive association between PR and systemic inflammation.[45-47] Although PR as a prognostic marker was mostly studied in patient populations receiving clopidogrel, newer studies show that high PR is still present with newer P2Y12 blockers.[30,48,49] These studies revealed that the interindividual variability in response to prasugrel and ticagrelor was reduced compared with that in response to clopidogrel, but still present.[28,30] A prospective study on patients with ST elevation MI showed that the rates of on-treatment high PR defined as >208 PRU were similar at 2 hours of treatment between ticagrelor and prasugrel (46.2% and 34.6%, respectively).[28]

The results of the abovementioned trials suggest that PR is a good marker for risk of CVD events among patients who have undergone PCI.[40,43,50] High PR is associated with substantial hazard of subsequent thrombotic events. In prediction models, high PR improves net reclassification index proving to be a good prognostic marker. In ADAPT-DES trial, a PR>208 PRU was able to reclassify the risk for ST for 35% of patients when they were classified by tertiles of risk. In this trial the area under the curve for PR>208 PRU for prediction of definite or probable ST was 0.62.[40] In the meta-analysis by Brar et al. a cutoff point of 230 had an net discrimination improvement (NRI) of 0.23 for ST risk.[43]

PR and Antiplatelet Therapy Selection

PR was also evaluated in large studies as a possible biomarker to guide the antiplatelet treatment. In Gauging Responsiveness With a VerifyNow Assay–Impact on Thrombosis and Safety (GRAVITAS) study, 2214 patients with high PR (>235 PRU) at 12–24 h after PCI with DES were randomized to either standard dose of clopidogrel or 600-mg loading followed by 150-mg daily after PCI.[50] The primary outcome was a 6-months composite of cardiovascular death, nonfatal MI, and ST. This trial failed to show a difference between the two arms (HR, 1.01; 95% CI, 0.58–1.76).[50] The overall event rate was lower than what was used for power calculation; therefore it is believed that this trial could have been underpowered.[51] Subsequent time-dependent analyses of the GRAVITAS patient population have shown that a PR < 208 PRU was actually associated with less events; however, only a small fraction of patients treated with high-dose clopidogrel achieved a PR < 208 PRU.[50] In the Assessment by a Double Randomization of a Conventional Antiplatelet Strategy vs. a Monitoring-Guided Strategy for Drug-Eluting Stent Implantation and of Treatment Interruption vs. Continuation One Year After Stenting trial, 2440 patients were randomized to either drug adjustment if high PR reactivity was found according to platelet function monitoring (150-mg clopidogrel daily) or conventional treatment (75-mg clopidogrel daily). The primary endpoint was a composite of death, MI, stroke, or urgent revascularization at 1 year.[22] The trial showed no difference in primary outcome between the two arms (HR, 1.13; 95% CI, 0.98–1.29). Finally, Testing Platelet Reactivity in Patients Undergoing Elective Stent Placement on Clopidogrel to Guide Alternative Therapy With Prasugrel (TRIGGER-PCI) study randomized post-PCI stable CAD patients with high PR > 208 PRU to either clopidogrel or prasugrel.[52] This trial was terminated prematurely due to low events rate.[52] A non-prespecified interim analysis of TRIGGER-PCI shows that the prasugrel arm had a more significant decrease in PR from a median of 245 PRU at baseline to 80 PRU than clopidogrel arm which decreased from 249 PRU at baseline to 241 PRU (P < .001). No conclusion could be drawn regarding the clinical use of this trial due to extremely low event rates.[52]

The availability of the two newer antiplatelet drugs has prompted evaluation of the change in the PR that occurs with escalating therapy from clopidogrel to ticagrelor or prasugrel.[52-64] SWitching Anti-Platelet (SWAP) study included patients receiving clopidogrel therapy after ACS. In this patient population, change of therapy to prasugrel was associated with reduction in PR that was maintained at 1 week.[60] Similarly, A Study of the Antiplatelet Effects Comparing Ticagrelor (Ticag. - AZD6140) With Clopidogrel (Clop.) Responder and Non-responders (RESPOND) study showed decreased PR among patients who were treated with clopidogrel and were switched to ticagrelor later.[61] The SWAP2 study showed that switching from ticagrelor to prasugrel resulted in PR that was higher at 7 days with significant differences noted as soon as 24 h after the switch.[65] Other trials also showed consistent decreased PR associated with changing therapy from clopidogrel to either ticagrelor or prasugrel; however, no randomized trial has so far shown that targeting PR by changing therapy impacts clinical events. The latest trial

Testing Responsiveness to Platelet Inhibition on Chronic Antiplatelet Treatment For Acute Coronary Syndromes Trial (TROPICAL ACS) tested whether de-escalation of therapy in early maintenance phase based on PR impacts outcomes. In this trial, 2610 patients were randomized either to conventional treatment with prasugrel or de-escalation of therapy to clopidogrel based on PR testing. There was no difference in composite of death, MI, or stroke between the groups (5% vs. 3%; P = 0.0115 for noninferiority) or in bleeding academic research consortium 2 (BARC2) or greater bleeding (5% vs. 6%; P = .23).[66]

PR and Bleeding

Although the newer P2Y12 antagonists have shown superiority in reducing CVD events, they are also associated with a higher risk of bleeding.[23,24] Therefore the role of PR in preventing bleeding by de-escalating therapy has been evaluated.[67,68] Multiple small observational studies have shown association between low PR and bleeding.[49,57,69-73] The inverse association between PR and bleeding was further confirmed in the large ADAPT-DES trial. In this trial a value < 208 PRU was associated with higher rate of bleeding (HR: 0.73; 95% CI, 0.61–0.89).[40,74] De-escalation of therapy from newer P2Y12 inhibitors to clopidogrel has consistently been associated with subsequent increase in PR. This finding should be interpreted with caution because the increase in PR did not consistently translate into decreased bleeding in all trials, and none of these trials were statistically powered to detect a difference in clinical outcomes.[61,62,75-79] Table 13.4 summarizes some of these trials. The latest trial TROPICAL ACS described earlier did not show reduction in bleeding events after PR guided de-escalation of therapy from prasugrel to clopidogrel.[66]

Guidelines and Recommendations for PR Testing

PR measured with various platelet function assays was shown to be a good marker for risk prediction for CVD events in patients receiving PCI. Persistent high PR in patients who have received PCI and are treated with antiplatelet therapy is associated with high CVD event rates. Attempts to modify risk of CVD after PCI by targeting PR with higher dose clopidogrel therapy have failed to show benefit in clinical trials. No trial has shown that intervening on PR has resulted in better clinical outcomes; however, several studies suggest that escalation of therapy from clopidogrel to newer P2Y12 antagonists is associated with decreased PR, and other studies showed superiority of newer P2Y12 antagonists in preventing recurrent CVD events.[23,24] The current american college of cardiology/american heart association (ACC/AHA) guidelines

TABLE 13.4
Platelet Reactivity Cutoff Associated With Ischemic and Bleeding Events

Reference	Assay Used for Platelet Function Testing	Cutoff for Ischemic Events	Ischemic Endpoint	Cutoff for Bleeding Events	Bleeding Endpoint
Campo et al. [86]	VerifyNow (PRU)	>238 PRU	Death, MI, stroke	<85	TIMI
Sibbing et al. [69]	Multiple assay analyzer ADP-induced aggregation units (AU)	>46	Stent Thrombosis	<19	TIMI major
Gurbel et al. [61]	Thrombelastography; platelet mapping; assay ADP-induced; platelet-fibrin clot; strength, mm	>47	Death, stent thrombosis, MI, stroke	<31	TIMI major
Bonello et al. [49]	VASP-PRI	≥50%	Cardiovascular death, MI, ST	<16%	Minor and major bleed

ADP, adenosine diphosphonate; *MI*, myocardial infarction; *ST*, stent thrombosis ; *VASP-PRI*, vasodilator stimulated phosphoprotein-platelet reactivity index.

give a class IIb recommendation for platelet function testing in patients at high risk for poor outcomes. The clinician should assess individual risk of each patient and decide the appropriateness of PR testing on case-by-case basis. The patients who are most likely to benefit are those, after PCI, who are at high risk for subsequent events such as patients with ACS or patients who have had ST. The guidelines also recommend that patients treated with clopidogrel who were found to have high PR alternative agents such as prasugrel or ticagrelor may be considered (class IIb). Routine platelet function testing carries a class III recommendation.[80] Currently there are no recommendations for using PR to predict bleeding or to guide therapy with the goal to reduce bleeding events.

GENETIC TESTING
Genetic Testing and CVD Risk Prediction

The association between CYP2C19 polymorphism and CVD outcomes has been tested in large-scale trials.[36,37,81,82] TRial to assess Improvement in Therapeutic Outcomes by optimizing platelet InhibitioN with prasugrel Thrombolysis In Myocardial Infarction 38 (TRITON TIMI 38) enrolled 13,608 patients with ACS who underwent PCI and were subsequently treated with clopidogrel. Of all, 1477 patients had undergone genetic testing, and the CYP2C19 reduced-function allele was present in 30% of the patients and was associated with increased risk of composite endpoint of cardiovascular death, nonfatal MI, or nonfatal stroke (HR, 1.53; 95% CI, 1.07–2.19). The risk of ST in these patients was increased by 3 times.[36] In the French Registry on Acute ST-Elevation and Non-ST-Elevation Myocardial Infarction study, patients with acute MI

receiving clopidogrel were included. Among the 1535 patients who underwent PCI, the patients with two CYP2C19 loss-of-function alleles had 3.58 times higher rates of subsequent CVD events than those with none (95% CI, 1.71–7.51).[37] Similar results were reproduced by Sibbing et al. who showed that CYP2C19*2 carrier status was associated with a significant increased risk of ST at 30 days in patients undergoing PCI.[82] Risk of events was also shown to be proportional with the number of alleles carried. A meta-analysis by Mega et al. showed an incremental risk of major adverse cardiac events (MACE) with one (HR, 1.55; 95% CI, 1.11–2.17; *P*=0.01) and two (HR, 1.76; 95% CI, 1.24–2.50; *P*=0.002) reduced-function CYP2C19 alleles, when compared with noncarriers. Similar trends were noticed for ST.[83]

Although prasugrel is also metabolized by liver, studies have shown that its metabolism is not affected by the presence of CYP2C19 reduced-function alleles. In the TRITON TIMI 38 trial, plasma concentrations of active drug metabolite and platelet inhibition in response to prasugrel were tested in 238 healthy subjects, and no significant attenuation of the pharmacokinetic or pharmacodynamic response to prasugrel was observed. In those patients with ACS who were treated with prasugrel, no significant associations were found between any of the tested cytochrome P450 (CYP) genotypes and risk of cardiovascular death, MI, or stroke.[36] Additional analyses have also evaluated the impact of CYP2C19 allele in patients treated with ticagrelor. In the study of platelet inhibition and patient outcomes (PLATO) trial of 10,285 patients, the primary outcome composite of cardiovascular death, MI, or stroke at 12 months occurred less often with ticagrelor regardless of CYP2C19 genotype.[84]

Guidelines and Recommendations for Genetic Testing

As reviewed previously, CYP2C19 has proven itself as a good prognostic marker for subsequent CVD in patients who are treated with clopidogrel after PCI for stable CAD or ACS. Data are less supportive of its benefit in medically managed patients.[85] Large clinical trials have shown that CYP2C19 carrier status does not appear to have any influence on patients treated with prasugrel or ticagrelor.[36,84] These findings led to the current ACC/AHA guideline recommendation that genetic testing may be considered to identify whether patients are at risk for poor clinical outcomes due to inadequate metabolism of clopidogrel (class IIb).[80] Switching clopidogrel to a more potent P2Y12 inhibitor (prasugrel or ticagrelor) is recommended if a patient is identified to be poorly metabolizing clopidogrel by genetic testing (class IIb).[80] ACC/AHA guidelines recommend against-routine genetic testing (class III recommendation).[80]

Future Directions

Several other trials are ongoing and are intended to determine whether tailoring antiplatelet therapy based on CYP2C19 genotyping would provide any benefit. The Tailored Antiplatelet Initiation to Lesson Outcomes Due to Decreased Clopidogrel Response After Percutaneous Coronary Intervention (NCT01742117) trial enrolls 5270 patients undergoing PCI for either ACS or stable CAD. The patients will be randomized to either conventional management or CYP2C19 genotype–based antiplatelet therapy approach with escalation of therapy to ticagrelor 90 mg bid if carrier status is identified. The primary endpoint will be a composite of cardiovascular mortality, nonfatal MI, nonfatal stroke, severe recurrent ischemia, and ST. The Dutch POPular Genetics (Cost-effectiveness of CYP2C19 Genotype Guided Treatment With Antiplatelet Drugs in Patients With ST-segment-elevation Myocardial Infarction Undergoing Immediate PCI With Stent Implantation: Optimization of Treatment, NCT01761786) is another trial that enrolls 2700 patients with ST segment elevation myocardial infarction (STEMI) and randomize them to either conventional prasugrel/ticagrelor therapy or to a CYP2C19 genotype-guided treatment. In the genotyping group, noncarrier patients receive clopidogrel and carriers will receive prasugrel or ticagrelor. Primary clinical benefit outcome will be a composite of death, MI, definite ST, stroke, and PLATO major bleeding at 1 year. Safety and cost-effectiveness will also be analyzed.

CONCLUSION

Assessing biomarkers after administering antiplatelet drugs has provided valuable information on the way patients respond to a treatment which is a cornerstone of managing ACS and is in fact a requisite treatment for patients undergoing intracoronary stenting. Despite the intuitive appeal of this concept, however, the randomized trials that to date have been working on measurements of platelet response to therapy have not shown a clinical benefit to these assessments. The trials to date have been based on phenotypic responses to various measurements of platelet aggregation. The next generation of trials will focus on genotypic assessment of the hepatic enzymes that govern this response.

REFERENCES

1. Alexopoulos D, Xanthopoulou I, Deftereos S, et al. In-hospital switching of oral P2Y12 inhibitor treatment in patients with acute coronary syndrome undergoing percutaneous coronary intervention: prevalence, predictors and short-term outcome. *Am Heart J.* 2014;167(1):68–76.e2.
2. Clemmensen P, Grieco N, Ince H, et al. MULTInational non-interventional study of patients with ST-segment elevation myocardial infarction treated with PRimary Angioplasty and Concomitant use of upstream antiplatelet therapy with prasugrel or clopidogrel–the European MULTIPRAC Registry. *Eur Heart J Acute Cardiovasc Care.* 2015;4(3):220–229.
3. Levine GN, Bates ER, Blankenship JC, et al. 2015 ACC/AHA/SCAI focused update on primary percutaneous coronary intervention for patients with ST-elevation myocardial infarction: an update of the 2011 ACCF/AHA/SCAI guideline for percutaneous coronary intervention and the 2013 ACCF/AHA guideline for the management of ST-elevation myocardial infarction. *J Am Coll Cardiol.* 2016;67(10):1235–1250.
4. Valgimigli M, Bueno H, Byrne RA, et al. 2017 ESC focused update on dual antiplatelet therapy in coronary artery disease developed in collaboration with EACTS: the Task Force for dual antiplatelet therapy in coronary artery disease of the European Society of Cardiology (ESC) and of the European Association for Cardio-Thoracic Surgery (EACTS). *Eur Heart J.* 2017.
5. Zhang J, Zhang K, Gao ZG, et al. Agonist-bound structure of the human P2Y12 receptor. *Nature.* 2014;509(7498):119–122.
6. Angiolillo DJ. The evolution of antiplatelet therapy in the treatment of acute coronary syndromes: from aspirin to the present day. *Drugs.* 2012;72(16):2087–2116.
7. Franchi F, Angiolillo DJ. Novel antiplatelet agents in acute coronary syndrome. *Nat Rev Cardiol.* 2015;12(1):30–47.

8. Angiolillo DJ, Fernandez-Ortiz A, Bernardo E, et al. Variability in individual responsiveness to clopidogrel: clinical implications, management, and future perspectives. *J Am Coll Cardiol.* 2007;49(14):1505–1516.

9. Storey RF, Newby LJ, Heptinstall S. Effects of P2Y(1) and P2Y(12) receptor antagonists on platelet aggregation induced by different agonists in human whole blood. *Platelets.* 2001;12(7):443–447.

10. Savi P, Herbert JM. Clopidogrel and ticlopidine: P2Y12 adenosine diphosphate-receptor antagonists for the prevention of atherothrombosis. *Semin Thromb Hemost.* 2005;31(2):174–183.

11. Farid NA, Kurihara A, Wrighton SA. Metabolism and disposition of the thienopyridine antiplatelet drugs ticlopidine, clopidogrel, and prasugrel in humans. *J Clin Pharmacol.* 2010;50(2):126–142.

12. Farid NA, Payne CD, Small DS, et al. Cytochrome P450 3A inhibition by ketoconazole affects prasugrel and clopidogrel pharmacokinetics and pharmacodynamics differently. *Clin Pharmacol Ther.* 2007;81(5):735–741.

13. Bernlochner I, Morath T, Brown PB, et al. A prospective randomized trial comparing the recovery of platelet function after loading dose administration of prasugrel or clopidogrel. *Platelets.* 2013;24(1):15–25.

14. Price MJ, Walder JS, Baker BA, et al. Recovery of platelet function after discontinuation of prasugrel or clopidogrel maintenance dosing in aspirin-treated patients with stable coronary disease: the recovery trial. *J Am Coll Cardiol.* 2012;59(25):2338–2343.

15. Husted S, van Giezen JJ. Ticagrelor: the first reversibly binding oral P2Y12 receptor antagonist. *Cardiovasc Ther.* 2009;27(4):259–274.

16. Gurbel PA, Bliden KP, Butler K, et al. Randomized double-blind assessment of the ONSET and OFFSET of the antiplatelet effects of ticagrelor versus clopidogrel in patients with stable coronary artery disease: the ONSET/OFFSET study. *Circulation.* 2009;120(25):2577–2585.

17. Wiviott SD, Braunwald E, McCabe CH, et al. Prasugrel versus clopidogrel in patients with acute coronary syndromes. *N Engl J Med.* 2007;357(20):2001–2015.

18. Wallentin L, Becker RC, Budaj A, et al. Ticagrelor versus clopidogrel in patients with acute coronary syndromes. *N Engl J Med.* 2009;361(11):1045–1057.

19. Levine GN, Bates ER, Bittl JA, et al. 2016 ACC/AHA guideline focused update on duration of dual antiplatelet therapy in patients with coronary artery disease: a report of the American College of Cardiology/American Heart Association Task Force on Clinical Practice Guidelines. *J Thorac Cardiovasc Surg.* 2016;152(5):1243–1275.

20. Sherwood MW, Wiviott SD, Peng SA, et al. Early clopidogrel versus prasugrel use among contemporary STEMI and NSTEMI patients in the US: insights from the National Cardiovascular Data Registry. *J Am Heart Assoc.* 2014;3(2):e000849.

21. Bueno H, Sinnaeve P, Annemans L, et al. Opportunities for improvement in anti-thrombotic therapy and other strategies for the management of acute coronary syndromes: insights from EPICOR, an international study of current practice patterns. *Eur Heart J Acute Cardiovasc Care.* 2016;5(1):3–12.

22. Michelson AD, Frelinger 3rd AL, Braunwald E, et al. Pharmacodynamic assessment of platelet inhibition by prasugrel vs. clopidogrel in the TRITON-TIMI 38 trial. *Eur Heart J.* 2009;30(14):1753–1763.

23. Storey RF, Angiolillo DJ, Patil SB, et al. Inhibitory effects of ticagrelor compared with clopidogrel on platelet function in patients with acute coronary syndromes: the PLATO (PLATelet inhibition and patient Outcomes) PLATELET substudy. *J Am Coll Cardiol.* 2010;56(18):1456–1462.

24. Gurbel PA, Bliden KP, Hiatt BL, O'Connor CM. Clopidogrel for coronary stenting: response variability, drug resistance, and the effect of pretreatment platelet reactivity. *Circulation.* 2003;107(23):2908–2913.

25. Collet JP, Cuisset T, Range G, et al. Bedside monitoring to adjust antiplatelet therapy for coronary stenting. *N Engl J Med.* 2012;367(22):2100–2109.

26. Michelson AD, Frelinger 3rd AL, Furman MI. Current options in platelet function testing. *Am J Cardiol.* 2006;98(10A):4N–10N.

27. Bonello L, Tantry US, Marcucci R, et al. Consensus and future directions on the definition of high on-treatment platelet reactivity to adenosine diphosphate. *J Am Coll Cardiol.* 2010;56(12):919–933.

28. Alexopoulos D, Xanthopoulou I, Gkizas V, et al. Randomized assessment of ticagrelor versus prasugrel antiplatelet effects in patients with ST-segment-elevation myocardial infarction. *Circ Cardiovasc Interv.* 2012;5(6):797–804.

29. Gurbel PA, Erlinge D, Ohman EM, et al. Platelet function during extended prasugrel and clopidogrel therapy for patients with ACS treated without revascularization: the TRILOGY ACS platelet function substudy. *JAMA.* 2012;308(17):1785–1794.

30. Parodi G, Valenti R, Bellandi B, et al. Comparison of prasugrel and ticagrelor loading doses in ST-segment elevation myocardial infarction patients: RAPID (Rapid Activity of Platelet Inhibitor Drugs) primary PCI study. *J Am Coll Cardiol.* 2013;61(15):1601–1606.

31. Lin G, Yi L, Zhang K, et al. Implementation of cell samples as controls in national proficiency testing for clopidogrel therapy-related CYP2C19 genotyping in China: a novel approach. *PLoS One.* 2015;10(7):e0134174.

32. Marin F, Gonzalez-Conejero R, Capranzano P, Bass TA, Roldan V, Angiolillo DJ. Pharmacogenetics in cardiovascular antithrombotic therapy. *J Am Coll Cardiol.* 2009;54(12):1041–1057.

33. Goldstein JA. Clinical relevance of genetic polymorphisms in the human CYP2C subfamily. *Br J Clin Pharmacol.* 2001;52(4):349–355.

34. Aleil B, Ravanat C, Cazenave JP, Rochoux G, Heitz A, Gachet C. Flow cytometric analysis of intraplatelet VASP phosphorylation for the detection of clopidogrel resistance in patients with ischemic cardiovascular diseases. *J Thromb Haemost.* 2005;3(1):85–92.

35. von Beckerath N, Pogatsa-Murray G, Wieczorek A, Sibbing D, Schomig A, Kastrati A. Correlation of a new point-of-care test with conventional optical aggregometry for the assessment of clopidogrel responsiveness. *Thromb Haemost.* 2006;95(5):910–911.

36. Mega JL, Close SL, Wiviott SD, et al. Cytochrome p-450 polymorphisms and response to clopidogrel. *N Engl J Med.* 2009;360(4):354–362.

37. Simon T, Verstuyft C, Mary-Krause M, et al. Genetic determinants of response to clopidogrel and cardiovascular events. *N Engl J Med.* 2009;360(4):363–375.

38. Roberts JD, Wells GA, Le May MR, et al. Point-of-care genetic testing for personalisation of antiplatelet treatment (RAPID GENE): a prospective, randomised, proof-of-concept trial. *Lancet.* 2012;379(9827):1705–1711.

39. Erlinge D, James S, Duvvuru S, et al. Clopidogrel metaboliser status based on point-of-care CYP2C19 genetic testing in patients with coronary artery disease. *Thromb Haemost.* 2014;111(5):943–950.

40. Stone GW, Witzenbichler B, Weisz G, et al. Platelet reactivity and clinical outcomes after coronary artery implantation of drug-eluting stents (ADAPT-DES): a prospective multicentre registry study. *Lancet.* 2013;382(9892):614–623.

41. Ahn SG, Lee SH, Yoon JH, et al. Different prognostic significance of high on-treatment platelet reactivity as assessed by the VerifyNow P2Y12 assay after coronary stenting in patients with and without acute myocardial infarction. *JACC Cardiovasc Interv.* 2012;5(3):259–267.

42. Park DW, Ahn JM, Song HG, et al. Differential prognostic impact of high on-treatment platelet reactivity among patients with acute coronary syndromes versus stable coronary artery disease undergoing percutaneous coronary intervention. *Am Heart J.* 2013;165(1):34–42.e1.

43. Brar SS, ten Berg J, Marcucci R, et al. Impact of platelet reactivity on clinical outcomes after percutaneous coronary intervention. A collaborative meta-analysis of individual participant data. *J Am Coll Cardiol.* 2011;58(19):1945–1954.

44. Reny JL, Berdague P, Poncet A, et al. Antiplatelet drug response status does not predict recurrent ischemic events in stable cardiovascular patients: results of the Antiplatelet Drug Resistances and Ischemic Events study. *Circulation.* 2012;125(25):3201–3210.

45. Tantry US, Bliden KP, Suarez TA, Kreutz RP, Dichiara J, Gurbel PA. Hypercoagulability, platelet function, inflammation and coronary artery disease acuity: results of the Thrombotic RIsk Progression (TRIP) study. *Platelets.* 2010;21(5):360–367.

46. Gori AM, Cesari F, Marcucci R, et al. The balance between pro- and anti-inflammatory cytokines is associated with platelet aggregability in acute coronary syndrome patients. *Atherosclerosis.* 2009;202(1):255–262.

47. Bernlochner I, Steinhubl S, Braun S, et al. Association between inflammatory biomarkers and platelet aggregation in patients under chronic clopidogrel treatment. *Thromb Haemost.* 2010;104(6):1193–1200.

48. Alexopoulos D, Xanthopoulou I, Gkizas V, et al. Response to letter regarding article, "Randomized assessment of ticagrelor versus prasugrel antiplatelet effects in patients with ST-segment-elevation myocardial infarction. *Circ Cardiovasc Interv.* 2013;6(2):e29.

49. Bonello L, Mancini J, Pansieri M, et al. Relationship between post-treatment platelet reactivity and ischemic and bleeding events at 1-year follow-up in patients receiving prasugrel. *J Thromb Haemost.* 2012;10(10):1999–2005.

50. Price MJ, Berger PB, Teirstein PS, et al. Standard- vs high-dose clopidogrel based on platelet function testing after percutaneous coronary intervention: the GRAVITAS randomized trial. *JAMA.* 2011;305(11):1097–1105.

51. Gurbel PA, Tantry US. An initial experiment with personalized antiplatelet therapy: the GRAVITAS trial. *JAMA.* 2011;305(11):1136–1137.

52. Trenk D, Stone GW, Gawaz M, et al. A randomized trial of prasugrel versus clopidogrel in patients with high platelet reactivity on clopidogrel after elective percutaneous coronary intervention with implantation of drug-eluting stents: results of the TRIGGER-PCI (Testing platelet reactivity in patients undergoing elective stent placement on clopidogrel to guide alternative therapy with prasugrel) study. *J Am Coll Cardiol.* 2012;59(24):2159–2164.

53. Lhermusier T, Lipinski MJ, Drenning D, et al. Switching patients from clopidogrel to prasugrel in acute coronary syndrome: impact of the clopidogrel loading dose on platelet reactivity. *J Interv Cardiol.* 2014;27(4):365–372.

54. Mayer K, Schulz S, Bernlochner I, et al. A comparative cohort study on personalised antiplatelet therapy in PCI-treated patients with high on-clopidogrel platelet reactivity. Results of the ISAR-HPR registry. *Thromb Haemost.* 2014;112(2):342–351.

55. Nuhrenberg TG, Trenk D, Leggewie S, et al. Clopidogrel pretreatment of patients with ST-elevation myocardial infarction does not affect platelet reactivity after subsequent prasugrel-loading: platelet reactivity in an observational study. *Platelets.* 2013;24(7):549–553.

56. Koul S, Andell P, Martinsson A, et al. A pharmacodynamic comparison of 5 anti-platelet protocols in patients with ST-elevation myocardial infarction undergoing primary PCI. *BMC Cardiovasc Disord.* 2014;14:189.

57. Alexopoulos D, Galati A, Xanthopoulou I, et al. Ticagrelor versus prasugrel in acute coronary syndrome patients with high on-clopidogrel platelet reactivity following percutaneous coronary intervention: a pharmacodynamic study. *J Am Coll Cardiol.* 2012;60(3):193–199.

58. Sardella G, Calcagno S, Mancone M, et al. Pharmacodynamic effect of switching therapy in patients with high on-treatment platelet reactivity and genotype variation with high clopidogrel Dose versus prasugrel: the RESET GENE trial. *Circ Cardiovasc Interv.* 2012;5(5):698–704.

59. Diodati JG, Saucedo JF, French JK, et al. Effect on platelet reactivity from a prasugrel loading dose after a clopidogrel loading dose compared with a prasugrel loading dose alone: transferring from clopidogrel loading dose to prasugrel loading dose in acute coronary syndrome patients (TRIPLET): a randomized controlled trial. *Circ Cardiovasc Interv.* 2013;6(5):567–574.

60. Angiolillo DJ, Saucedo JF, Deraad R, et al. Increased platelet inhibition after switching from maintenance clopidogrel to prasugrel in patients with acute coronary syndromes: results of the SWAP (SWitching Anti Platelet) study. *J Am Coll Cardiol.* 2010;56(13):1017–1023.

61. Gurbel PA, Bliden KP, Butler K, et al. Response to ticagrelor in clopidogrel nonresponders and responders and effect of switching therapies: the RESPOND study. *Circulation.* 2010;121(10):1188–1199.

62. Lhermusier T, Voisin S, Murat G, et al. Switching patients from clopidogrel to novel P2Y12 receptor inhibitors in acute coronary syndrome: comparative effects of prasugrel and ticagrelor on platelet reactivity. *Int J Cardiol.* 2014;174(3):874–876.

63. Parodi G, De Luca G, Bellandi B, et al. Switching from clopidogrel to prasugrel in patients having coronary stent implantation. *J Thromb Thrombol.* 2014;38(3):395–401.

64. Cuisset T, Gaborit B, Dubois N, et al. Platelet reactivity in diabetic patients undergoing coronary stenting for acute coronary syndrome treated with clopidogrel loading dose followed by prasugrel maintenance therapy. *Int J Cardiol.* 2013;168(1):523–528.

65. Angiolillo DJ, Curzen N, Gurbel P, et al. Pharmacodynamic evaluation of switching from ticagrelor to prasugrel in patients with stable coronary artery disease: results of the SWAP-2 study (Switching anti platelet-2). *J Am Coll Cardiol.* 2014;63(15):1500–1509.

66. Sibbing D, Aradi D, Jacobshagen C, et al. Guided de-escalation of antiplatelet treatment in patients with acute coronary syndrome undergoing percutaneous coronary intervention (TROPICAL-ACS): a randomised, open-label, multicentre trial. *Lancet.* 2017;390(10104):1747–1757.

67. Tantry US, Bonello L, Aradi D, et al. Consensus and update on the definition of on-treatment platelet reactivity to adenosine diphosphate associated with ischemia and bleeding. *J Am Coll Cardiol.* 2013;62(24):2261–2273.

68. Thomas MR, Angiolillo DJ, Bonaca MP, et al. Consistent platelet inhibition with ticagrelor 60 mg twice-daily following myocardial infarction regardless of diabetes status. *Thromb Haemost.* 2017;117(5):940–947.

69. Sibbing D, Schulz S, Braun S, et al. Antiplatelet effects of clopidogrel and bleeding in patients undergoing coronary stent placement. *J Thromb Haemost.* 2010;8(2):250–256.

70. Mokhtar OA, Lemesle G, Armero S, et al. Relationship between platelet reactivity inhibition and non-CABG related major bleeding in patients undergoing percutaneous coronary intervention. *Thromb Res.* 2010;126(2):e147–e149.

71. Patti G, Pasceri V, Vizzi V, Ricottini E, Di Sciascio G. Usefulness of platelet response to clopidogrel by point-of-care testing to predict bleeding outcomes in patients undergoing percutaneous coronary intervention (from the Antiplatelet Therapy for Reduction of Myocardial Damage during Angioplasty-Bleeding Study). *Am J Cardiol.* 2011;107(7):995–1000.

72. Tsukahara K, Kimura K, Morita S, et al. Impact of high-responsiveness to dual antiplatelet therapy on bleeding complications in patients receiving drug-eluting stents. *Circ J.* 2010;74(4):679–685.

73. Parodi G, Bellandi B, Venditti F, et al. Residual platelet reactivity, bleedings, and adherence to treatment in patients having coronary stent implantation treated with prasugrel. *Am J Cardiol.* 2012;109(2):214–218.

74. Stuckey TD, Kirtane AJ, Brodie BR, et al. Impact of aspirin and clopidogrel hyporesponsiveness in patients treated with drug-eluting stents: 2-year results of a prospective, multicenter registry study. *JACC Cardiovasc Interv.* 2017;10(16):1607–1617.

75. Pourdjabbar A, Hibbert B, Chong AY, et al. A randomised study for optimising crossover from ticagrelor to clopidogrel in patients with acute coronary syndrome. The CAPITAL OPTI-CROSS Study. *Thromb Haemost.* 2017;117(2):303–310.

76. Wiviott SD, Trenk D, Frelinger AL, et al. Prasugrel compared with high loading- and maintenance-dose clopidogrel in patients with planned percutaneous coronary intervention: the Prasugrel in Comparison to Clopidogrel for Inhibition of Platelet Activation and Aggregation-Thrombolysis in Myocardial Infarction 44 trial. *Circulation.* 2007;116(25):2923–2932.

77. Montalescot G, Sideris G, Cohen R, et al. Prasugrel compared with high-dose clopidogrel in acute coronary syndrome. The randomised, double-blind ACAPULCO study. *Thromb Haemost.* 2010;103(1):213–223.

78. Kerneis M, Silvain J, Abtan J, et al. Switching acute coronary syndrome patients from prasugrel to clopidogrel. *JACC Cardiovasc Interv.* 2013;6(2):158–165.

79. Deharo P, Pons C, Pankert M, et al. Effectiveness of switching 'hyper responders' from Prasugrel to Clopidogrel after acute coronary syndrome: the POBA (Predictor of Bleeding with Antiplatelet drugs) SWITCH study. *Int J Cardiol.* 2013;168(5):5004–5005.

80. Levine GN, Bates ER, Blankenship JC, et al. 2011 ACCF/AHA/SCAI guideline for percutaneous coronary intervention: a report of the American College of Cardiology Foundation/American heart association Task Force on practice guidelines and the society for cardiovascular angiography and interventions. *Catheter Cardiovasc Interv.* 2013;82(4):E266–E355.

81. Collet JP, Hulot JS, Pena A, et al. Cytochrome P450 2C19 polymorphism in young patients treated with clopidogrel after myocardial infarction: a cohort study. *Lancet.* 2009;373(9660):309–317.

82. Sibbing D, Stegherr J, Latz W, et al. Cytochrome P450 2C19 loss-of-function polymorphism and stent thrombosis following percutaneous coronary intervention. *Eur Heart J.* 2009;30(8):916–922.

83. Mega JL, Simon T, Collet JP, et al. Reduced-function CY-P2C19 genotype and risk of adverse clinical outcomes among patients treated with clopidogrel predominantly for PCI: a meta-analysis. *JAMA.* 2010;304(16):1821–1830.

84. Wallentin L, James S, Storey RF, et al. Effect of CYP2C19 and ABCB1 single nucleotide polymorphisms on outcomes of treatment with ticagrelor versus clopidogrel for acute coronary syndromes: a genetic substudy of the PLATO trial. *Lancet.* 2010;376(9749):1320–1328.

85. Doll JA, Neely ML, Roe MT, et al. Impact of CYP2C19 metabolizer status on patients with ACS treated with prasugrel versus clopidogrel. *J Am Coll Cardiol.* 2016;67(8):936–947.

86. Campo G, Parrinello G, Ferraresi P, et al. Prospective evaluation of on-clopidogrel platelet reactivity over time in patients treated with percutaneous coronary intervention relationship with gene polymorphisms and clinical outcome. *J Am Coll Cardiol.* 2011;57(25):2474–2483.

CHAPTER 14

Biomarkers in the Management of Venous Thromboembolism

TERESA L. CARMAN, MD

INTRODUCTION

A biomarker is broadly considered to be an externally observed medical sign that can be objectively and accurately measured, is reproducible, and is reflective of a normal biologic process, pathologic state, or response to treatment. The use of biomarkers is indicated to predict, impact, or influence the incidence or outcome of a disease state.[1] Venous thromboembolism (VTE), including deep vein thrombosis (DVT) and pulmonary embolism (PE), is a relatively common clinical condition. Defects in blood coagulation, irritation of the vessel wall and surrounding tissues, and interruption of normal blood flow have been referred to as Virchow's triad.[2] Indeed many identifiable clinical and biologic risks for VTE can be attributed to alterations in these 3 components. The incidence of VTE is increasing and follows myocardial infarction and stroke as the third most common cardiovascular disease. It is estimated that 2,000,000 cases of DVT and up to 300,000 deaths from PE occur annually in the United States.[3] Data from the Atherosclerosis Risk in Communities (ARIC) study suggests the life-time risk for VTE in an individual aged 45 years is approximately 8%. Risk is higher in African-American and obese individuals.[4] Recognizing the impact of VTE, the Surgeon General issued a "Call to Action to Prevent Deep Vein Thrombosis and Pulmonary Embolism" in 2008.[5] Identifying ways to better prevent and reduce the risk of VTE was the focus of this effort. Both clinical and laboratory biomarkers can be used to impact VTE including opportunities to predict disease probability, effect clinical outcomes, and determine the risk of recurrence (Table 14.1).

CLINICAL BIOMARKERS IN VTE

Cancer and cancer treatment, recent surgery, medical hospital admission, travel, trauma, orthopedic injury or immobilization, systemic inflammation, hormonal therapy, varicose veins, inherited and acquired thrombophilia, and pregnancy or recent delivery are identified clinical conditions that increase VTE risk. Although associated with VTE and imposing risk, these are not measurable biomarkers. Clinical biomarkers associated with VTE and recurrent VTE include age, height, and obesity. In addition, male gender, technically not a biomarker, is a binary clinical variable for VTE recurrence that should not be overlooked.

VTE is uncommon in children and usually associated with other clinical risks. In adults, the incidence of VTE increases with age and is estimated at 1–2 per 1000 person-years.[3,6–8] In most studies, the incidence in young women aged 18–39 years generally outpaces that in men.[3,8] This is felt to be related predominantly because of child-bearing and contraception. Using several cohorts from the Framingham Heart Study, Puurunen et al. examined the incidence of VTE over 2 decades. In a multivariable model, the hazard ratio (HR) per 10-year increase in age was 1.69 (95% confidence interval [CI], 1.48–1.92).[9] The Iowa Women's Health Study prospectively followed up >40,000 women; using International Classification of Diseases, Ninth Revision, codes as reported in Medicare hospitalization discharge records, they identified 2137 incident VTE events during 19 years of follow-up. Overall, the VTE rate increased from 2.93 per 1000 person-years in patients aged 65–69 years to 5.82 per 1000 person-years in patients aged >85 years.[10] An increased incidence in men compared to women has been demonstrated in some but not all population-based studies.[8] The Framingham Heart Study cohorts demonstrated a higher age-adjusted incidence rate (IR) in men than in women; 23.5 of 10,000 (95% CI, 19.7–27.4) versus 17.5 of 10,000 (95% CI, 14.7–20.4) (P<.05).[9] However, in the Alberta-Venous Thromboembolism (AB-VTE) population-based study and a Norwegian population-based study, the IR was higher in women than in men.[3,7]

Age has also been demonstrated to increase the risk for VTE recurrence. Lauber et al. followed up 991 patients older than 65 years and demonstrated a cumulative incidence of recurrence of 14.8% at 3 years.[11] The Prolong study enrolled patients from 30 centers in

TABLE 14.1
Biomarkers for Venous Thromboembolism

CLINICAL BIOMARKERS

1. Age
   a. increased risk across advancing decades
   b. increased risk for recurrent VTE

2. Height
   a. increased risk for first VTE
   b. increased risk for recurrent VTE

3. Body mass index (BMI)
   a. increased risk for first VTE
   b. unclear impact on recurrent VTE
   c. lower BMI associated with increased bleeding risk
   d. lower BMI associated with increased risk for mortality

4. Gender
   a. possible increased risk for first VTE in men
   b. increased risk for recurrent VTE in men

LABORATORY BIOMARKERS

1. D-Dimer
   a. normal D-dimer or age-adjusted D-dimer can exclude the need for additional imaging
   b. used to determine feasibility of withholding anti-coagulation after completion of therapy

2. Soluble P-selectin
   a. Investigative biomarker for the diagnosis of venous thromboembolism

3. Non–O blood group
   a. associated with venous thromboembolism
   b. increased risk for recurrent venous thromboembolism

4. troponin T (TnT) and hs-TnT
   a. when elevated, associated with short-term mortality and mortality from pulmonary embolism

5. Brain natriuretic peptide (BNP) and NT-pro-BNP
   a. when elevated, associated with short-term mortality and mortality from pulmonary embolism and adverse events

Italy. The Prolong extension study reported outcomes for 608 patients. The HR for recurrence for age >65 years compared with that for <65 years was 2.3 (95% CI, 1.4–3.8; P = .001). For each 10-year increase in age, there was an increase in risk for recurrence off anticoagulation; adjusted HR for recurrence was 1.021 (95% CI, 1.002–1.039; P = .033).[12] In another population-based study, Spencer et al., in addition to finding a lower 3-year recurrence rate (9.5%), did not identify

a similar increased risk with advancing age.[13] The absolute mechanisms responsible for increased VTE risk with advancing age are unknown, but speculation surrounds the attributable, associated clinical risks. As the population ages there are increasing trends toward obesity, surgery, hospitalizations, and medical illness including cancer. Although this would account for the increased risk of provoked VTE, contributors associated with seemingly idiopathic events remain unknown.

Height is a risk factor for VTE as well as for recurrent VTE. From 1999 to 2004, the Multiple Environmental and Genetic Assessment (MEGA) case-control study enrolled patients with a history of VTE and followed them up for an average 5 years. In 4464 patients compared with 5803 controls, men with a height >200 cm had a 3.8-fold increased risk for VTE compared with men 166–170 cm tall. In women a more modest association was identified with a 1.5-fold increased risk (95% CI, 0.7–3.4) for women of height >185 cm compared with women 166–170 cm tall.[14] The Iowa Women's Health Study using self-reported biophysical data found that women with a height >66 in. demonstrated an adjusted HR of 1.86 (95% CI, 1.54–2.16) compared with women of height <62 in.[10] In a Norwegian population study of >26,000 individuals, the age-adjusted HR per 10-cm height was 1.34 (95% CI, 1.09–1.64). Men of height >181 cm had an HR of 1.99 (95% CI, 1.36–2.93) compared with men of height <173 cm. However, the impact of height in women with VTE was not confirmed (HR, 1.06; 95% CI, 0.86–1.31). These trends for both men and women held true for both provoked and unprovoked VTE.[15] Independent of height, longer leg length has also been shown to increase VTE risk.[16]

The case-controlled MEGA trial also demonstrated an increased risk for recurrent VTE in men with a height >200 cm, with the HR for recurrent VTE being 3.7 (95% CI, 1.4–10.0), compared with men 166–170 cm tall. For women with a height of 186–190 cm, the HR for recurrence was 3.0 (95% CI, 0.9–9.4) compared with women whose height was 166–170 cm.[14] In women older than 65 years, the Iowa Women's Health Study documented an HR of 1.76 (95% CI, 1.16–2.68) for women of height >66 in. compared with women of height <62 in.[17] Although the association seems fairly consistent, the mechanism underlying the increased risk related to height remains unknown. It has been suggested that height has been attributed to increased hydrostatic pressure, increased number of venous valves, and even increased surface area of the veins.

The impact of height combined with other VTE biomarker risks is variable. The Tromsø study is a Norwegian population study including >26,000 Norwegian individuals, in which investigators did not identify an interaction between height and factor V Leiden, prothrombin G21210A, and non–O blood group alleles.[18] The Longitudinal Investigation of Thromboembolism Etiology (LITE) study identified an increased risk with height; the adjusted relative risk (RR) for the tallest individuals in the fourth quartile was 1.5 (95% CI, 1.1–1.9). However, no interaction between height and hemostasis or inflammation was noted.[19] Several studies have demonstrated a synergistic effect between obesity and height relative to increasing risk for VTE including the Tromsø study. Investigators demonstrated a fivefold increased risk for tall, obese men compared with men with a normal weight and short stature. Tall, obese women had a nearly threefold increased risk compared with normal-weight, short-statured women.[20]

Obesity has been identified as a risk for VTE. Many models of DVT prophylaxis risk stratification and recurrent VTE risk assessment include some measure of obesity. In 2002 the LITE investigators using cohorts from the Cardiovascular Health Study (CHS) and ARIC study identified body mass index (BMI) as a VTE risk factor. After adjusting for age, gender, and race, a BMI > 30 kg/m^2 had an HR of 2.27 (95% CI, 1.57–3.28) compared with a BMI < 25 kg/m^2. BMI demonstrated an increasing risk for VTE, BMI of <25 kg/m^2, 25 to <30 kg/m^2, 30 to <35 kg/m^2, 35 to <40 kg/m^2, and >40 kg/m^2 were associated with an HR of 1.0, 1.47, 2.23, 1.52, and 2.71, respectively (P < .001 for the trend). This association was stronger for idiopathic events than for provoked VTE.[21] Similarly, the Tromsø study investigators demonstrated increased risk based on BMI measurements but also identified waist circumference (WC) as a better predictor for VTE. In women with a WC > 85 cm and in men with WC > 95 cm, a 1.9-fold and 2.8-fold increased risk for VTE, respectively, was observed.[22] VTE is uncommon in children; however, in one study, obese adolescents (BMI > 95th percentile) were more likely to develop VTE while admitted than normal-weight adolescents (BMI < 85th percentile), odds ratio (OR) 2.1 (95% CI, 1.1–4.2).[23]

Along with weight and BMI, other anthropometric measurements of body composition have been associated with VTE. After adjusting for age, race, and gender, the LITE study demonstrated increased RR across quartiles for weight, BMI, WC, hip circumference, and waist-hip ratio.[19] In similar fashion a Danish population-based study of >54,000 individuals also demonstrated a positive association of weight, BMI, waist and hip circumference, and body fat mass with VTE in both men and women with increased risk across quartiles for all measurements.[24]

The association of BMI with recurrent VTE has generated mixed results. In one study of nearly 1000 elderly patients aged >65 years with a history of VTE, BMI was not associated with recurrent VTE. As expected in an elderly population, recurrence rates were high; at 3 years, recurrence for patients with BMI < 25 kg/m^2 was 17.6%, 11.5% for BMI 25 to <30 kg/m^2, and 16.9% for BMI > 30 kg/m^2 (P = .09).[25] Other investigators have also failed to identify an association between BMI and recurrent VTE. In a Dutch population, after adjusting for age and gender, patients who were overweight (BMI 25–30 kg/m^2) had an HR for recurrence of 1.05 (95% CI, 0.88–1.27), and patients who were obese (BMI > 30 kg/m^2) had an HR of 0.94 (95% CI, 0.74–1.19) compared with the normal-weight patients (BMI < 25 kg/m^2).[26] With obesity increasing in the population and approaching a health crisis, it is unclear whether this has or will impact VTE rates. The effect of obesity on risk should be reflected in preventive strategies, and the influence of obesity on duration of therapy should be weighed against the risk of persistent anticoagulation.

As previously stated, gender is not truly a biomarker, but it is a binary variable, and there is considerable data suggesting a difference in VTE between men and women. The incident risk for VTE in men and women has been somewhat variable in different trials.[3,7-9] In most trials, however, men demonstrate a higher risk for recurrent VTE than women. In 2004 Kyrle et al. published follow-up data on 826 patients with a first VTE event. Overall, 102 of 826 (12%) developed recurrent thromboembolism. Recurrent events occurred in 20% (74/373) of men and 6% (28/453) of women (P < .001). The RR for recurrence was 3.6 for men compared with that for women.[27] In the Prolong extension study, the recurrence rate was higher in men than in women with an unadjusted HR of 1.7 (95% CI, 1.1–2.7; P = .027).[12] A meta-analysis published in 2011 included 2554 patients with a first episode of VTE. There were 193 recurrences in men during 30,046 years of follow-up and 97 recurrences in 33,182 years of follow-up in women. In patients with unprovoked VTE, men had a 2.2-fold higher risk of recurrence than women.[28] Not all studies have confirmed the increased risk for recurrence in men; the Worcester VTE Study evaluated multiple clinical variables and did not identify male gender as a short- or long-term risk for recurrence.[29]

Many practitioners focus on laboratory biomarkers to determine length of anticoagulation and risk for recurrence. However, the clinical risk related to age, gender, and obesity should not be overlooked. Indeed, all of the validated VTE recurrent risk-prediction tools, HERDOO2, DASH, and the Vienna prediction model, include one or more of these variables as part of the tool to help determine recurrence risk (Fig. 14.1A).[30-32]

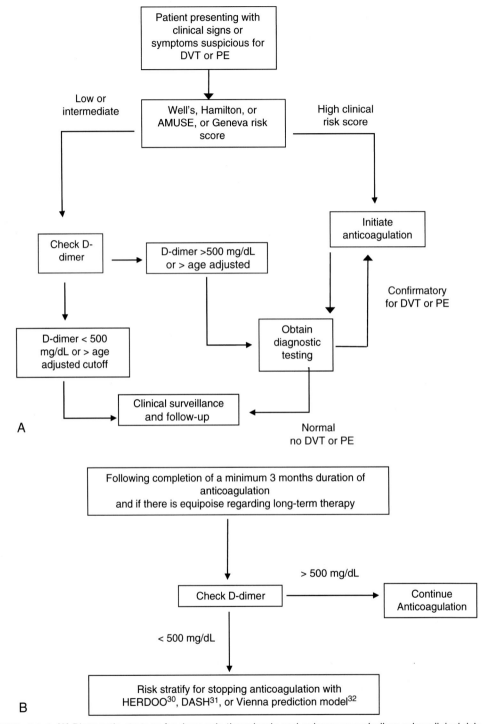

FIG. 14.1 **(A)** Diagnostic strategy for deep vein thrombosis and pulmonary embolism using clinical risk stratification and D-dimer biomarker testing. **(B)** Use of D-dimer and clinical risk strategies to determine if withholding anticoagulation is clinically feasible before stopping anticoagulation.

LABORATORY BIOMARKERS FOR VTE

D-dimer is a soluble degradation product that is produced during the plasmin-mediated breakdown of cross-linked fibrin. D-dimer is only produced by the formation and subsequent degradation of terminally cross-linked fibrin. Therefore it serves as an indirect marker of thrombosis acknowledging the activation of both the coagulation and fibrinolytic systems.[33] There are three different types of D-dimer assays in use: (1) whole blood agglutination, (2) enzyme-linked immunosorbent assays or enzyme-linked immunofluorescent assays, and (3) latex agglutination assays. There is a significant variability between assays and results that are not comparable between assays.[34,35] Therefore understanding the performance, cut-points, and limitations of the assay(s) in use within an individual institution is imperative.[33]

Baseline elevated D-dimer levels are associated with an increased risk of thrombosis. Data from the population-based ARIC study demonstrated that the incidence of VTE increased as the baseline concentration of D-dimer increased across quintiles. At the lowest quintile the IR was 1.7 per 1000 person-years, and at the highest quintile, the IR was 5.2 per 1000 person-years. The adjusted HR for VTE in the highest quintile of D-dimer was 3.2 compared with the lowest quintile.[36] The limiting clinical issue with D-dimer remains that levels are increased in thrombosis but also in other clinical conditions. D-dimer increases with age, surgery or trauma, pregnancy and peripartum, cancer, disseminated intravascular coagulation, infection or sepsis, and in other inflammatory disorders. Therefore D-dimer lacks specificity for VTE. Thus D-dimer cannot be used as a diagnostic assay, and its use is limited to VTE exclusion.

Clinical signs and symptoms for DVT and PE are neither sensitive nor specific. The Hamilton score, Amsterdam Maastricht Utrecht Study on Thromboembolism (AMUSE) score, and the Well's score can be used to calculate a clinical pretest probability for DVT, whereas the Well's rule and Geneva score are used for PE.[37–41] D-Dimer is part of the AMUSE score, and when used along with the other risk scores as part of a risk stratification process, it can safely identify low-risk patients in whom DVT and PE can be excluded without the need for additional radiologic imaging.[42–44] The American College of Chest Physician guidelines recommend using a strategy of clinical classification and pretest risk assessment, followed by D-dimer assessment to determine whether additional radiologic testing is warranted in low-risk to intermediate-risk patients with suspected DVT.[45] In patients with a low clinical pretest probability for DVT or PE, a normal D-dimer safely excludes VTE. A recent meta-analysis including 4 trials that investigated the use of the Well's criteria and D-dimer in patients with suspected PE demonstrated the pooled incidence of PE to be 0.34%, negative predictive value (NPV) 99.7% (95% CI, 99%–99.9%).[46] It is important to note that the false-negative rate of D-dimer for VTE is variable based on the assay used. Therefore, high-risk patients are appropriate for imaging regardless of the D-dimer result.

The typical cutoff for D-dimer in trials has been <500 µg/L. Use of an age-adjusted D-dimer (age × 10 µg/L) in patients aged >50 years has been proposed to increase specificity of testing. In a cohort of >1300 consecutive patients, Schouten et al. investigated 2 different strategies for using D-dimer in older patients. They evaluated the age-adjusted D-dimer strategy in patients older than 50 years (age × 10 µg/L) as well as a cutoff of 750 µg/L in patients aged >60 years.[47] Of 647 patients with a low clinical prediction score, 272 (42%) had a D-dimer < 500 µg/L, excluding DVT without the need for further testing. Using the age-adjusted D-dimer, they were able to exclude VTE in 309 patients; therefore, an additional 5.7% of patients were excluded. Using the fixed D-dimer cutoff of <750 µg/L in patients aged >60 years, DVT was excluded in 307 patients, an additional 5.4% of patients. In patients over the age of 80 years, age-adjusted D-Dimer excluded 35.5% of patients compared with 21% using the D-dimer cutoff of <500 µg/L.[47] The Age-Adjusted D-Dimer Cutoff Levels to Rule Out Pulmonary Embolism (ADJUST-PE) trial was a multicentered European trial evaluating more than 3000 patients presenting to the emergency department with suspected PE. D-dimer <500 µg/L excluded PE in 887 patients. An additional 337 patients had a D-dimer >500 µg/L but less than their calculated age-adjusted D-dimer cutoff. In these patients, only one patient was diagnosed with PE during a 3-month follow-up.[48] Most importantly, using an age-adjusted D-dimer strategy in patients over the age of 75 years increased the number of patients in whom PE could be excluded from 6.4% to 29.7% avoiding additional imaging in 157 patients without affecting the testing sensitivity.[48] A recent meta-analysis included 5 studies with 13 cohorts and approximately 12,500.[49] Overall, the use of the age-adjusted D-dimer improved specificity of the test at all age groups >50 years with a nonsignificant decrease in sensitivity which remained >97%.[49]

D-dimer may be used to help determine the duration of anticoagulation in some patients (Figure 14.1B). Especially for patients with nonprovoked VTE, determining the duration of therapy may be particularly challenging. Current guidelines suggest that in patients with low or moderate bleeding risk, extended duration of therapy may be appropriate.[50] However, this is not always acceptable to patients.

Palereti et al. examined 619 patients with idiopathic VTE who had completed a minimum of 3 months of anticoagulation. Thirty days after stopping anticoagulation, 227 patients had an abnormal D-dimer, 105 were assigned to resume anticoagulation, and 122 continued in follow-up without anticoagulation. Overall, 24 of 385 (6.2%) patients with a normal D-dimer remaining off anticoagulation had a recurrent event compared with 18 of 120 (15%) patients with a positive D-dimer remaining off anticoagulation. Only 2 of 103 (2%) with a positive D-dimer on anticoagulation had recurrence. Recurrence was significantly higher for patients with an abnormal D-dimer who remained off anticoagulation in whom the adjusted HR was 4.26 (P = .02) and 2.27 (P = .02) for comparisons with patients with an elevated D-dimer resuming anticoagulation and patients with a normal D-dimer remaining off anticoagulation, respectively.[51] The PROLONG II study examined the use of serial D-dimer measurements over a year after cessation of anticoagulation in patients with idiopathic VTE who completed 6 months of anticoagulation therapy.[52] Patients were followed up for up to 13 months after completing therapy, and D-dimer was tested every 2 months throughout follow-up. A total of 336 patients had a normal D-dimer at baseline, and anticoagulation was stopped. At the 30-day follow-up, 85 patients had a positive D-dimer, and anticoagulation was resumed. The remaining 243 patients were followed off anticoagulation. In patients with a normal D-dimer at 90 days and in whom the D-dimer remained normal or was abnormal only once during follow-up, the incidence of recurrent VTE at 13 months was 4.6% compared with 22.6% in patients with an abnormal D-dimer at T90 (P = .003).[52] It is important to note that in this population is stable, but a significant rate of 10%–15% of patients had a positive D-dimer at each visit throughout the follow-up period.[52]

Patients at high risk for VTE still require imaging. However, the use of D-dimer to exclude VTE in low-risk patients has been well popularized and should be part of most emergency department and outpatient risk-prediction strategies. Similar to other clinical biomarkers, a positive D-dimer is considered in the validated tools available to help predict risk of recurrence.[30–32] Positive D-dimer at the completion of the intended duration of therapy should encourage the practitioner to extend therapy given the risk of recurrence. Serial D-dimer measurements after stopping anticoagulation may be favored if there would be consideration given to reinitiating therapy or changing ongoing secondary prophylaxis strategies. Although D-dimer is commonly measured in most laboratories, the assays are

not interchangeable, and knowledge of the local assays is important when using them in VTE strategies.

P-selectin is a cell surface adhesion molecule stored in the α-granules of platelets and in the Weibel-Palade bodies of endothelial cells. The protein is functionally active in both its membrane-bound form and when released into plasma, the soluble form (sP-selectin). P-selectin glycoprotein ligand-1 (PSGL-1) is predominantly found on leukocytes. The interaction between endothelial and platelet P-selectin and leukocyte PSGL-1 has been shown to facilitate leukocyte recruitment and adhesion to the endothelium and platelets occurring at the site of thrombosis and vascular injury. Both sP-selectin and membrane-bound P-selectin induce tissue factor expression on monocytes and presumably contribute to the production of tissue factor–bearing monocyte-derived microparticles (TF-MMPs). In turn these TF-MMPs bind to P-selectin on platelets contributing in a positive fashion to further thrombus growth.[53] P-selectin has a role as a biomarker for VTE, and inhibition of P-selectin may be exploited as a therapeutic option.

Ramacciotti et al. investigated P-selectin along with other biomarkers of VTE in 62 patients with confirmed DVT, 116 patients with leg pain but no DVT on imaging, and 30 healthy controls.[54] Well's criteria[43] was recorded for all patients enrolled. Soluble P-selectin was higher in patients with DVT than in patients without, 87.3 ± 44 ng/mL versus 53.4 ± 24 ng/mL, respectively (P < .0001). Using a cut-point of 90 ng/mL, P-selectin demonstrated a sensitivity of 28% and specificity of 96% for diagnosing DVT. When the same cut-point was combined with the Well's score > 2, the sensitivity and specificity was 33% and 95%, respectively, for the diagnosis of DVT. The positive predictive value (PPV) was 100%. Importantly when a cut-point of 60 ng/mL and Well's score < 2 was used, these criteria could exclude DVT with a sensitivity of 99%, specificity of 33%, and negative predictive value 96%.[54] An additional study carried out within the same institution demonstrated different results. Two hundred thirty-four patients were included in the lower extremity DVT (LE-DVT) group, and 45 patients were included in the upper extremity DVT (UE-DVT) group. Compression ultrasound was positive for DVT in 112 of 234 patients in the LE-DVT group and 32 of 45 patients in the UE-DVT group. In patients with documented LE-DVT, P-selectin was higher than that in patients without DVT (77.2 ng/mL [95% CI, 70.7–83.8] versus 54.5 ng/mL [95% CI, 49.9–59.2] [P < .001]). Using the predetermined cutoff of 90 ng/mL and Well's score > 2, this study demonstrated a specificity of 97.5% and a PPV of 91% for the diagnosis of DVT. Using a sP-selectin < 60 ng/mL and Well's score < 2, the sensitivity was 91%, and

NPV was 79%. Traditional use of D-dimer < 0.5 mg/L and Well's score < 2 performed better with an NPV of 95%. There was no difference in sP-selectin between patients with UE-DVT and patients without, 59.2 ng/mL (95% CI, 49.2–69.1) versus 50.0 ng/mL (95% CI, 34.3–65.7), respectively, (*P*=.3). The role of sP-selectin in UE-DVT therefore remains uncertain.[55] sP-selectin is also increased in patients with acute coronary syndrome. This would further limit its use in evaluating patients with suspected PE. In addition, there is no rapid assessment or point-of-care test for sP-selectin. So, although sP-selectin may improve diagnostic testing strategies and further eliminate unnecessary testing, widespread use is unlikely.

Non–O blood group (A, AB, and B) is another commonly available laboratory biomarker for VTE. In a Scandinavian population of over 1,000,000 blood donors with 13.6 million person-years of follow-up non–O blood group donors demonstrated a higher incidence of both arterial and venous thromboembolic events. Compared with type O blood group, the incidence rate ratio (IRR) for DVT was 1.92 (95% CI, 1.8–2.05), 1.75 for PE (95% CI, 1.64–1.86), and 2.22 for pregnancy-related events (95% CI, 1.76–2.78). In people with VTE, IRR decreased with age, and IRR was generally higher in men than in women.[56] This incident risk as well as a risk for recurrence has been confirmed in multiple trials.[57-60] In addition, several studies have confirmed excess VTE risk when non–ABO blood groups are associated with concomitant risk factors such as thrombophilia or hormone therapy.[57,59,61] The VTE risk associated with non–O blood groups likely explains some of the apparently idiopathic VTE. The actual impact relative to most at-risk groups is unknown. Whether screening for non–O blood groups is warranted in high-risk patients or assists with decisions regarding extended VTE prophylaxis has yet to be determined.

BIOMARKERS FOR VTE RISK STRATIFICATION

Biomarkers may also be used to help risk stratify patients with respect to outcomes in VTE. As noted previously, biomarkers are differentiated from clinical predictors of outcomes. Clinical predictors for worse outcomes include massive PE at presentation, cancer, and ongoing immobilization with neurologic disease.[62]

Clinical Biomarkers

The Registro Informatizado de la Enfermedad Trombo-Embólica registry prospectively enrolled patients with VTE from 94 international centers. The investigators published a short-term analysis of 8845 patients to determine whether weight impacted the acute management phase of VTE. Overall, patients with a weight <50 kg had increased risk for bleeding (OR, 2.2) compared with patients weighing 50–100 kg. Clinical outcomes with respect to bleeding and recurrent VTE were similar in patients with a weight >100 kg compared with patients weighing 50–100 kg.[63] The same investigators studied the relationship between BMI and mortality and suggested BMI may be inversely related to mortality in VTE.[64] A study including >10,000 patients demonstrated increased mortality rates in underweight patients compared with that in normal-weight patients and lower mortality in overweight and obese patients. When survival was adjusted for age, DVT or PE presentation, cancer, renal dysfunction, and idiopathic VTE, the RR for death was 2.1 (95% CI, 1.5–2.7) in patient with $BMI < 18.5 \text{ kg/m}^2$ compared with that in the reference group ($18.5–24.9 \text{ kg/m}^2$). In obese patients, $BMI > 30 \text{ kg/m}^2$, overall mortality was 4.2% compared with 12% in the reference group (RR, 0.5; 95% CI, 0.4–0.6). Notably, fatal PE was also lower in obese and overweight patients with OR 0.4 and 0.6, respectively.[64]

Risk stratification in PE plays a key role in management. Patient presenting with hypotension or overt shock are considered massive or high-risk patients. They are at significant risk for poor clinical outcomes and in whom thrombolysis may be considered. In normotensive patients with confirmed PE, most authors recommend using the pulmonary embolism severity index (PESI) or the simplified PESI (sPESI) for initial risk stratification to determine which patient are at low or intermediate risk for a poor outcome.[65] For low-risk patients, early discharge or outpatient therapy may be appropriate. By further risk stratifying intermediate-risk patients using echocardiography and laboratory biomarkers including cardiac troponin I (cTnI), cardiac troponin T (cTnT), brain natriuretic peptide (BNP), and N-terminal-pro-BNP (NT-pro-BNP), we can secure insight into which patients are at increased risk for in-hospital decompensation or mortality. In addition, one can be alerted to patients at risk for decompensation and in whom endovascular or reperfusion therapy may be warranted.[65-67]

In one meta-analysis, elevated troponin (either cTnT or cTnI) was associated with short-term mortality (OR, 5.24) as well as death from PE (OR, 9.44).[68] The high-sensitivity troponin T (hs-TnT) assay has also been shown to have good prognostic sensitivity as well as high negative predictive value. Lankeit et al. examined the use of hs-TnT in 526 normotensive PE patients. In 127 patients with a sPESI of 0 and hs-TnT < 14 pg/mL, none had identified adverse events at 30 days.

In 241 patients with sPESI > 1 and hs-TnT > 14 pg/mL, 10.4% had adverse events at 30 days, mortality was 9.5%, and 6-month mortality was 15.8% (P < .001). Overall sensitivity was 100% and specificity was 26% for the combination of sPESI > 1 and hs-TnT > 14 pg/mL.[69] In addition to VTE risk stratification, hs-TNT has been associated with increased VTE risk. Using stored samples from the ARIC and CHS cohorts, the LITE investigators demonstrated that elevated hs-TNT was associated with increased incidence of VTE over an 8- to 10-year follow-up. Based on a pooled analysis, participants with hs-TNT in the highest quintile (hs-TNT > 13 ng/L) had an HR of 1.98 (95% CI, 1.36–2.87) compared with patients with hs-TNT < 3 ng/L. Interestingly, the risk was greater for provoked VTE (HR, 2.27; 95% CI, 1.43–3.59) but not for unprovoked VTE (HR, 0.84; 95% CI, 0.38–1.82).[70]

Both BNP and NT-pro-BNP have been shown to be elevated in many different clinical conditions including right and left ventricular dysfunction, renal disease, chronic pulmonary disease, and advancing age. BNP is released in response to myocardial stretch. Right ventricular (RV) dysfunction is known to contribute to the morbidity and mortality associated with PE. Although NT-pro-BNP is typically associated with left ventricular dysfunction and heart failure, Pasha et al. demonstrated the association between NT-pro-BNP and computed tomography (CT)-measured decrease in RV ejection fraction, as well as higher RV end-diastolic volume.[71] No correlation was found for left ventricular ejection fraction or end-diastolic volume. It has been demonstrated by several meta-analyses that increased BNP or NT-pro-BNP is associated with increased risk of all-cause mortality, PE-related mortality, as well as serious adverse events.[72,73]

Although associated with mortality and adverse outcomes, both BNP and NT-pro-BNP have a low PPV in PE. However, the NPV is high, and patients with a normal BNP or NT-pro-BNP are at low risk for adverse events.[65] In general, both troponin and BNP demonstrate a high negative predictive value for adverse outcomes in PE patients, and when normal, patients may be considered low risk and early discharge or outpatient PE management may be an option.

CONCLUSION

VTE is a relatively common clinical condition. Clinical and laboratory biomarkers have been demonstrated to play a role in identifying patients at risk for VTE, for predicting recurrence of VTE, and predicting risk of adverse outcomes associated with VTE and anticoagulation therapy. The 2008 Surgeon General's call to action

challenged the medical community to find better ways to prevent and reduce the risk of VTE.[5] Using the available therapies and validated risk-stratification tools along with appropriate biomarkers, we should begin to be able to make an impact on this task.

REFERENCES

1. Strimbu K, Tavel JA. What are biomarkers? *Curr Opin HIV AIDS*. 2010;5(6):463–466.
2. Kumar DR, Hanlin E, Glurich I, et al. Virchow's contribution to the understanding of thrombosis and cellular biology. *Clin Med Res*. 2010;8(3–4):168–172.
3. Alotaibi GS, Wu C, Senthilselvan A, McMurtry MS. Secular trends in incidence and mortality of acute venous thromboembolism: the AB-VTE population-based study. *Am J Med*. 2016;129(8):879.e19–e25.
4. Bell EJ, Lutsey PL, Basu S, et al. Lifetime risk of venous thromboembolism in two cohort studies. *Am J Med*. 2016;126:339.e19–e26.
5. Office of the Surgeon General (US). *National Heart, Lung, and Blood Institute (US). The Surgeon General's Call to Action to Prevent Deep Vein Thrombosis and Pulmonary Embolism*. Rockville (MD): Office of the Surgeon General (US); 2008. Available from: https://www.ncbi.nlm.nih.gov/books/NBK44178/.
6. Huang W, Goldberg RJ, Anderson FA, et al. Secular trends in occurrence of acute venous thromboembolism: the Worcester venous thromboembolism study (1985–2009). *Am J Med*. 2014;127(9):829–839.
7. Næss IA, Christiansen SC, Romundstad P, et al. Incidence and mortality of venous thrombosis; a population-based study. *J Thromb Haemost*. 2007;5:692–699.
8. Heit JA, Spencer FA, White RH. The epidemiology of venous thromboembolism. *J Thromb Thrombolysis*. 2016; 41:3–14.
9. Puurunen MK, Gona P, Larson MG, et al. Epidemiology of venous thromboembolism in the Framingham heart study. *Thromb Res*. 2016;145:27–33.
10. Lutsey PL, Virnig BA, Durham SB, et al. Correlates and consequences of venous thromboembolism: the Iowa Women's Health Study. *Am J Public Health*. 2010;100:1506–1513.
11. Lauber S, Limacher A, Tritschler T, et al. Predictors and outcomes of recurrent venous thromboembolism in elderly patients. *Am J Med*. 2018;131:703.e7–e16.
12. Cosmi B, Legnani C, Tosetto A, et al. Sex, age, and normal post-anticoagulation D-dimer as risk factors for recurrence after idiopathic venous thromboembolism in the Prolong study extension. *J Thromb Haemost*. 2010;8:1933–1942.
13. Spencer FA, Gurwitz JH, Schulman S, et al. Venous thromboembolism in older adults: a community-based study. *Am J Med*. 2014;127:530–537.
14. Flinterman LE, van Hylckama Vlieg A, Rosendaal FR, et al. Body height, mobility, and risk of first and recurrent venous thromboembolism. *J Thromb Haemost*. 2015;13:548–554.

15. Brækkan SK, Borch KH, Mathiesen EB, et al. Body height and risk of venous thromboembolism. The Tromsø Study. *Am J Epidemiol.* 2010;171:1109–1115.

16. Lutsey PL, Cushman M, Heckbert SR, et al. Longer legs are associated with greater risk of incident venous thromboembolism independent of total body height: the Longitudinal Investigation of Thromboembolism Etiology (LITE). *Thromb Haemost.* 2011;106:113–120.

17. Lutsey PL, Folsom AR. Taller women are at greater risk of recurrent venous thromboembolism: the Iowa Women's Health Study. *Am J Hematol.* 2012;87:716–717.

18. Horvei LD, Brækkan SK, Smith EN, et al. Joint effects of prothrombotic genotypes and body height on the risk of venous thromboembolism: the Tromsø study. *J Thromb Haemost.* 2017;16:83–89.

19. Cushman M, O'Meara ES, Heckbert SR, et al. Body size measures, hemostatic and inflammatory markers and risk of venous thrombosis: the longitudinal investigation of thromboembolism etiology. *Thromb Res.* 2016;144: 127–132.

20. Borcht KH, Nyegaard C, Hansen JB, et al. Joint effects of obesity and body height on the risk of venous thromboembolism: the Tromsø Study. *Arterioscler Thromb Vasc Biol.* 2011;31:1439–1444.

21. Tsai AW, Cushman M, Rosamond WD, et al. Cardiovascular risk factors and venous thromboembolism. *Arch Intern Med.* 2002;162:1182–1189.

22. Borch KH, Brækkan SK, Mathiesen EB, et al. Anthropometric measures of obesity and risk of venous thromboembolism. The Tromsø Study. *Arterioscler Thromb Vasc Biol.* 2010;30:121–127.

23. Stokes S, Breheny P, Radulescu A, Radulescu VC. Impact of obesity on the risk of venous thromboembolism in an inpatient pediatric population. *Pediatr Hematol Oncol.* 2014;31(5):475–480.

24. Severinsen MT, Kristensen SR, Johnsen SP, et al. Anthropometry, bodyfat, and venous thromboembolism. A Danish follow-up study. *Circulation.* 2009;120:1850–1857.

25. Mueller C, Limacher A, Méan M, et al. Obesity is not associated with recurrent venous thromboembolism in elderly patients: results from the prospective SWITCO65+ cohort study. *PLoS One.* 2017;12(9):e0184868.

26. Vučković BA, Cannegieter SC, van Hylckama Vlieg A, et al. Recurrent venous thromboembolism related to overweight and obesity results from the MEGA follow-up study. *J Thromb Haemost.* 2017;15:1430–1435.

27. Kyrle PA, Minar E, Bialonczyk C, et al. The risk of recurrent venous thromboembolism in men and women. *N Engl J Med.* 2004;350:2558–2563.

28. Douketis J, Tosetto A, Marcucci M, et al. Risk of recurrence after venous thromboembolism in men and women: a patient level meta-analysis. *BMJ.* 2011;342:d813.

29. Huang W, Goldberg RJ, Anderson FA, et al. Occurrence and predictors of recurrence after a first episode of acute venous thromboembolism: population-based Worcester Venous Thromboembolism Study. *J Thromb Thrombolysis.* 2016;41:525–538.

30. Rodger MA, Kahn SR, Wells PS, et al. Identifying unprovoked thromboembolism patients at low risk for recurrence who can discontinue anticoagulant therapy. *CMAJ.* 2008;179(5):417–426.

31. Tosetto A, Iorio A, Marcucci M, et al. Predicting disease recurrence in patients with previous unprovoked venous thromboembolism: a proposed prediction score (DASH). *J Thromb Haemost.* 2012;10:1019–1025.

32. Eichinger S, Heinze G, Jandeck LM, et al. Risk assessment of recurrence in patients with unprovoked deep vein thrombosis or pulmonary embolism: the Vienna prediction model. *Circulation.* 2010;121:1630–1636.

33. Weitz JI, Fredenburgh JC, Eikelboom JW. A test in context: D-dimer. *J Am Coll Cardiol.* 2017;70:2411–2420.

34. DiNisio M, Squizzato A, Rutjes AW, et al. Diagnostic accuracy of D-dimer test for exclusion of venous thromboembolism: a systematic review. *J Thromb Haemost.* 2007;5:296–304.

35. Stein PD, Hull RD, Patel KC, et al. D-dimer for the exclusion of acute venous thrombosis and pulmonary embolism: a systematic review. *Ann Intern Med.* 2004;140:589–602.

36. Folsom AR, Alonso A, George KM, et al. Prospective study of plasma D-dimer and incident venous thromboembolism: the Atherosclerosis Risk in Communities (ARIC) Study. *Thromb Res.* 2015;136:781–785.

37. Büller HR, Ten Cate-Hoek AJ, Hoes AW, et al. Safely ruling out deep venous thrombosis in primary care. *Ann Intern Med.* 2009;150:229–235.

38. Wells PS, Anderson DR, Bormanis J, et al. Value of assessment of pretest probability of deep-vein thrombosis in clinical judgement. *Lancet.* 1997;350:1795–1798.

39. Subramaniam RM, Chou T, Heath R, Allen R. Importance of pretest probability score and D-dimer assay before sonography for lower limb deep venous thrombosis. *AJR Am J Roentgenol.* 2006;186:206–212.

40. Gibson NS, Sohne M, Kruip MJ, et al. Further validation and simplification of the Wells clinical decisions rule in pulmonary embolism. *Thromb Haemost.* 2008;99:229–234.

41. Le Gal G, Righini M, Roy PM, et al. Prediction of pulmonary embolism in the emergency department: the revised Geneva Score. *Ann Intern Med.* 2006;144:165–171.

42. Anderson DR, Kovacs MJ, Kovacs G, et al. Combined use of the clinical assessment and D-dimer to improve the management of patients presenting to the emergency department with suspected deep vein thrombosis (the EDITED Study). *J Thromb Haemost.* 2003;1:645–651.

43. Wells PS, Anderson DR, Rodger M, et al. Evaluation of D-dimer in the diagnosis of suspected deep vein thrombosis. *N Engl J Med.* 2003;349:1227–1235.

44. Crawford F, Andreas A, Welch K, et al. D-dimer test for excluding the diagnosis of pulmonary embolism. *Cochrane Database Syst Rev.* 2016;(8):CD010864.

45. Bates SM, Jaeschke R, Stevens SM, et al. Diagnosis of DVT. Antithrombotic therapy and prevention of thrombosis, 9th ed: American College of chest physicians evidence-based clinical practice guidelines. *Chest.* 2012;141(suppl 2): e315S–e418S.

46. Pasha SM, Klok FA, Snoep JD, et al. Safety of excluding acute pulmonary embolism based on an unlikely clinical probability by the Well's rule and normal D-dimer concentration: a meta-analysis. *Thromb Res*. 2010;125:e123–e127.

47. Schouten HJ, Koek HL, Oudega R, et al. Validation of two age dependent D-dimer cut-off values for exclusion of deep vein thrombosis in suspected elderly patients in primary care: retrospective, cross-sectional, diagnostic analysis. *BMJ*. 2012;344:e2985.

48. Righini M, Van Es J, Den Exter PL, et al. Age-adjusted D-dimer cutoff levels to rule out pulmonary embolism: the ADJUST-PE study. *JAMA*. 2014;311:1117–1124.

49. Schouten HJ, Geersing GJ, Koek HL, et al. Diagnostic accuracy of conventional or age adjusted D-dimer cut-off values in older patients with suspected venous thromboembolism: a systematic review and meta-analysis. *BMJ*. 2013;346:f2492.

50. Kearon C, Akl EA, Ornelas J, et al. Antithrombotic therapy for VTE disease: CHEST guidelines and expert panel report. *Chest*. 2016;149:315–352.

51. Palareti G, Cosmi B, Legnani C, et al. D-dimer testing to determine duration of anticoagulation therapy. *N Engl J Med*. 2006;355:1780–1789.

52. Cosmi B, Legnani C, Tosetto A, et al. Usefulness of repeated D-dimer testing after stopping anticoagulation for as first episode of unprovoked venous thromboembolism: the PROLONG II prospective study. *Blood*. 2010;115:481–488.

53. André P. P-selectin in haemostasis. *Br J Haematol*. 2004;126:298–306.

54. Ramacciotti E, Blackburn S, Hawley AE, et al. Evaluation of soluble P-selectin as a marker for the diagnosis of deep venous thrombosis. *Clin Appl Thromb Hemost*. 2011;17:425–431.

55. Vandy FC, Stabler C, Eliassen AM, et al. Soluble P-selectin for the diagnosis of lower extremity deep venous thrombosis. *J Vasc Surg Venous Lymphat Disord*. 2013;1:1117–1125.

56. Vasan SK, Rostgaard K, Majeed A, et al. ABO blood group and risk of thromboembolic and arterial disease. A study of 1.5 million blood donors. *Circulation*. 2016;133:1449–1457.

57. Spiezia L, Campello E, Bon M, et al. ABO blood groups and the risk of venous thrombosis in patients with inherited thrombophilia. *Blood Transfus*. 2013;11:250–253.

58. Wolpin BM, Kabrhel C, Varraso R, et al. Prospective study of ABO blood type and the risk of pulmonary embolism in two large cohort studies. *Thromb Haemost*. 2010;104:962–971.

59. Ohira T, Cushman M, Tsai MY, et al. ABO blood group, other risk factors and incidence of venous thromboembolism: the Longitudinal Investigation of Thromboembolism Etiology (LITE). *J Thromb Haemost*. 2007;5:1455–1461.

60. Gándara E, Kovacs MJ, Kahn SR, et al. Non-OO blood type influences the risk of recurrent venous thromboembolism. A cohort study. *Thromb Haemost*. 2013;110:1172–1179.

61. Canonico M, Olié V, Carcaillon L, et al. Synergism between non-O blood group and oral estrogen in the risk of venous thromboembolism among menopausal women: the ESTHER study. *Thromb Haemost*. 2008;99:246–248.

62. Laporte S, Mismetti P, Décousus H, et al. Clinical predictors for fatal pulmonary embolism in 15 520 patients with venous thromboembolism. Findings from the Registro Informatizade de la Enfermedad TromboEmbolica venosa (RIETE) Registry. *Circulation*. 2008;117:1711–1716.

63. Barba R, Marco J, Martín-Alvarez H, et al. The influence of extreme body weight on clinical outcome of patients with venous thromboembolism: findings from a prospective registry (RIETE). *J Thromb Haemost*. 2005;3:856–862.

64. Barba R, Zapatero A, Losa JE, et al. Body mass index and mortality in patients with acute venous thromboembolism: findings from the RIETE registry. *J Thromb Haemost*. 2008;6:595–600.

65. Giannitsis E, Katus HAS. Biomarkers for clinical decision-making in the management of pulmonary embolism. *Clin Chem*. 2017;63:91–100.

66. Konstantinides SV, Barco S, Lankeit M, Meyer G. Management of pulmonary embolism: an update. *J Am Coll Cardiol*. 2016;67:976–990.

67. Meyer G, Planquette B, Sanchez O. Pulmonary embolism: whom to discharge and whom to thrombolyze? *J Thromb Haemost*. 2015;13(suppl 1):S252–S258.

68. Becattini C, Vedovati MC, Agnelli G, et al. Prognostic value of troponins in acute pulmonary embolism: a meta-analysis. *Circulation*. 2007;116:427–433.

69. Lankeit M, Jiménez D, Kostrubiec M, et al. Predictive value of the high-sensitivity troponin T assay and the simplified pulmonary embolism severity index in hemodynamically stable patients with acute pulmonary embolism. A prospective validation study. *Circulation*. 2011;124:2716–2724.

70. Folsom AR, Lutsey PL, Nambi V, et al. Troponin T, NT-proBNP, and venous thromboembolism: the longitudinal investigation of thromboembolism etiology (LITE). *Vasc Med*. 2014;19:33–41.

71. Pasha SM, Klok FA, van der Bijl N, et al. NT-pro-BNP levels in patients with acute pulmonary embolism are correlated to right but not left ventricular volume and function. *Thromb Haemost*. 2012;108:367–372.

72. Lega JC, Lacasse Y, Lakhal L, Provencher S. Natriuretic peptidews and troponins in pulmonary embolism: a meta-analysis. *Thorax*. 2009;64:869–875.

73. Bajaj A, Rathor P, Sehgal V, et al. Prognostic value of biomarkers in acute non-massive pulmonary embolism: a systematic review and meta-analysis. *Lung*. 2015;193:639–651.

CHAPTER 15

Metabolomics, Proteomics, and Genomics: An Introduction to a Clinician

ZHE WANG, MSC • BING YU, PHD

INTRODUCTION

Cardiovascular disease (CVD) remains to be a major global public-health challenge and the leading cause of mortality globally.[1] A key factor in the fight against CVD is to enhance our understanding of its pathophysiological processes. High-throughput omics technologies have revolutionized CVD research. The omics cascade starts from genomics (e.g., genes), followed by transcriptomics (e.g., RNA transcripts), proteomics (e.g., proteins), and finally the ultimate downstream product, metabolomics (e.g., metabolites) (Fig. 15.1). The advent of omics, including genotyping arrays, proteomics, and metabolomics, alone and in combination, offers unique opportunities to advance the knowledge of molecular mechanisms for CVD and the needs for clinics (Fig. 15.2).

Genomics of CVD studies the impact of DNA variation on CVD and its risk factors. Over the past decades, remarkable progress has been made in identifying and functionally characterizing genetic variants that are associated with multiple CVD conditions.[2,3] Proteomics, which studies systematic profiling of proteins, provides opportunities for unbiased discovery of novel markers to improve disease diagnostic or predictive accuracy. Proteins in the circulatory system mirror an individual's physiology. The recent high-throughput proteomics technology allows rapid identification of clinically relevant biomarkers and has been applied in studies of CVD, aging, and other diseases.[4–9] Metabolomics systematically studies small-molecule metabolites found in biologic samples such as cells, biofluids, tissues, or organisms. These small-molecule metabolites are thought to represent intermediates that profile biological status closely related to phenotypes.[10] Therefore the metabolome may provide a more accurate estimation of a disease status than that provided by genome or proteome, making metabolomics a powerful tool for revealing pathologic or etiologic pathways to complex diseases such as CVD and for monitoring treatment efficacy.

In this chapter, we first summarize the recent advances of genomics on CVD and then focus on various methodological and technological aspects related to proteomics and metabolomic profiling. We also present the integrated omics studies carried out to date on CVD, discussing the potential links that integrate metabolic and genetic studies of some common CVD, including blood pressure/hypertension, coronary heart disease, stroke, and heart failure (HF).

GENOMICS AND CVD

CVD encompasses a range of conditions, including hypertension, coronary heart disease, stroke, and HF, most of which are heritable. Enormous effort has been invested in understanding the relationship between genetic variants responsible for this heritability, including candidate gene, genome-wide association, whole-exome sequencing, and most recent whole-genome sequencing (WGS) approaches.

Candidate gene approach focuses on prespecified genes of interest, such as the causal genes for Mendelian disease. A few Mendelian disease genes have been shown to be associated with CVD,[11–21] including *LDLR* and *APOB* for severe hypercholesterolemia[12,13]; *PCSK9* for familial hypobetalipoproteinemia;[14] and *TNNT2* for hypertrophic cardiomyopathy.[20]

In contrast to candidate gene approach, genome-wide association study (GWAS) scans the entire genome for common single nucleotide polymorphisms (SNPs). SNP is a genetic variation in a single nucleotide which occurs at a specific position in the genome. In most GWASs, bi-allelic SNPs (i.e., two alleles) at appreciable degree within a population are analyzed (e.g., minor

Biomarkers in Cardiovascular Disease. https://doi.org/10.1016/B978-0-323-54835-9.00015-6

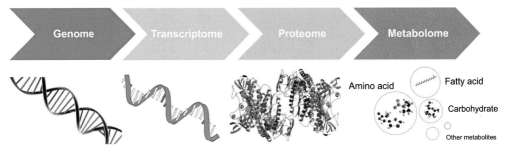

FIG. 15.1 The omics cascade

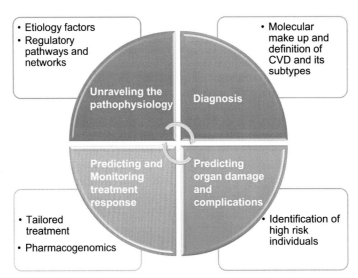

FIG. 15.2 Applications of omics technologies in cardiovascular disease research and clinical needs. *CVD*, cardiovascular disease.

allele frequency > 1%). Early GWASs identified multiple common SNPs for CVD; however, the proportion of variance explained by those SNPs was small, and the causal variants were not clear.[22] The accumulated experience and relative lack of success of initial efforts to identify novel causal variants lead to the formation of collaborative consortia on multiple CVDs to promote novel findings. Table 15.1 provides information on CVD international consortia and their hallmark GWAS work in revealing the common SNPs of specific disease.

With the emerging whole-exome sequencing technology, additional low-frequency and rare variants have been identified on CVD, including blood pressure/hypertension,[23] myocardial infarction,[24] and stroke.[25,26] Whole-exome sequencing is a genomic technique to sequence all protein-coding genes in a genome, which generates detailed catalogs of genetic variation in the protein-coding regions (i.e., both common and low-frequency/rare SNPs). For common complex traits (i.e., lipid levels), studies have demonstrated that low-frequency/rare variants tend to have more deleterious effects, which may be valuable for clinical studies to unravel protective null alleles that can serve as targets for pharmaceutical intervention. For example, targeted sequencing identified loss-of-function (LoF) variants in *PCSK9* that occur in about 3% of the population.[14] Such variants are associated with a low LDL cholesterol level. It has been reported that Black carriers of one of two mutations in *PCSK9* (Y142X and C679X) and White carriers of *PCSK9* R46LL allele have reduced susceptibilities to myocardial infarction,[14,27] implicating *PCSK9* as an attractive therapeutic target. Recent large randomized control trials have

TABLE 15.1
International Consortiums on Cardiovascular Diseases

Consortium	Full Name	Website	Key Paper[a]
ICBP	International Consortium for Blood Pressure	https://www.ncbi.nlm.nih.gov/projects/gap/cgi-bin/study.cgi?study_id=phs000585.v2.p1	Ehret G. B., 2016[112]
CARDIoGRAM-plusC4D	Coronary ARtery DIsease Genome-wide Replication and Meta-analysis (CARDIoGRAM) plus The Coronary Artery Disease (C4D) Genetics Consortium	http://www.cardiogramplusc4d.org/	Nikpay, M., 2015[113]
ISGC	International Stroke Genetics Consortium	http://www.strokegenetics.org/	Neurology Working Group of the CHARGE Consortium, 2016[114]
HERMES	**HE**art Failu**R**e **M**olecular **E**pidemiology for Therapeutic Target**S**	http://www.hermesconsortium.org/	Ongoing

[a]Most recent published hallmark paper: first author, year, and reference number.

shown that using PCSK9 inhibitor on a background of statin therapy can lower LDL cholesterol levels and further reduce the risk of cardiovascular events.[28]

Most recently, WGS, which allows for a comprehensive view of the sequence of the human genome, has been implemented in CVD research. Morrison et al.[29] applied integrated methodologic steps to interrogate WGS data to characterize the genetic architecture of heart- and blood-related traits. Aggregate tests of low frequency and rare variation identified multiple motifs that were associated with two CVD risk factors, namely, lipoprotein(a) and cardiac troponin T levels, and demonstrated the use of WGS data for characterizing the genetic architecture of complex traits.

PROTEOMICS AND CVD

Proteomic Profiling: Approaches and Technological Platform

The earliest approaches for protein detection were electrophoresis and liquid chromatography. They were widely used in plasma proteomic measures before mass spectrometry (MS); however, the resolution of these two methods is limited to the most abundant proteins.[30] MS is a powerful tool for systematic detection of the full set of proteins present in body fluid, e.g., plasma.[31,32] However, MS-based plasma proteomic profiling is challenging for a few reasons, including difficulty to capture high abundance proteins and lack of reproducible, robust, and high-throughput proteomic workflows.[30] Instead, multiplexed affinity

methods have been increasingly applied for plasma proteomics.[33] Affinity-based or targeted assays were developed based on antibodies to target specific proteins[34] and currently are the gold standard for clinical protein analysis. Examples of important immunoassays for CVD research include troponins and natriuretic peptides.[35] Affinity-based immunoassays overcome the limitations for detection of low-abundance proteins and high sample throughput. However, they cannot discover proteins that are not targeted by the assay and can potentially be influenced by coding DNA variants on epitope structures and affinity of reagents. Recently, single-stranded DNA aptamers have been developed as alternative affinity reagents to antibodies to overcome the limitations of immunoassays.[36] Single-stranded DNA aptamers are nucleotides of ~50 base pairs in length which are selected for their ability to bind target proteins or peptides with high specificity and affinity.[37]

The Proteomics Biomarkers for CVD

Although there is a long history for proteomics research, studies in human beings are still limited. For CVD, most proteomic studies to date have been based on experimental models.[38–40] With the advent of commercially available aptamer microarrays, population cohort studies are emerging to explore proteomic profiling of CVD. We highlight the major findings in the following sections and expect that a wave of studies will produce multiple candidate proteins for further testing, as well as genomics influence on human proteome, in the near future.

One of the first proteomics studies on CVD using an aptamer assay was published for risk prediction. Ganz et al. derived and validated a nine-protein score to predict 4-year probability risk of myocardial infarction, stroke, HF, and all-cause death among patients with CHD, using large-scale analysis of circulating proteins.[8] Assessment of circulating biomarkers to predict adverse CVD events among at-risk patients is clinically important. The nine proteins, including troponin I, matrix metalloproteinase-12, and angiopoietin-2, were combined into a score that was reproducibly associated with an increased risk of adverse events. The authors reported that the performance of this risk score was better than the Framingham Risk Score, but still, it only achieved modest discrimination (area under the receiver operating characteristic curve [AUC] at 0.70 compared with 0.64 for a clinical score) highlighting the complexities of clinical risk prediction.

Another landmark study published at about the same time used aptamer-based proteomic platform to identify early protein biomarkers of myocardial injury. Ngo et al.[41] reported that 217 proteins were significantly changed in the peripheral vein blood among patients who underwent alcohol septal ablation for hypertrophic cardiomyopathy, a model of planned myocardial injury in which each patient serves as his/her own biological control.[42] Seventy-nine out of 217 proteins were validated in an independent cohort, including Dickkopf-related protein 4 (a WNT pathway inhibitor) and cripto (a growth factor important in cardiac development). Out of 217, 156 significant proteins were associated with Framingham Risk Score, including aminoacylase 1 and trigger factor 2. The authors also developed a novel workflow integrating DNA-based immunoaffinity with MS to analytically validate aptamer specificity. The scalability of this approach was examined by Jacob et al. using an expanded proteomic platform to investigate a broader range of human proteins for myocardial injury.[43] Despite the promising results, further work is warranted to characterize the clinical relevance of these proteomic markers.

A recent study explored plasma proteome in relationship with the survival of pulmonary arterial hypertension (PAH). Rhodes et al.[44] reported that 20 proteins differentiated survivors and nonsurvivors in patients with idiopathic or heritable PAH. Nine proteins, including interleukin-1 receptor-like 1 (IL1R1/ST2), tissue inhibitors of metalloproteinases (TIMP-1 and TIMP-2), plasminogen, apolipoprotein-E (ApoE), erythropoietin, complement factor H and factor D, and insulin-like growth factor–binding protein-1, were independent of plasma N-terminal pro-brain natriuretic peptide (NT-pro-BNP), a classic biomarker correlating PAH survival. The functions of these proteins relate to, but are not limited to, myocardial stress, inflammation, pulmonary vascular cellular dysfunction, and structural dysregulation. A cutoff-based score using the panel of nine proteins improved AUC from 0.83 (for REVEAL risk score[45]) to 0.91 and reclassification indices without detriment to calibration. Identification of circulating proteins among patients with PAH, independent of existing clinical assessments, might have a use in clinical management and the evaluation of new therapies.

Future Directions

The emerging proteomics technologies open for an unbiased discovery of novel biomarkers, biomarker profiles, and therapeutic targets. The initial studies largely focused on high-risk individuals with existing CVD conditions. There is a need for accurate cardiovascular risk prediction in the general population. By applying proteomics to large population cohorts, ongoing efforts aim to discover novel cardiovascular biomarkers and highlight potential pathways. Furthermore, genomics findings on proteomic markers are largely focused on well-know proteins, such as troponins, NT-pro-BNP, and lipoprotein particles. Deep integration of genomics and proteomics in the future may provide additional novel cardiovascular biomarkers and characterize the genetic and environmental determinants of protein profiles.

METABOLOMICS AND CVD

Metabolomic Profiling: Approaches and Technological Platform

The human metabolome includes thousands of small-molecule metabolites,[46] but the total number of possibly detectable metabolites is unknown, and the entire metabolome has yet to be fully covered. There are two major distinct technological approaches, "untargeted" and "targeted", for metabolite measurements.[47,48] The scope of these two types of analysis is different, and they both have advantages and disadvantages. The targeted metabolomic approaches enable the absolute quantification of metabolites in the sample. However, it does not enable the discovery of unknown compounds, as it means to measure an a priori defined group of chemically characterized metabolites (e.g., lipids). In contrast, the untargeted metabolomic approaches aim to analyze all the measurable analytes in a sample including unknown chemicals. There are concerns about the semiquantitative nature of the untargeted approach (i.e., lack of absolute quantification), but it has notable advantages for detecting and semiquantifying (relative quantification) as many metabolites as possible in a biological sample. Therefore untargeted approaches are especially useful for finding novel mechanisms or biomarkers, whereas targeted approaches are great tools for follow-up pathway analyses because of a higher degree of sensitivity and easy identification of compounds. Several review papers have described and contrasted these platforms and approaches.[49,50]

At present, there are two major instrument platforms for measuring metabolite levels in biological samples, namely nuclear magnetic resonance (NMR) and chromatography and MS-based metabolic profiling.[51-53] Both techniques enable high-throughput profiling of large numbers of metabolites simultaneously within a sample, whereas each has unique analytical strengths and weaknesses. NMR spectroscopy technique identifies metabolites by chemical shifts in resonance frequency and provides detailed information about solution-state molecular structures based on atom-centered nuclear interactions.[54] NMR spectroscopy has several advantages, including that it is robust, requires minimal sample preparation, costs low per measurement, has high reproducibility, and has the nondiscriminating and nondestructive nature of the technique.[55,56] However, NMR spectroscopy has a limited sensitivity and can only detect metabolites at medium-to-high levels of abundance although NMR spectroscopy is also quantitative.[47] Alternatively, MS-based metabolomics identifies metabolites based on their mass to charge ratio (m/z) and provides highly selective and sensitive quantitative analyses.[57] Although samples can be infused directly into the mass spectrometer, the more common procedure is initially separating metabolites using chromatography (gas chromatography, liquid chromatography, or ultra-performance liquid chromatography) to facilitate further analyte identification and quantification.[58] Techniques based on different platforms (such as gas chromatography–MS and liquid chromatography-MS [LC-MS]) are better at detecting specific metabolites, making the integration of these techniques desirable to comprehensively study the metabolome. Moreover, such parallel utilization of these serial platforms provides a high sensitivity in identifying and analyzing metabolite components with concentrations as low as femtomolar range.[59]

The Metabolomic Biomarkers for CVD

Large-scale metabolomic profiling, for instance "metabolome-wide" studies, may identify metabolic changes occurring in the process of organ damage even before the appearance of disease and thereby may lead to early identification of individuals at high risk of developing disease including CVD given that a very interesting aspect of metabolomics research is to search for metabolites that could be used as clinical biomarkers of CVD. In addition, the identification of metabolomic risk profiles has the potential to improve risk stratification and explain risk disparities of CVD, for example, the substantial sex and race differences in the burden of CVD.[60] It is generally accepted that metabolite levels are the reflections of gene functional activities and environmental exposures,[61,62] making metabolome an ideal intermediate to better understand the pathophysiology and biological pathways involved in the genesis of clinical CVD events. Moreover, different clinical responses to therapy may result in different metabolite profiles, and hence metabolomic profiling could be used to identify response to therapy and improve the precision of medical management of CVD. In the past few years, various epidemiology studies using metabolomics have successfully linked metabolite levels to the etiology and progression of CVD and its risk factors in multiple ethnicities.[63-71]

Hypertension

Hypertension is an important worldwide public-health challenge[72] as it is a leading risk factor for cardiovascular diseases [73] and overall mortality.[74,75] Animal studies using hypertensive rats have pointed to metabolites, such as succinate and free fatty acids and their role in blood pressure regulation.[76,77] Recent advances in metabolomic techniques enable large-scale human studies, which showed promise in identifying metabolites that are causally linked to the pathogenesis of hypertension.[66,68] In a population of normotensive Blacks who were followed up for over 10 years, a 1-SD difference in serum metabolite 4-hydroxyhippurate (a product of gut microbial fermentation) was associated with 17% higher risk of developing hypertension.[66] Within the same study, the authors also identified a sex steroid pattern that was significantly associated with 72% higher risk (highest vs. lowest quintile) of developing hypertension. One recent study identified the association between hexadecanedioate (a dicarboxylic acid) levels with hypertension and mortality in human and demonstrated that oral hexadecanedioate intake increased blood pressure as well as vascular response to noradrenaline in Wistar-Kyoto rats.[68]

One of the most important potentials of metabolomics research in hypertension may be the monitoring of treatment responses. It was demonstrated that changes in metabolomic profiles in response to hydrochlorothiazide treatment differed between ethnicities and were able to predict treatment success.[78] In addition, the recent development in assays for comprehensive monitoring of drug metabolites in urine has already been introduced into clinical practice to assess adherence to therapy.[79] The most recent study carried out to search for metabolic biomarkers of antihypertensive drug responsiveness compared metabolic profiles of four different antihypertensive drugs and, in turn, provided supportive evidence that linked fatty acid metabolism to human hypertension.[80]

Coronary heart disease

Tang et al. has demonstrated that circulating trimethylamine-N-oxide (TMAO) is a significant predictor for atherosclerosis, with the gut microbiome being a critical factor regulating this process.[81] A previous study has observed higher circulating levels of choline, betaine, and TMAO in individuals suffering CVD events using untargeted MS-based metabolomics approaches.[71] The catabolism of dietary betaine and choline by intestinal microbes leads to TMAO production. TMAO may promote the progression of atherosclerosis through interfering with reverse cholesterol transport, which subsequently increases the risk of cardiovascular events.[81]

Metabolomic profiling also has identified markers predicting incident CHD events, such as myocardial infarction, unstable angina, and CAD.[63,64,67,69,70] For example, Ganna et al. conducted an untargeted LC-MS analysis and successfully identified three metabolites protectively associated with lower CHD risk (lysophosphatidylcholine 18:1 and 18:2, and sphingomyelin 28:1), and 1 metabolite (monoglyceride 18:2) associated with higher CHD risk in meta-analyses of the discovery and validation samples.[67] However, in the follow-up analysis using Mendelian randomization, only a weak positive causal effect was observed for the association between monoglyceride 18:2 and CHD. In another prospective study that combined CHD and ischemic stroke using CVD as their main outcome, the authors analyzed 68 targeted metabolites including lipids, amino acids, and others in a discovery cohort and subsequently two separate replication cohorts.[70] In meta-analyses of these three cohorts, five metabolites were identified: (1) phenylalanine and (2) monounsaturated fatty acid were associated with higher risk of CVD; and (3) polyunsaturated fatty acids, (4) ω-6 fatty acid, and (5) docosahexaenoic acid were associated with lower risk of CVD.

Stroke

The study of metabolites related with stroke is becoming increasingly more important as a way to broaden our knowledge of the pathological changes that occur in cerebrovascular disease. Because many studies included stroke as one of the CVD event and studied them together as we discussed previously,[64,70,71] the number of metabolomic studies primarily focusing on linking metabolites to stroke is limited. In a Korean population, an NMR-based metabolomic approach was used to identify potential biomarkers of stroke in patients with cerebral infarction, which characterized metabolic pathways of cerebral infarction by anaerobic glycolysis, folic acid deficiency, and hyperhomocysteinemia.[82] Metabolites in relation to the progression and treatment of ischemic stroke, the most common type of stroke, have also been studied.[83,84] For example, in a study of transient ischemic attack patients, novel biomarkers of stroke recurrence was identified and replicated using metabolomic analysis, which improves the predictive power of conventional predictors such as diabetes scale and large-artery atherosclerosis.[84]

Heart failure

Despite the variety of pathophysiological factors contributing to the development and progression in HF, a long-standing concept is that the failing heart has impaired oxidative phosphorylation, depressed oxygen consumption, and compromised ATP production.[85] As a result of the profound changes that occur in energy metabolism during HF, many studies using metabolomic analyses have reported that metabolomics profiles changed among HF patients or differed across patients with different severities of HF.[65,86–89]

As previously reviewed elsewhere, the regulation of myocardial fatty acid β-oxidation and the alterations in fatty acid β-oxidation can contribute to HF.[90] Metabolomic studies have observed that multiple fatty acids altered in the blood and/or urine of HF patients, especially changes in acylcarnitine profiles.[91,92] Hunter et al.[91] identified that circulating long-chain acylcarnitines were increased in HF patients compared with non-HF controls and were greater in HF with reduced ejection fraction than in HF with preserved ejection fraction (HFpEF). Another study that used metabolomic profiling in a subset of HF patients showed that circulating C16 and C18:1 acylcarnitines were increased in patients with end-stage HF and associated with increased risk for mortality and hospitalization of HF.[92] Most recently, a prognostic metabolite profile (PMP) was derived and validated based on quantification of acylcarnitines along with amino acids and organic

TABLE 15.2
Published Review Papers on Metabolomics and Cardiovascular Diseases

First Author	Year	Journal	References
Griffin, J. L.	2011	Nature Reviews Cardiology	115
Rhee, E. P.	2012	Clinical Chemistry	49
Shah, S. H.	2012	Circulation	59
Dona, A. C.	2016	European Journal of Preventive Cardiology	116
Hunter, W. G.	2016	Current Heart Failure Reports	117
Ussher, J. R.	2016	Journal of the American College of Cardiology	118
Ruiz-Canela, M.	2017	Journal of the American Heart Association	94

acids in HF patients. Thirteen metabolite PMPs were derived where low PMPs were related to survival incremental beyond conventional predictors.[93] In addition, there are other metabolites alteration (such as amino acids and ketone bodies) that have been observed in the development of HF.[86–88] All suggest that metabolomic profiling has significant diagnostic and prognostic value for managing HF.

A recently published systematic review summarized 12 articles that have prospectively assessed the association between circulating metabolomics profile and risk of CVD events[94] and showed remarkable heterogeneous results and approaches, suggesting that the standardization of metabolomics profiling platforms, data analysis approaches, and study design is critical. A list of major published review papers on metabolomics and cardiovascular diseases was summarized in Table 15.2.

Future Directions

Metabolomic profiles provide significant insights into biological and pathophysiological pathways that may be altered during the progression of CVD. However, metabolomic profiling performed on blood or urine samples cannot inform us with organ-specific pathophysiological processes. For complex diseases such as CVD, molecular changes that occur within the heart may provide more precise information than the changes across all the organs. Therefore, future assessment of metabolism at the organ levels may supplement the measurements of changes in metabolites in blood or urine samples. Nevertheless, metabolomic signatures in blood or urine can often lead to hypothesis generation, and such hypothesis can be further verified using experimental animal study and/or causal instrument, which ultimately will enhance our understanding of disease pathophysiology.

GENOMIC-METABOLOMIC FINDINGS ON CVD

Metabolomics has been integrated with other 'omic' technologies, such as genomics, to identify novel biological pathways and understand hidden disease mechanisms. For example, linking metabolomics to CVD and identifying relevant genetic loci for CVD-related metabolites opens the possibilities of novel biomarker discovery and hypothesis testing in understanding the etiological pathways to CVD. In addition, metabolomics may serve as a bridge that enables the discovery of formerly undetected associations between genes, metabolic pathways, and disease. In this section, we first highlighted the recent genetic findings for human metabolome, and then reviewed the integration of genomic-metabolomic findings on CVD.

GWAS Findings and Post-GWAS Era

In the past few years, numerous studies have used both traditional GWAS and whole-exome/genome sequencing analyses to map genetic variations on human plasma, serum, and urine metabolites, highlighting the influence of genetic variations on human metabolome among multiple ethnicities.[95–108] Hundreds of common genetic variants on multiple human metabolites have been reported,[97–102] and a Web-based tool, Metabolomics GWAS server, is available to facilitate access to the results (http://mips.helmholtz-muenchen.de/proj/GWAS/gwas/). Of note, this resource was based on results from European ancestry population only.[97,100]

Recent studies focusing on rare and low-frequency variants with marked functional consequences demonstrated a large cumulative effect on metabolite levels. Studies have reported additional variants that modulate metabolite levels independently of the GWAS hits using exome arrays and a targeted analytical approach for exome sequence.[103–105] Most recently, three studies have assessed the impact of rare and low-frequency variants captured by WGS on human metabolome,[106–108] including both European and African ancestries.

Integrated Genomic-Metabolomic Findings

Ever since the first GWAS with metabolomics study was conducted by Gieger et al.,[96] hundreds of genetic loci have been showed to be associated with one or multiple metabolites so far, and many of them can be further linked to clinically relevant factors of developing CVD. An early example of integrating genomics and metabolomics to promote additional findings for CVD is the story of *FADS1*. Using metabolites as the intermediate phenotypes, *FADS1* was identified as a risk locus for multiple phospholipids, key components of serum lipids.[96] At that time, the association of *FADS1* variants and lipid levels was not strong enough to reach genome-wide significance. Two years later, with significantly increased sample sizes, a GWAS on lipid parameters confirmed the prediction of *FADS1* being a lipid risk locus.[109]

In addition to common variants identified by GWASs, sequencing analyses on rare/low-frequency functional variants and metabolite levels combined with follow-up CVD events can help establish a paradigm for defining the pathophysiology of disease. For example, in a whole-exome sequencing study of African-American population, Yu et al. identified a LoF variant in *SLCO1B1* that was associated with increased levels, a metabolite, which for the first time, was reported for its relationship with HF risk.[105] Hexadecanedioate, a long-chain dicarboxylic acid, was also reported to be significantly associated with increased blood pressure and mortality.[68,105] The aforementioned genetics and metabolomics evidences together implicated a potential pathway for HF.

The integration of genetics and metabolomics can be particularly useful in the context of a focused pathway analysis. We discussed earlier how TMAO linked host metabolism with microbiome metabolism and its association with atherosclerosis and risk of cardiovascular events. Follow-up animal studies have now demonstrated that the *FMO3* gene contributes to variations of TMAO levels in mice. Specifically, there was a relationship between *FMO3* gene expression and plasma TMAO levels, and the mice that expressed *FMO3*, in turn, had increased susceptibility to atherosclerosis.[108]

The integrated approach can also be helpful in monitoring the drug response. In the subsection of metabolomics and hypertension, we highlighted that metabolite profiles that change in response to treatment with hydrochlorothiazide were able to predict treatment success.[78] The authors integrated their metabolomics findings with genomic data and thus identified genetic markers that predicted response to hydrochlorothiazide.[110]

CONCLUSION

Single biomarkers are not sufficient to interpret or characterize complex biological phenomena such as CVD, and new multiomics approaches recognize the importance of characterizing and integrating the interrelation—genomic, proteomic, and metabolomic "fingerprint" of disease and preclinical disease states. In the emerging "systems biology" area, a more comprehensive approach integrating not only genomics and metabolomics but also epigenetics and transcriptomics together provided an accurate picture of biological pathways. A recent system-based study analyzing gene variations, metabolic quantitative trait loci, expression quantitative trait loci, and metabolomics together identified a novel pathway of endoplasmic reticulum (ER) stress in CVD pathogenesis.[111] This ER stress pathway, represented by elevated levels of circulating short-chain dicarboxylacylcarnitine metabolites, would not have been identified from a single platform approach. In the future the integration of data from multiple techniques could help identify pathways that are involved in disease progression, improve early diagnosis, and personalize treatment plan. We expect that comprehensive network linking genetic susceptibility to proteomic and metabolomics changes of CVD will be established.

REFERENCES

1. Organization WH. World health statistics 2017: monitoring health for the SDGs. *Sustain Dev Goals Geneva WHO*. 2017.
2. McCarthy MI, MacArthur DG. Human disease genomics: from variants to biology. *Genome Biol*. 2017;18(1):20.
3. O'Donnell CJ, Nabel EG. Genomics of cardiovascular disease. *N Engl J Med*. 2011;365(22):2098–2109.
4. Menni C, Kiddle SJ, Mangino M, et al. Circulating proteomic signatures of chronological age. *J Gerontol a Biol Sci Med Sci*. 2015;70(7):809–816.
5. De Groote MA, Sterling DG, Hraha T, et al. Discovery and validation of a six-marker serum protein signature for the diagnosis of active pulmonary tuberculosis. *J Clin Microbiol*. 2017;55(10):3057–3071.
6. Ostroff RM, Mehan MR, Stewart A, et al. Early detection of malignant pleural mesothelioma in asbestos-exposed individuals with a noninvasive proteomics-based surveillance tool. *PLoS One*. 2012;7(10):e46091.

7. Hathout Y, Brody E, Clemens PR, et al. Large-scale serum protein biomarker discovery in Duchenne muscular dystrophy. *Proc Natl Acad Sci U. S. A.* 2015;112(23):7153–7158.

8. Ganz P, Heidecker B, Hveem K, et al. Development and validation of a protein-based risk score for cardiovascular outcomes among patients with stable coronary heart disease. *JAMA.* 2016;315(23):2532–2541.

9. Williams SA, Murthy AC, DeLisle RK, et al. Improving assessment of drug safety through proteomics: early detection and mechanistic characterization of the unforeseen harmful effects of torcetrapib. *Circulation.* 2017;117:028213.

10. Villas-Bôas SG, Mas S, Åkesson M, Smedsgaard J, Nielsen J. Mass spectrometry in metabolome analysis. *Mass Spect Rev.* 2005;24(5):613–646.

11. Abifadel M, Varret M, Rabès J-P, et al. Mutations in PCSK9 cause autosomal dominant hypercholesterolemia. *Nat Genet.* 2003;34:154.

12. Brown MS, Goldstein JL. A receptor-mediated pathway for cholesterol homeostasis. *Science.* 1986;232(4746):34–47.

13. Garcia CK, Wilund K, Arca M, et al. Autosomal recessive hypercholesterolemia caused by mutations in a putative LDL receptor adaptor protein. *Science.* 2001;292(5520):1394–1398.

14. Cohen JC, Boerwinkle E, Mosley THJ, Hobbs HH. Sequence variations in PCSK9, low LDL, and protection against coronary heart disease. *N Engl J Med.* 2006;354(12):1264–1272.

15. Soria LF, Ludwig EH, Clarke HR, Vega GL, Grundy SM, McCarthy BJ. Association between a specific apolipoprotein B mutation and familial defective apolipoprotein B-100. *Proc Natl Acad Sci U. S. A.* 1989;86(2):587–591.

16. Musunuru K, Pirruccello JP, Do R, et al. Exome sequencing, ANGPTL3 mutations, and familial combined hypolipidemia. *N Engl J Med.* 2010;363(23):2220–2227.

17. Bonne G, Carrier L, Bercovici J, et al. Cardiac myosin binding protein-C gene splice acceptor site mutation is associated with familial hypertrophic cardiomyopathy. *Nat Genet.* 1995;11(4):438–440.

18. Geisterfer-Lowrance AA, Kass S, Tanigawa G, et al. A molecular basis for familial hypertrophic cardiomyopathy: a beta cardiac myosin heavy chain gene missense mutation. *Cell.* 1990;62(5):999–1006.

19. Carrier L, Hengstenberg C, Beckmann JS, et al. Mapping of a novel gene for familial hypertrophic cardiomyopathy to chromosome 11. *Nat Genet.* 1993;4(3):311–313.

20. Kimura A, Harada H, Park JE, et al. Mutations in the cardiac troponin I gene associated with hypertrophic cardiomyopathy. *Nat Genet.* 1997;16(4):379–382.

21. Olson TM, Doan TP, Kishimoto NY, Whitby FG, Ackerman MJ, Fananapazir L. Inherited and de novo mutations in the cardiac actin gene cause hypertrophic cardiomyopathy. *J Mol Cell Cardiol.* 2000;32(9):1687–1694.

22. Manolio TA, Collins FS, Cox NJ, et al. Finding the missing heritability of complex diseases. *Nature.* 2009;461(7265):747–753.

23. Yu B, Pulit SL, Hwang S-J, et al. Rare exome sequence variants in CLCN6 reduce blood pressure levels and hypertension risk. *Circ Cardiovasc Genet.* 2016;9(1):64–70.

24. Do R, Stitziel NO, Won H-H, et al. Exome sequencing identifies rare LDLR and APOA5 alleles conferring risk for myocardial infarction. *Nature.* 2015;518(7537):102–106.

25. Carrera C, Jimenez-Conde J, Derdak S, et al. Whole exome sequencing analysis reveals TRPV3 as a risk factor for cardioembolic stroke. *Thrombosis Haemostasis.* 2016;116(6):1165–1171.

26. Auer PL, Nalls M, Meschia JF, et al. Rare and coding region genetic variants associated with risk of ischemic stroke: the NHLBI exome sequence project. *JAMA Neurol.* 2015;72(7):781–788.

27. Kathiresan SA. PCSK9 missense variant associated with a reduced risk of early-onset myocardial infarction. *N Engl J Med.* 2008;358(21):2299–2300.

28. Sabatine MS, Giugliano RP, Keech AC, et al. Evolocumab and clinical outcomes in patients with cardiovascular disease. *N Engl J Med.* 2017;376(18):1713–1722.

29. Morrison AC, Huang Z, Yu B, et al. Practical approaches for whole-genome sequence analysis of heart- and blood-related traits. *Am J Human Genet.* 2017;100(2):205–215.

30. Gerszten RE, Accurso F, Bernard GR, et al. Challenges in translating plasma proteomics from bench to bedside: update from the NHLBI Clinical Proteomics Programs. *Am J Physiol Lung Cell Mol Physiol.* 2008;295(1):L16–L22.

31. Aebersold R, Mann M. Mass spectrometry-based proteomics. *Nature.* 2003;422(6928):198–207.

32. Udeshi ND, Mertins P, Svinkina T, Carr SA. Large-scale identification of ubiquitination sites by mass spectrometry. *Nat Protoc.* 2013;8(10):1950–1960.

33. Solier C, Langen H. Antibody-based proteomics and biomarker research - current status and limitations. *Proteomics.* 2014;14(6):774–783.

34. Ellington AA, Kullo IJ, Bailey KR, Klee GG. Antibody-based protein multiplex platforms: technical and operational challenges. *Clin Chem.* 2010;56(2):186–193.

35. Vasan R. Biomarkers of cardiovascular disease: molecular basis and practical considerations. *Circulation.* 2006;113(19):2335.

36. Taussig MJ, Schmidt R, Cook EA, Stoevesandt O. Development of proteome-wide binding reagents for research and diagnostics. *Proteomics Clin Appl.* 2013;7(11–12):756–766.

37. Rohloff JC, Gelinas AD, Jarvis TC, et al. Nucleic acid ligands with protein-like side chains: modified aptamers and their use as diagnostic and therapeutic agents. *Mol Ther Nucleic Acids.* 2014;3:e201.

38. Loffredo FS, Steinhauser ML, Jay SM, et al. Growth differentiation factor 11 is a circulating factor that reverses age-related cardiac hypertrophy. *Cell.* 2013;153(4):828–839.

39. Walker RG, Poggioli T, Katsimpardi L, et al. Biochemistry and biology of GDF11 and myostatin: similarities, differences, and questions for future investigation. *Circ Res.* 2016;118(7):1125–1141; discussion 42.

40. Schafer MJ, Atkinson EJ, Vanderboom PM, et al. Quantification of GDF11 and myostatin in human aging and cardiovascular disease. *Cell Metab.* 2016;23(6):1207–1215.

41. Ngo D, Sinha S, Shen D, et al. Aptamer-based proteomic profiling reveals novel candidate biomarkers and pathways in cardiovascular disease. *Circulation.* 2016;134(4):270–285.

42. Lewis GD, Wei R, Liu E, et al. Metabolite profiling of blood from individuals undergoing planned myocardial infarction reveals early markers of myocardial injury. *J Clin Invest.* 2008;118(10):3503–3512.

43. Jacob J, Ngo D, Finkel N, et al. Application of large scale aptamer-based proteomic profiling to "planned" myocardial infarctions. *Circulation.* 2017.

44. Rhodes CJ, Wharton J, Ghataorhe P, et al. Plasma proteome analysis in patients with pulmonary arterial hypertension: an observational cohort study. *Lancet Respir Med.* 2017.

45. Benza RL, Miller DP, Gomberg-Maitland M, et al. Predicting survival in pulmonary arterial hypertension: insights from the registry to evaluate early and long-term pulmonary arterial hypertension disease management (REVEAL). *Circulation.* 2010;122(2):164–172.

46. Wishart DS, Jewison T, Guo AC, et al. HMDB 3.0—the human metabolome database in 2013. *Nucleic Acids Res.* 2013;41(Database issue):D801–D807.

47. Lewis GD, Asnani A, Gerszten RE. Application of metabolomics to cardiovascular biomarker and pathway discovery. *J Am Coll Cardiol.* 2008;52(2):117–123.

48. Koal T, Deigner H-P. Challenges in mass spectrometry based targeted metabolomics. *Curr Mol Med.* 2010;10(2):216–226.

49. Rhee EP, Gerszten RE. Metabolomics and cardiovascular biomarker discovery. *Clin Chem.* 2012;58(1):139–147.

50. Bain JR, Stevens RD, Wenner BR, Ilkayeva O, Muoio DM, Newgard CB. Metabolomics applied to diabetes research: moving from information to knowledge. *Diabetes.* 2009;58(11):2429–2443.

51. German JB, Hammock BD, Watkins SM. Metabolomics: building on a century of biochemistry to guide human health. *Metabolomics.* 2005;1(1):3–9.

52. Watson AD. Thematic review series: systems biology approaches to metabolic and cardiovascular disorders. Lipidomics: a global approach to lipid analysis in biological systems. *J Lipid Res.* 2006;47(10):2101–2111.

53. Dettmer K, Aronov PA, Hammock BD. Mass spectrometry-based metabolomics. *Mass Spectrometry Rev.* 2007;26(1):51–78.

54. Marion D. An introduction to biological NMR spectroscopy. *Mol Cell Proteomics.* 2013;12(11):3006–3025.

55. Soininen P, Kangas AJ, Würtz P, Suna T, Ala-Korpela M. Quantitative serum nuclear magnetic resonance metabolomics in cardiovascular epidemiology and genetics. *Circ Cardiovasc Genet.* 2015;8(1):192–206.

56. Markley JL, Brüschweiler R, Edison AS, et al. The future of NMR-based metabolomics. *Curr Opin Biotechnol.* 2017;43:34–40.

57. Lei Z, Huhman DV, Sumner LW. Mass spectrometry strategies in metabolomics. *J Biol Chem.* 2011;286(29):25435–25442.

58. Kind T, Wohlgemuth G, Lee DY, et al. FiehnLib: mass spectral and retention index libraries for metabolomics based on quadrupole and time-of-flight gas chromatography/mass spectrometry. *Anal Chem.* 2009;81(24):10038–10048.

59. Shah SH, Kraus WE, Newgard CB. Metabolomic profiling for the identification of novel biomarkers and mechanisms related to common cardiovascular diseases. *Circulation.* 2012;126(9):1110–1120.

60. National Center for Health Statistics. *Health, United States, 2015: With Special Feature on Racial and Ethnic Health Disparities;* 2016.

61. Greef Jvd, Stroobant P, Heijden Rvd. The role of analytical sciences in medical systems biology. *Curr Opin Chem Biol.* 2004;8(5):559–565.

62. Ordovas JM. Nutrigenetics, plasma lipids, and cardiovascular risk. *J Am Diet Assoc.* 2006;106(7):1074–1081.

63. Shah SH, Sun J-L, Stevens RD, et al. Baseline metabolomic profiles predict cardiovascular events in patients at risk for coronary artery disease. *Am Heart J.* 2012;163(5):844–850.e1.

64. Rizza S, Copetti M, Rossi C, Cianfarani MA, Zucchelli M, Luzi A, et al. Metabolomics signature improves the prediction of cardiovascular events in elderly subjects. *Atherosclerosis.* 2014;232(2):260–264.

65. Zheng Y, Yu B, Alexander D, et al. Associations between metabolomic compounds and incident heart failure among African Americans: the ARIC Study. *Am J Epidemiol.* 2013:kwt004.

66. Zheng Y, Yu B, Alexander D, et al. Metabolomics and incident hypertension among blacks. *Hypertension.* 2013;113:01166.

67. Ganna A, Salihovic S, Sundström J, et al. Large-scale metabolomic profiling identifies novel biomarkers for incident coronary heart disease. *PLoS Genet.* 2014;10(12):e1004801.

68. Menni C, Graham D, Kastenmüller G, et al. Metabolomic identification of a novel pathway of blood pressure regulation involving hexadecanedioate. *Hypertension.* 2015;66(2):422–429.

69. Vaarhorst AAM, Verhoeven A, Weller CM, Böhringer S, Göraler S, Meissner A, et al. A metabolomic profile is associated with the risk of incident coronary heart disease. *Am Heart J.* 2014;168(1):45–52.e7.

70. Würtz P, Havulinna AS, Soininen P, et al. Metabolite profiling and cardiovascular event risk. *Circulation.* 2015;131(9):774–785.

71. Wang Z, Klipfell E, Bennett BJ, et al. Gut flora metabolism of phosphatidylcholine promotes cardiovascular disease. *Nature.* 2011;472(7341):57–63.

72. Kearney PM, Whelton M, Reynolds K, Muntner P, Whelton PK, He J. Global burden of hypertension: analysis of worldwide data. *Lancet.* 2005;365(9455):217–223.

73. Wolf-Maier K, Cooper RS, Banegas JR, et al. Hypertension prevalence and blood pressure levels in 6 european countries, Canada, and the United States. *JAMA.* 2003;289(18):2363–2369.

74. Gu Q, Burt VL, Paulose-Ram R, Yoon S, Gillum RF. High blood pressure and cardiovascular disease mortality risk among U.S. Adults: the third national health and nutrition examination survey mortality follow-up study. *Ann Epidemiol.* 2008;18(4):302–309.

75. Lawes CM, Hoorn SV, Law MR, Elliott P, MacMahon S, Rodgers A. Blood pressure and the global burden of disease 2000. Part II: estimates of attributable burden. *J Hypertens.* 2006;24(3):423–430.

76. Lu Y, A J, Wang G, et al. Gas chromatography/time-of-flight mass spectrometry based metabonomic approach to differentiating hypertension- and age-related metabolic variation in spontaneously hypertensive rats. *Rapid Commun Mass Spectrom.* 2008;22(18):2882–2888.

77. Fujiwara M, Arifuku K, Ando I, Nemoto T. Pattern recognition analysis for classification of hypertensive model rats and diurnal variation using 1H-NMR spectroscopy of urine. *Anal Sci.* 2005;21(11):1259–1262.

78. Rotroff DM, Shahin MH, Gurley SB, et al. Pharmacometabolomic assessments of atenolol and hydrochlorothiazide treatment reveal novel drug response phenotypes. *CPT Pharm Syst Pharmacol.* 2015;4(11):669–679.

79. Tomaszewski M, White C, Patel P, et al. High rates of non-adherence to antihypertensive treatment revealed by high-performance liquid chromatography-tandem mass spectrometry (HP LC-MS/MS) urine analysis. *Heart.* 2014;100(11):855–861.

80. Hiltunen TP, Rimpelä JM, Mohney RP, Stirdivant SM, Kontula KK. Effects of four different antihypertensive drugs on plasma metabolomic profiles in patients with essential hypertension. *PLoS One.* 2017;12(11):e0187729.

81. Tang WW, Hazen SL. The contributory role of gut microbiota in cardiovascular disease. *J Clin Investig.* 2014;124(10):4204.

82. Jung JY, Lee H-S, Kang D-G, et al. 1H-NMR-based metabolomics study of cerebral infarction. *Stroke.* 2011;110:598789.

83. Tang H, Tang Y, Li N-G, et al. Comparative metabolomic analysis of the neuroprotective effects of scutellarin and scutellarein against ischemic insult. *PLoS One.* 2015;10(7):e0131569.

84. Jové M, Mauri-Capdevila G, Suárez I, et al. Metabolomics predicts stroke recurrence after transient ischemic attack. *Neurology.* 2015;84(1):36–45.

85. Neubauer S. The failing heart—an engine out of fuel. *N Engl J Med.* 2007;356(11):1140–1151.

86. Cheng M-L, Wang C-H, Shiao M-S, et al. Metabolic disturbances identified in plasma are associated with outcomes in patients with heart failure: diagnostic and prognostic value of metabolomics. *J Am Coll Cardiol.* 2015;65(15):1509–1520.

87. Zordoky BN, Sung MM, Ezekowitz J, et al. Metabolomic fingerprint of heart failure with preserved ejection fraction. *PLoS One.* 2015;10(5):e0124844.

88. Wang J, Li Z, Chen J, et al. Metabolomic identification of diagnostic plasma biomarkers in humans with chronic heart failure. *Mol Biosyst.* 2013;9(11):2618–2626.

89. Deidda M, Piras C, Dessalvi CC, et al. Metabolomic approach to profile functional and metabolic changes in heart failure. *J Transl Med.* 2015;13(1):297.

90. Lopaschuk GD, Ussher JR, Folmes CD, Jaswal JS, Stanley WC. Myocardial fatty acid metabolism in health and disease. *Physiol Rev.* 2010;90(1):207–258.

91. Hunter WG, Kelly JP, McGarrah RW, et al. Metabolomic profiling identifies novel circulating biomarkers of mitochondrial dysfunction differentially elevated in heart failure with preserved versus reduced ejection fraction: evidence for shared metabolic impairments in clinical heart failure. *J Am Heart Assoc.* 2016;5(8):e003190.

92. Ahmad T, Kelly JP, McGarrah RW, et al. Prognostic implications of long-chain acylcarnitines in heart failure and reversibility with mechanical circulatory support. *J Am Coll Cardiol.* 2016;67(3):291–299.

93. Lanfear DE, Gibbs JJ, Li J, et al. Targeted metabolomic profiling of plasma and survival in heart failure patients. *JACC Heart Fail.* 2017;5(11):823–832.

94. Ruiz-Canela M, Hruby A, Clish CB, Liang L, Martínez-González MA, Hu FB. Comprehensive metabolomic profiling and incident cardiovascular disease: a systematic review. *J Am Heart Assoc.* 2017;6(10):e005705.

95. Illig T, Gieger C, Zhai G, et al. A genome-wide perspective of genetic variation in human metabolism. *Nat Genet.* 2009;42(2):507.

96. Gieger C, Geistlinger L, Altmaier E, et al. Genetics meets metabolomics: a genome-wide association study of metabolite profiles in human serum. *PLoS Genet.* 2008;4(11):e1000282.

97. Suhre K, Shin S-Y, Petersen A-K, et al. Human metabolic individuality in biomedical and pharmaceutical research. *Nature.* 2011;477(7362). https://doi.org/10.1038/nature10354.

98. Kettunen J, Tukiainen T, Sarin AP, et al. Genome-wide association study identifies multiple loci influencing human serum metabolite levels. *Nat Genet.* 2012:44.

99. Rhee EP, Ho JE, Chen M-H, et al. A genome-wide association study of the human metabolome in a community-based cohort. *Cell Metab.* 2013;18(1):130–143.

100. Shin S-Y, Fauman EB, Petersen A-K, et al. An atlas of genetic influences on human blood metabolites. *Nat Genet.* 2014;46(6):543–550.

101. Yu B, Zheng Y, Alexander D, Morrison AC, Coresh J, Boerwinkle E. Genetic determinants influencing human serum metabolome among African Americans. *PLoS Genet.* 2014;10(3):e1004212.

102. Draisma HHM, Pool R, Kobl M, et al. Genome-wide association study identifies novel genetic variants contributing to variation in blood metabolite levels. *Nat Commun.* 2015;6:7208.

103. Demirkan A, Henneman P, Verhoeven A, et al. Insight in genome-wide association of metabolite quantitative traits by exome sequence analyses. *PLoS Genet.* 2015;11(1):e1004835.

104. Rhee EP, Yang Q, Yu B, et al. An exome array study of the plasma metabolome. *Nat Commun.* 2016;7:12360.

105. Yu B, Li AH, Metcalf GA, et al. Loss-of-function variants influence the human serum metabolome. *Sci Adv.* 2016;2(8):e1600800.

106. Yu B, de Vries PS, Metcalf GA, et al. Whole genome sequence analysis of serum amino acid levels. *Genome Biol.* 2016;17(1):237.

107. Long T, Hicks M, Yu H-C, et al. Whole-genome sequencing identifies common-to-rare variants associated with human blood metabolites. *Nat Genet.* 2017;49(4):568–578.

108. de Vries PS, Yu B, Feofanova EV, et al. Whole-genome sequencing study of serum peptide levels: the Atherosclerosis Risk in Communities study. *Hum Mol Genet.* 2017;26(17):3442–3450.

109. Teslovich TM, Musunuru K, Smith AV, et al. Biological, clinical and population relevance of 95 loci for blood lipids. *Nature.* 2010:466.

110. Shahin MH, Gong Y, McDonough CW, et al. A genetic response score for hydrochlorothiazide use. *Hypertension.* 2016;116:07328.

111. Kraus WE, Muoio DM, Stevens R, et al. Metabolomic quantitative trait loci (mQTL) mapping implicates the ubiquitin proteasome system in cardiovascular disease pathogenesis. *PLoS Genet.* 2015;11(11):e1005553.

112. Ehret GB, Ferreira T, Chasman DI, et al. The genetics of blood pressure regulation and its target organs from association studies in 342,415 individuals. *Nat Genet.* 2016;48(10):1171–1184.

113. Nikpay M, Goel A, Won H-H, et al. A comprehensive 1,000 Genomes-based genome-wide association meta-analysis of coronary artery disease. *Nat Genet.* 2015;47(10):1121–1130.

114. Neurology Working Group of the Cohorts for H, Aging Research in Genomic Epidemiology Consortium tSGN, The International Stroke Genetics C. Identification of additional risk loci for stroke and small vessel disease: a meta-analysis of genome-wide association studies. *Lancet Neurol.* 2016;15(7):695–707.

115. Griffin JL, Atherton H, Shockcor J, Atzori L. Metabolomics as a tool for cardiac research. *Nat Rev Cardiol.* 2011;8(11):630–643.

116. Dona AC, Coffey S, Figtree G. Translational and emerging clinical applications of metabolomics in cardiovascular disease diagnosis and treatment. *Eur J Prevent Cardiol.* 2016;23(15):1578–1589.

117. Hunter WG, Kelly JP, McGarrah RW, Kraus WE, Shah SH. Metabolic dysfunction in heart failure: diagnostic, prognostic, and pathophysiologic insights from metabolomic profiling. *Curr Heart Failure Rep.* 2016;13(3):119–131.

118. Ussher JR, Elmariah S, Gerszten RE, Dyck JR. The emerging role of metabolomics in the diagnosis and prognosis of cardiovascular disease. *J Am Coll Cardiol.* 2016;68(25):2850–2870.

CHAPTER 16

Future Directions in the Use of Biomarkers for Prevention of Cardiovascular Disease

ANUM SAEED, MD • CHRISTIE M. BALLANTYNE, MD

INTRODUCTION

Over the past 3 decades, significant advances in both assessment and treatment of cardiovascular disease (CVD) risk have led to reductions in age-adjusted CVD. Nevertheless, CVD remains a leading cause of morbidity across the United States.[1] The discovery of novel biomarkers that may be used to improve risk assessment for both atherosclerotic CVD and heart failure (HF) and to guide therapy remains a vital area of investigation.

In 2001 a working group of the National Institutes of Health standardized the definition of the word biomarker (biological marker) as "a characteristic that is objectively measured and evaluated as an indicator of normal biological processes, pathogenic processes, or pharmacologic responses to a therapeutic intervention".[2] In the current chapter, we explore emerging clinical uses and application of biomarkers in CVD risk prediction, diagnosis, and treatment, as well as highlight some innovative technologies that may facilitate newer biomarker discovery and validation.

BACKGROUND

The process of atherosclerosis confers a lifelong risk. Fatty streaks can form in the aorta within the first decade of life in humans,[3] yet the first clinical cardiovascular event (myocardial infarction, HF, or stroke) may not appear until many decades later. Atherogenesis in the arterial walls is a complex process.[4] Chronic exposure to metabolic and hemodynamic risk factors, for example, hypercholesterolemia, hypertension, oxidative stress, and proinflammatory mediators, leads to modifications in endothelial cell phenotype. Risk factor exposure is associated with changes in the extracellular matrix, enabling entry of cholesterol-containing low-density lipoprotein (LDL) particles into the arterial wall.[5,6] Changes in cell adhesion molecules, chemoattractants, and the extracellular matrix also allow leukocytes to enter the arterial wall and become macrophages, with further secretion of cytokines, chemokines, and growth factors and phagocytosis of modified LDL particles, and transition into "foam cells." Foam cells are a constituent of fatty streaks, the earliest lesion of atherosclerosis.

CVD RISK ASSESSMENT: PARADIGM SHIFTS

As mentioned previously, the process of atherosclerotic CVD hinges on a lifelong exposure to risk factors, development of subclinical disease, and ultimately progression to clinical events. The integral need for a personalized CVD risk assessment approach using a combination of biomarkers, genetic markers, and imaging for primordial, primary, and secondary prevention from CVD events has recently been highlighted.[7] The use of biomarkers is the central aspect of the emerging multimodality approach in CVD risk assessment as well as management[7,8] and has a key role in the era of precision medicine.[9]

Currently, more than 35 biomarkers representing various CVD processes are used in clinical practice for primary or secondary prevention of CVD events.[10] Among these are biomarkers for prediction and management of HF (e.g., brain natriuretic peptide [BNP], N-terminal prohormone of BNP [NT-pro-BNP], atrial natriuretic peptide) and biomarkers specific to myocardial "injury" or "damage" (e.g., troponin T or I, high-sensitivity troponin T or I, creatinine phosphokinase isoenzyme MB). CVD biomarkers can be specific to the pathological processes they represent, such as inflammation (e.g., C-reactive protein [CRP] and interleukin-6), oxidative stress (e.g., isoprostanes), and metabolic pathways (e.g., lipoprotein(a), LDL, high-density lipoprotein, apolipoprotein B-100, and homocysteine). Acute changes in certain biomarkers, for example,

Biomarkers in Cardiovascular Disease. https://doi.org/10.1016/B978-0-323-54835-9.00016-8

troponins or BNP, are routinely used to assess for acute coronary heart disease events including acute coronary syndromes and decompensated HF.

Clinicians routinely use dichotomized "cut points" or "thresholds" for traditional risk factors, but emerging evidence indicates that risk factors assessed as "normal" for one individual may not be optimal to prevent a first or recurrent CVD event in another individual.[7] Efforts are needed to focus not only on primary or secondary prevention from CVD events but also on primordial prevention, i.e., prevention of risk factor development.

Recently, Fernández-Friera et al.[11] showed that in a young-to-middle-aged cohort of 1779 men and women without prevalent CVD, traditional risk factors, or medications, approximately one-half of the subjects had subclinical atherosclerosis as evaluated by ultrasonography or coronary calcium imaging.[11] In a subgroup analysis of the same study, ~38% (n = 740) had optimal risk factors (blood pressure < 120/80 mm Hg, fasting glucose < 100 mg/dL, hemoglobin A1C < 5.7%, total cholesterol < 200 mg/dL) but detectable plaque.[11] This study highlights the need for personalized CVD risk assessment that extends beyond traditional risk factor thresholds. Use of novel biomarkers, including genomic scores,[12] may help ascertain an individual's lifetime risk for developing CVD risk factors or CVD events.

BIOMARKERS TO ASSESS FOR GLOBAL CVD EVENTS

In current recommendations, risk stratification is based 10-year atherosclerotic CVD risk calculated by the Pooled Cohort Equation (PCE).[13] However, the PCE does not account for HF hospitalization, a common event in the general population.[1] HF is also the leading CVD event in older adults without established CVD and a leading condition in the health-care expenditure in the United States.[1] In 2010 there were ~1 million hospitalizations for HF, with 71% in individuals aged ≥65 years and 53% in those aged ≥75 years.[14] Given the expected rise in HF incidence in Americans,[15,16] the need for HF prevention has recently been highlighted.[17] Robust associations of NT-pro-BNP with risk prediction and prognosis for clinical HF have been reported.[18,19] Therefore the ability to detect natriuretic peptides and derivatives with high-sensitivity assays, with or without imaging, may enable a more sophisticated approach for HF prevention in clinical cardiology practice.[20]

Multiple studies, including the Atherosclerosis Risk in Communities (ARIC) study, have shown the incremental value of candidate biomarkers and other diagnostic modalities in prediction of coronary heart disease events, stroke, and HF hospitalization,[21-25] and an increasing number of risk prediction and assessment models now include global CVD risk scores, including coronary heart disease, stroke, and HF.[25-27]

BIOMARKERS FOR RISK ASSESSMENT IN OLDER ADULTS

Although older individuals have the highest absolute risk for CVD events, application of the 2013 American College of Cardiology/American Heart Association (ACC/AHA) cholesterol guidelines[28] and the 2017 ACC/AHA hypertension management guidelines[29] remains challenging in clinical practice for this group. Both guidelines use the PCE, which, as noted, excludes HF hospitalization and estimates 10-year risk, which may not be the most relevant time frame for older individuals. In addition, the PCE is limited to individuals aged 40–79 years.

The association of traditional risk factors with atherosclerotic CVD events may be less robust in older adults,[30] which may be secondary to the high prevalence of traditional risk factors in older adults. Hence comprehensive risk assessment in these individuals may warrant use of additional measures beyond traditional risk factors.

Recently, we have shown the incremental benefit of adding three candidate biomarkers, namely, high-sensitivity cardiac troponin T, NT-pro-BNP, and high-sensitivity CRP (hs-CRP), to the PCE[25] for global CVD (coronary heart disease, stroke, and HF hospitalization) risk assessment in the ARIC study population (mean age of 75 years) over a short term of ~4 years. Each biomarker significantly increased the C-statistic when added to the PCE model. Collectively, the largest improvement in risk prediction metrics was seen with the addition of all three candidate biomarkers to traditional risk factors compared with the PCE (Δ area under the receiver operating characteristic curve [AUC], 0.103; category-free net reclassification index [NRI], 0.484; and integrated discrimination index [IDI], 0.075).[25] A model that included age, gender, race, and the three biomarkers also performed better than the PCE (ΔAUC, 0.091; category-free NRI, 0.355; IDI, 0.068) in predicting the global CVD risk in older adults over the short-term follow-up. The association of traditional risk factors with global CVD events appears to diminish with increasing age,[25] and therefore, better assessment with a biomarker-based approach may improve risk classification, with clinical implications.

These important observations require validation in other cohorts, and a prospective randomized clinical trial will be necessary to evaluate the clinical effectiveness of a biomarker-based approach for CVD risk assessment and determination of initiation/intensity of pharmacotherapy in older adults. Furthermore, the cost-effectiveness of a CVD prevention method based on biomarkers has not yet been validated.

BIOMARKERS: BENCHMARKS FOR COST-EFFECTIVENESS OF NEWER THERAPEUTIC AGENTS

Biomarkers may also provide a practical measure for determining which individuals are most likely to benefit from expensive newer therapies such as proprotein convertase subtilisin/kexin type 9 inhibitors, for which combined absolute risk, baseline LDL cholesterol, and drug price have been suggested to guide patient selection.[31] Such an approach may be useful in negotiating insurance restrictions and improving access to these agents[32,33] for appropriate patients.[34]

A similar strategy may be plausible for therapies that directly target specific biomarkers such as apolipoproteins[35-37] and cytokines.[38,39] A subanalysis from the Canakinumab Anti-Inflammatory Thrombosis Outcomes Study concluded that individuals allocated to canakinumab who achieved hs-CRP concentrations <2 mg/L had a 25% reduction in the primary endpoint of major adverse CVD events (multivariable adjusted hazard ratio, 0.75; 95% confidence interval, 0.66–0.85; $P < .0001$) compared with no significant response in those with hs-CRP unchanged from baseline.[40] Similar results were seen for secondary outcomes in the study.

Therefore, using an approach based on quantified change in a biomarker concentration may be helpful to direct expensive therapies to the appropriate patients. It is important to note, however, that the cost-effectiveness of such an approach has not been analyzed.

BIOMARKERS IN CLINICAL TRIALS

The time period between the development of a clinical therapeutic agent and its transition into patient care remains long. Depending on the phase, clinical trials are slow for several reasons, including need to access long-term safety of therapeutic agents, complex trial designs, and use of clinical endpoints such as mortality or hospitalization to meet regulatory approval or reimbursements. The use of biomarkers as surrogate endpoints in clinical trials has long been used to reduce clinical trial duration and sample size and enables accelerated approval and availability of new therapies.[2] Biomarkers may be used both for patient selection and to assess the response to therapy in selected patient groups. Improvements in assay sensitivity and imaging techniques, combined with advances in our understanding of the mechanisms by which biomarkers are involved in the pathophysiology of CVD, continue to expand the role of biomarkers in clinical trials.

There has been a recent trend toward using established biomarkers of cardiac myocyte injury or myocardial stretch in randomized clinical trials. Of note, the inflammatory pathway biomarker hs-CRP, myocardial stretch, BNP, and NT-pro-BNP have been widely used as entry criteria in randomized clinical trials enrolling individuals with or without prevalent CVD.[41-44]

Measurement of cardiac biomarkers alone or in combination with clinical outcomes such as hospitalization or mortality may, in the future, present alternative and novel endpoints for clinical trials, as tested recently in HF studies.[45] In an evaluation of 16 phase-3 chronic HF trials amassing 18 therapeutic comparisons in a total of 48,844 patients with median clinical endpoint follow-up of 28 months, Vaduganathan et al. concluded that changes in natriuretic peptide levels measured at a median of 4 months after randomization were not correlated with longer term treatment effects on all-cause mortality ($r = 0.12$; $P = .63$) but were modestly correlated with HF hospitalizations ($r = 0.63$; $P = .008$).[45] The correlation improved when analyses were controlled for trials finished since 2010 ($r = 0.92$; $P = .0095$), using NT-pro-BNP assays ($r = 0.65$; $P = .06$), and evaluating inhibitors of the renin–angiotensin–aldosterone system ($r = 0.97$; $P = .0002$).

Indeed, there has been a call to initiate studies to answer important questions about the reliability of using biomarkers as surrogate endpoints in clinical trials of HF prevention.[46] As the medical community continues to develop the essential characteristics of biomarkers to qualify as surrogate endpoints in clinical trials,[2,47,48] the implementation of biomarkers as endpoints in future clinical trials remains promising.

PROTEOMICS: MORE BIOMARKERS ON THE HORIZON?

One of the major challenges involved in the development of CVD biomarkers is the complexity of the disease process. The development of microarrays, proteomics, and nanotechnology combined with data from the Human Genome Project[49] and HapMap Project[50] are revolutionizing the pathways for discovering and investigating biomarkers associated with CVD.

Studying simultaneously a large number of proteins in the plasma, the plasma proteome, is a new opportunity for recognizing novel pathways and biomarkers for profiling CVD risk and diagnosis. The human plasma proteome is a mixture of proteins derived from all tissues and representing a variety of metabolic pathways.[51] Therefore, the plasma proteome includes carrier proteins, immune system effectors (e.g., immunoglobulins and complement factors), tissue messengers (e.g., natriuretic peptides and interleukins), products of tissue damage (e.g., troponin and creatine kinase), and other proteins involved in CVD.

The heterogeneous structure of the plasma proteome and its large range in protein concentrations have been a barrier to perform a complete simultaneous profiling of large number of plasma proteins. Mass spectrometry is an extremely powerful tool but technically demanding and expensive.[52] Therefore, the current most widely used approach for clinical protein analysis is affinity-based, or targeted, assays. This approach recognizes specific protein targets through the use of monoclonal or polyclonal antibodies and then quantifies these proteins based on either the signal intensity of luminescent, fluorescent, enzymatic (i.e., enzyme-linked immunosorbent assays), or radioactive (radioimmunoassays) antibody-labeled reporters or light scattering of antibody-protein complexes (turbidimetry and nephelometry).

Advantages of using affinity-based assays include high sensitivity for many low-abundance proteins, high sample throughput, easy performance with relatively low-cost equipment, and a targeted analysis of a protein of interest.[53] However, this technique also has several important limitations that include limited protein discovery depending on specific assays used, lack of differentiation of posttranslational modifications and isoforms, potential variability in reagents, and thus, lack of standardization and reproducibility.[53]

However, novel technologies are being applied to improve affinity-based proteomic assays in CVD risk profiling. One of these approaches is to label antibodies with nucleic acids that can be amplified and quantified by the polymerase chain reaction (PCR)[53] and is referred to as immuno-PCR.[54] A commercialized version of immuno-PCR (Olink Bioscience, Uppsala, Sweden) referred to as proximity extension assay has been developed that measures up to 92 proteins in a very small sample volume.[55] Affinity reagents, such as modified nucleic acid aptamers, have been described as another alternative to address the limitations of immunoassays.[56] Oligonucleotide-based aptamers[57-59] interact with protein surfaces by their folding capability and have a high-binding affinity.[60] Recently, chemically modified aptamers with improved affinity[61] have been developed by a commercial platform (SomaLogic, Inc, Boulder, CO). This assay has been determined to identify and quantify more than 1300 proteins[60] with high sample throughput.[53] These modified aptamer microarrays have recently been used in population cohorts to derive and validate risk scores for coronary heart disease outcomes.[62] In 938 and 971 samples analyzed from the derivative and validation cohorts (individuals with stable coronary heart disease), respectively, a 9-protein risk score was evaluated for adverse clinical outcomes including myocardial infarction, stroke, HF, and all-cause death. Addition of the 9-protein risk score to the refit Framingham model improved the C-statistic by 0.09 (95% confidence interval, 0.06–0.12) in the derivation cohort and 0.05 (95% confidence interval, 0.02–0.09) in the validation cohort. Included among the 9 proteins associated with adverse clinical outcomes were troponin I, matrix metalloproteinase–12, and angiopoietin-2. Although the 9-protein risk score model outperformed the Framingham risk model for secondary atherosclerotic events in these individuals with a stable coronary heart disease, the discriminative accuracy was modest. In another study, torcetrapib, a drug that increased total mortality and atherosclerotic CVD events in clinical trials, was associated with an increase in the 9-protein risk score at 3 months, suggesting that this risk score may also be useful as a surrogate to assess response to new drugs.[63]

The use of these and other novel technologies in concert with high-yield detection systems such as mass spectrometry and genomics may ultimately improve identification of newer biomarkers and therapeutic targets.

CONCLUSIONS

A more precise identification of individuals at high risk for first or recurrent CVD events to optimize preventive measures and curtail CVD is the ultimate goal of the scientific/clinical community. Biological markers, or biomarkers, have important implications for CVD risk prediction/stratification, diagnosis, and prognosis. With advances in genomics, proteomics, and bioinformatics, numerous high-throughput biomarkers may become available for more thorough CVD risk profiling. With improvements in technology,

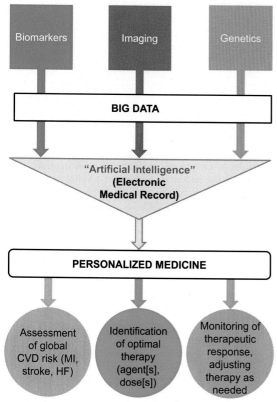

FIG. 16.1 Future Directions: Incorporating Biomarker, Imaging, and Genetic Data to Inform Personalized Medicine for Improved Risk Assessment and Optimal Therapy.

it is highly probable that the time from discovery to clinical approval of biomarkers for CVD will considerably shorten. However, before clinical application, standardization of assays, improvements in predictive models, and cost-effectiveness analyses will be necessary.

An approach using biomarkers, imaging, and genomics may be used to develop more precise tools for global CVD risk assessment, management, and individualized therapy within the near future. Currently, our ability to generate data is increasing faster than our ability to analyze data by traditional methods. In the future (Fig. 16.1) a more sophisticated version of the electronic medical record may enable data on an individual's biomarkers, imaging, and genetics to be processed through an analytical program that would probably include artificial intelligence to provide more accurate risk assessment for global CVD, more precise identification of optimal therapy, and longitudinal monitoring of response to therapy to direct prevention.

ACKNOWLEDGMENTS

The authors would like to acknowledge Kerrie Jara for her contribution in editing this chapter.

DISCLOSURES

Saeed: None.

Ballantyne received grant/research support from Abbott Diagnostic, Akcea, Amarin, Amgen, Esperion, Novartis, Regneron, Roche Diagnostic, and Sanofi-Synthelabo; has been a consultant for Abbott Diagnostic, Akcea, Amarin, Amgen, Astra Zeneca, Boehringer Ingelheim, Denka Seiken, Eli Lilly, Esperion, Gilead, Matinas BioPharma Inc, Merck, Novartis, Novo Nordisk, Regeneron, Roche Diagnostic, and Sanofi-Synthelabo. Provisional patent (patent no.: 61721475) entitled "Biomarkers to Improve Prediction of Heart Failure Risk" is filed by Baylor College of Medicine and Roche (V. Nambi, R. Hoogeveen, CM Ballantyne).

REFERENCES

1. Benjamin EJ, Virani SS, Callaway CW, et al. Heart disease and stroke statistics–2018 update: a report from the American Heart Association. *Circulation.* 2018;137: e67–e492.
2. Biomarkers Definitions Working Group. Biomarkers and surrogate endpoints: preferred definitions and conceptual framework. *Clin Pharmacol Ther.* 2001;69:89–95.
3. Lusis AJ. *Atheroscler Nat.* 2000;407:233–241.
4. Crea F, Libby P. Acute coronary syndromes: the way forward from mechanisms to precision treatment. *Circulation.* 2017;136:1155–1166.
5. Libby P, Ridker PM, Hansson GK. Progress and challenges in translating the biology of atherosclerosis. *Nature.* 2011;473:317–325.
6. Tabas I, Williams KJ, Boren J. Subendothelial lipoprotein retention as the initiating process in atherosclerosis: update and therapeutic implications. *Circulation.* 2007;116:1832–1844.
7. Nambi V, Bhatt DL. Primary prevention of atherosclerosis: time to take a selfie? *J Am Coll Cardiol.* 2017;70: 2992–2994.
8. Yu JT, Tan L, Hardy J. Apolipoprotein E in Alzheimer's disease: an update. *Annu Rev Neurosci.* 2014;37:79–100.
9. National Institutes of Health. Precision Medicine Initiative (PMI) Working Group. The Precision Medicine Initiative Cohort Program – Building a Research Foundation for 21st Century Medicine: Precision Medicine Initiative (PMI) Working Group Report to the Advisory Committee to the Director, NIH. http://www.nih.gov/sites/default/files/research-training/initiatives/pmi/pmi-working-group-report-20150917-2.pdf.
10. Vasan RS. Biomarkers of cardiovascular disease. *Circulation.* 2006;113:2335–2362.

11. Fernandez-Friera L, Fuster V, Lopez-Melgar B, et al. Normal LDL-cholesterol levels are associated with subclinical atherosclerosis in the absence of risk factors. *J Am Coll Cardiol.* 2017;70:2979–2991.

12. Khera AV, Emdin CA, Drake I, et al. Genetic risk, adherence to a healthy lifestyle, and coronary disease. *N Engl J Med.* 2016;375:2349–2358.

13. Goff Jr DC, Lloyd-Jones DM, Bennett G, et al. 2013 ACC/AHA guideline on the assessment of cardiovascular risk: a report of the American College of Cardiology/American Heart Association task force on practice guidelines. *Circulation.* 2013;129:S49–S73.

14. Hall M.J., Levant S., DeFrances C.J. Hospitalization for congestive heart failure: United States, 2000–2010. http://www.cdc.gov/nchs/data/databriefs/db108.pdf.

15. Bui AL, Horwich TB, Fonarow GC. Epidemiology and risk profile of heart failure. *Nat Rev Cardiol.* 2011;8:30–41.

16. Redfield MM, Jacobsen SJ, Burnett Jr JC, Mahoney DW, Bailey KR, Rodeheffer RJ. Burden of systolic and diastolic ventricular dysfunction in the community: appreciating the scope of the heart failure epidemic. *JAMA.* 2003;289:194–202.

17. Nambi V, Deswal A, Ballantyne CM. Prevention of "failure": is it a failure of prevention? *Circulation.* 2018;137:106–108.

18. Kistorp C, Raymond I, Pedersen F, Gustafsson F, Faber J, Hildebrandt P. N-terminal pro-brain natriuretic peptide, C-reactive protein, and urinary albumin levels as predictors of mortality and cardiovascular events in older adults. *JAMA.* 2005;293:1609–1616.

19. Wang TJ, Larson MG, Levy D, et al. Plasma natriuretic peptide levels and the risk of cardiovascular events and death. *N Engl J Med.* 2004;350:655–663.

20. Yancy CW, Jessup M, Bozkurt B, et al. 2017 ACC/AHA/HFSA focused update of the 2013 ACCF/AHA guideline for the management of heart failure: a report of the American College of cardiology/American Heart Association task force on clinical practice guidelines and the heart failure Society of America. *J Am Coll Cardiol.* 2017;70:776–803.

21. Nambi V, Liu X, Chambless LE, et al. Troponin T and N-terminal pro-B-type natriuretic peptide: a biomarker approach to predict heart failure risk–the atherosclerosis risk in communities study. *Clin Chem.* 2013;59:1802–1810.

22. Saunders JT, Nambi V, de Lemos JA, et al. Cardiac troponin T measured by a highly sensitive assay predicts coronary heart disease, heart failure, and mortality in the atherosclerosis risk in communities study. *Circulation.* 2011;123:1367–1376.

23. Yeboah J, Young R, McClelland RL, et al. Utility of nontraditional risk markers in atherosclerotic cardiovascular disease risk assessment. *J Am Coll Cardiol.* 2016;67:139–147.

24. Akintoye E, Briasoulis A, Afonso L. Biochemical risk markers and 10-year incidence of atherosclerotic cardiovascular disease: independent predictors, improvement in pooled cohort equation, and risk reclassification. *Am Heart J.* 2017;193:95–103.

25. Saeed A, Nambi V, Sun W, et al. Short-term global cardiovascular disease risk prediction in older adults. *J Am Coll Cardiol.* 2018;71:2527–2536.

26. D'Agostino RB, Vasan RS, Pencina MJ, et al. General cardiovascular risk profile for use in primary care: the Framingham Heart Study. *Circulation.* 2008;117:743–753.

27. de Lemos JA, Ayers CR, Levine B, et al. Multimodality strategy for cardiovascular risk assessment: performance in 2 population-based cohorts. *Circulation.* 2017;135:2119–2132.

28. Stone NJ, Robinson JG, Lichtenstein AH, et al. 2013 ACC/AHA guideline on the treatment of blood cholesterol to reduce atherosclerotic cardiovascular risk in adults: a report of the American College of Cardiology/American Heart Association Task Force on Practice Guidelines. *Circulation.* 2014;129:S1–S45.

29. Whelton PK, Carey RM, Aronow WS, et al. 2017 ACC/AHA/AAPA/ABC/ACPM/AGS/APhA/ASH/ASPC/NMA/PCNA guideline for the prevention, detection, evaluation, and management of high blood pressure in adults: a report of the American College of Cardiology/American Heart Association Task Force on Clinical Practice Guidelines. *Hypertension.* 2017.

30. Whelton SP, Roy P, Astor BC, et al. Elevated high-sensitivity C-reactive protein as a risk marker of the attenuated relationship between serum cholesterol and cardiovascular events at older age: the ARIC Study. *Am J Epidemiol.* 2013;178:1076–1084.

31. Annemans L, Packard CJ, Briggs A, Ray KK. 'Highest risk–highest benefit' strategy: a pragmatic, cost-effective approach to targeting use of PCSK9 inhibitor therapies. *Eur Heart J.* 2017. ehx710.

32. Whayne TF. Outcomes, access, and cost issues involving PCSK9 inhibitors to lower LDL-cholesterol. *Drugs.* 2018;78:287–291.

33. Cohen JD, Cziraky MJ, Jacobson TA, Maki KC, Karalis DG. Barriers to PCSK9 inhibitor prescriptions for patients with high cardiovascular risk: results of a healthcare provider survey conducted by the National Lipid Association. *J Clin Lipidol.* 2017;11:891–900.

34. Saeed A, Virani SS, Jones PH, Nambi V, Zoch D, Ballantyne CM. A simplified pathway to proprotein convertase subtilisin/kexin type 9 inhibitor prior authorization approval: a lipid clinic experience. *J Clin Lipidol.* 2017;11:596–599.

35. Schmitz J, Gouni-Berthold I. APOC-III antisense oligonucleotides: a new option for the treatment of hypertriglyceridemia. *Curr Med Chem.* 2018;25:1567–1576.

36. Pechlaner R, Tsimikas S, Yin X, et al. Very-low-density lipoprotein–associated apolipoproteins predict cardiovascular events and are lowered by inhibition of APOC-III. *J Am Coll Cardiol.* 2017;69:789–800.

37. Viney NJ, van Capelleveen JC, Geary RS, et al. Antisense oligonucleotides targeting apolipoprotein(a) in people with raised lipoprotein(a): two randomised, double-blind, placebo-controlled, dose-ranging trials. *Lancet.* 2016;388:2239–2253.

38. Ridker PM, Everett BM, Thuren T, et al. Antiinflammatory therapy with canakinumab for atherosclerotic disease. *N Engl J Med.* 2017;377:1119–1131.

39. Everett BM, Pradhan AD, Solomon DH, et al. Rationale and design of the Cardiovascular Inflammation Reduction Trial: a test of the inflammatory hypothesis of athero-thrombosis. *Am Heart J.* 2013;166:199–207.

40. Ridker PM, MacFadyen JG, Everett BM, Libby P, Thuren T, Glynn RJ. Relationship of C-reactive protein reduction to cardiovascular event reduction following treatment with canakinumab: a secondary analysis from the CANTOS randomised controlled trial. *Lancet.* 2018;391:319–328.

41. Ridker PM, Thuren T, Zalewski A, Libby P. Interleukin-1b inhibition and the prevention of recurrent cardiovascular events: rationale and design of the Canakinumab Anti-inflammatory Thrombosis Outcomes Study (CANTOS). *Am Heart J.* 2011;162:597–605.

42. McMurray JJ, Packer M, Desai AS, et al. Angiotensin-neprilysin inhibition versus enalapril in heart failure. *N Engl J Med.* 2014;371:993–1004.

43. O'Connor CM, Starling RC, Hernandez AF, et al. Effect of nesiritide in patients with acute decompensated heart failure. *N Engl J Med.* 2011;365:32–43.

44. Solomon SD, Zile M, Pieske B, et al. The angiotensin receptor neprilysin inhibitor LCZ696 in heart failure with preserved ejection fraction: a phase 2 double-blind randomised controlled trial. *Lancet.* 2012;380:1387–1395.

45. Vaduganathan M, Claggett B, Packer M, et al. Natriuretic peptides as biomarkers of treatment response in clinical trials of heart failure. *JACC Heart Fail.* 2018.

46. Januzzi Jr JL. Will biomarkers succeed as a surrogate endpoint in heart failure trials? *JACC Heart Fail.* 2018.

47. Cohn JN. Introduction to surrogate markers. *Circulation.* 2004;109:IV20–IV21.

48. Ibrahim NE, Gaggin HK, Konstam MA, Januzzi Jr JL. Established and emerging roles of biomarkers in heart failure clinical trials. *Circ Heart Fail.* 2016;9:e002528.

49. Lander ES, Linton LM, Birren B, et al. Initial sequencing and analysis of the human genome. *Nature.* 2001;409:860–921.

50. Abecasis GR, Altshuler D, Auton A, et al. A map of human genome variation from population-scale sequencing. *Nature.* 2010;467:1061–1073.

51. Ping P, Vondriska TM, Creighton CJ, et al. A functional annotation of subproteomes in human plasma. *Proteomics.* 2005;5:3506–3519.

52. Gerszten RE, Accurso F, Bernard GR, et al. Challenges in translating plasma proteomics from bench to bedside: update from the NHLBI Clinical Proteomics Programs. *Am J Physiol Lung Cell Mol Physiol.* 2008;295:L16–L22.

53. Smith JG, Gerszten RE. Emerging affinity-based proteomic technologies for large-scale plasma profiling in cardiovascular disease. *Circulation.* 2017;135:1651–1664.

54. Sano T, Smith CL, Cantor CR. Immuno-PCR: very sensitive antigen detection by means of specific antibody-DNA conjugates. *Science.* 1992;258:120–122.

55. Assarsson E, Lundberg M, Holmquist G, et al. Homogenous 96-plex PEA immunoassay exhibiting high sensitivity, specificity, and excellent scalability. *PLoS One.* 2014;9:e95192.

56. Taussig MJ, Schmidt R, Cook EA, Stoevesandt O. Development of proteome-wide binding reagents for research and diagnostics. *Proteomics Clin Appl.* 2013;7:756–766.

57. Reddy MM, Kodadek T. Protein "fingerprinting" in complex mixtures with peptoid microarrays. *Proc Natl Acad Sci U. S. A.* 2005;102:12672–12677.

58. Tuerk C, Gold L. Systematic evolution of ligands by exponential enrichment: RNA ligands to bacteriophage T4 DNA polymerase. *Science.* 1990;249:505–510.

59. Ellington AD, Szostak JW. In vitro selection of RNA molecules that bind specific ligands. *Nature.* 1990;346:818–822.

60. Gold L, Ayers D, Bertino J, et al. Aptamer-based multiplexed proteomic technology for biomarker discovery. *PLoS One.* 2010;5:e15004.

61. Rohloff JC, Gelinas AD, Jarvis TC, et al. Nucleic acid ligands with protein-like side chains: modified aptamers and their use as diagnostic and therapeutic agents. *Mol Ther Nucleic Acids.* 2014;3:e201.

62. Ganz P, Heidecker B, Hveem K, et al. Development and validation of a protein-based risk score for cardiovascular outcomes among patients with stable coronary heart disease. *JAMA.* 2016;315:2532–2541.

63. Williams SA, Murthy AC, DeLisle RK, et al. Improving assessment of drug safety through proteomics: early detection and mechanistic characterization of the unforeseen harmful effects of torcetrapib. *Circulation.* 2018;137:999–1010.

Index

Note: Page numbers followed by "f" indicate figures, "t" indicate tables.

Printed in the United States
By Bookmasters